Clinical Reasoning

Clinical Reasoning
Forms of Inquiry in a Therapeutic Practice

Cheryl Mattingly, PhD
University of Illinois
Chicago, Illinois
Department of Occupational Therapy

Maureen Hayes Fleming, EdD, OTR, FAOTA
Boston School of Occupational Therapy
Tufts University
Medford, Massachusetts
Director
Clinical Reasoning Institute

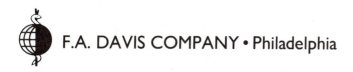
F.A. DAVIS COMPANY • Philadelphia

F. A. Davis Company
1915 Arch Street
Philadelphia, PA 19103

Printed in the United States of America

Last digit indicates print number: 10 9 8 7 6 5

Acquisitions Editor: Lynn Borders Caldwell
Production Editor: Arofan Gregory
Cover Design By: Steven Ross Morrone
Clinical Reasoning Logo Design By: Jodi Makovsky

As new scientific information becomes available through basic and clinical research, recommended treatments and drug therapies undergo changes. The author(s) and publisher have done everything possible to make this book accurate, up to date, and in accord with accepted standards at the time of publication. The authors, editors, and publisher are not responsible for errors or omissions or for consequences from application of the book, and make no warranty, expressed or implied, in regard to the contents of the book. Any practice described in this book should be applied by the reader in accordance with professional standards of care used in regard to the unique circumstances that may apply in each situation. The reader is advised always to check product information (package inserts) for changes and new information regarding dose and contraindications before administering any drug. Caution is especially urged when using new or infrequently ordered drugs.

Library of Congress Cataloging-in-Publication Data

Mattingly, Cheryl, 1951–
    Clinical reasoning : forms of inquiry in a therapeutic practice / Cheryl
Mattingly, Maureen Hayes Fleming.
      p. cm.
    Includes bibliographical references and index.
    ISBN 0-8036-5937-7
    1. Occupational therapy.   2. Medical logic.   I. Fleming, Maureen
Hayes, 1944– . II. Title.
RM735.M396   1993
616.8'515 — dc20
                                         93-31102
                                           CIP

Dedication

To Brian Vincent Hayes,
whose quick wit brightened the lives
of all who knew him.

Foreword

As the twentieth century draws to a close, it is natural for attention in many areas to turn to the future, and the field of health care is no exception. References to the dawning of a new age are abundant, and at least within American health care, there is an acute sense that profound change is underway. Thoughts have turned to the need to consider a system of health care delivery that renders services with the patient's interests in mind. Outcomes are being defined increasingly in social as well as biomedical terms.

During this renaissance, the process of coming to decide about how care ought to proceed for a particular patient is being transformed. The focus of concern has widened. There is recognition that intervention must go beyond defining a problem in biomechanical terms and following a diagnosis with a circumscribed list of procedural options. Providers now make reference to other considerations, often described as "the patient's quality of life." Occasionally, there is acknowledgment that the patient's participation in the care process is important, and that what and how the patient is thinking may influence the outcome of care.

To be sure, there have been many voices arguing for a change to the constricted paradigm of concern that has characterized traditional western medicine in the past. Many influential scholars have advocated changes in the way providers think about health and illness. Others have drawn our attention to the importance of considering how the patient experiences illness or disability within the context of his or her life. These ideas are not foreign to occupational therapy.

Occupational therapy's historian-laureate, Robert Bing, would argue that arriving at this turning point represents an evolutionary process of moral and humanistic ideology that began decades ago. Thus, it may not be a coincidence that this book, which has considerable relevance beyond occupational therapy, comes at this time. While the important ideas and ideals of occupational therapy have survived in the writings of scholars and in the culture of the profession over time, they have done so with muted influence, awkwardly co-existing within a biomedical environment that seems only begrudgingly to take the time to be concerned about the patient's engagement in life. During this time, many occupational therapists have struggled with their need to integrate seemingly incompatible ideals and procedures within their daily practices without a framework for understanding why this integration is so difficult.

In this book, Mattingly and Fleming offer very readable and engaging descriptions of how therapists work and think. They provide insights into the complexities of understanding the patient's story, and in doing so, make clear the immense importance of narrative (how people organize and interpret their lives through stories) to the clinical reasoning of occupational therapists. They reassure therapists who have experienced the difficulties and frustrations of entering the personal world of the patient within the structure of a biomedical environment that the inevitable tensions that result can be reconciled. Therapists are encouraged to recognize and respect that multiple types of considerations both characterize and are important to daily practice.

A major contribution of this book is its framework for understanding the complexities of practice, as well as the language it provides for communicating about these complexities. To use their terms, Mattingly and Fleming have helped to make the implicit or tacit aspects of practice more explicit. Perhaps in doing so they may also have unintentionally uncovered weaknesses in the current approaches to educating therapists. Their work suggests to me that therapy students could benefit from increased exposure to the concepts and tools of anthropology, philosophy, and phenomenology.

This book is the product of years of study and reflection. It provides an important and badly needed conceptual bridge between the technical and humanistic sides of occupational therapy practice. While its impact cannot be predicted, its importance cannot be denied. It should become required reading for every therapist and every therapy student.

In the years ahead, health care providers must endeavor to deliver services in ways that are smarter and softer. That is, providers must deliver those services that work best for a particular patient, and which have been selected in concert with the patient following a thorough consideration of his or her life circumstances. In this book, Mattingly and Fleming have made a landmark contribution toward achieving these goals. Thus, their book has substantial importance for health care as well as for occupational therapy.

Charles Christiansen

Acknowledgments

Several years ago a group of theorists and researchers in occupational therapy (including Charles Christiansen, Wendy Coster, Gary Kielhofner, Terry Litterest, and Joan Rogers) met to discuss the possibility of conducting an extensive study of clinical reasoning in occupational therapy. This effort was spearheaded by two members of the American Occupational Therapy Foundation, Nedra Gillette and Stephanie Hoover. This group met with Donald Schön at the Massachusetts Institute of Technology to discuss and begin to outline research designed to investigate clinical knowledge and expertise within the profession. Neither Maureen nor I were involved in this initial group but their efforts helped shape our work. We want to thank them.

Nedra Gillette deserves very special thanks. She has played an integral part in our work. She was a key organizer of the first group of theorists that initially formulated the research project. She recruited Cheryl Mattingly as a researcher for the project and then later introduced her to Maureen Fleming whom she recruited as research collaborator. She said she had an idea that we might work well together, initiating a research partnership that we expect will last a lifetime. She helped find the money to fund the original project, pushing for support from AOTA and AOTF for a highly innovative study that combined ethnographic methods with action research. In a very real sense she has been a partner in our research since the beginning. She spent many hours on Maureen Fleming's back porch and in Cheryl Mattingly's cramped Cambridge apartment watching research videotapes, combing through piles of transcribed data, and helping to devise coding schemes to categorize the data. She has been a co-presenter with us at various workshops and seminars on clinical reasoning and a co-writer of articles and book chapters. It is difficult to know how to thank Nedra sufficiently for the central role she has played in helping to make this project happen. Without her continual efforts, this book would never have been written.

This is a book that has been created, quite literally, by dozens of people. A few are acknowledged in the text itself. These are storytellers who have allowed us to use their cases throughout the book. But much of the data that provided the basis for our theory-making came from the initial Clinical Reasoning Study. As part of this study, a group of therapists and patients allowed us to follow them through treatment.

The patients will remain anonymous because we have promised confidentiality. However, we would like to acknowledge the therapists who participated. Seven senior therapists, including the department director, Deborah Yarett Slater, were extensively involved. We wish especially to thank them: Christa Czycholl, Cindy Mootz, Cathy Hill, Lizbeth Squires, Gwen Berkowsky, and Andrea Segel. As the study progressed, five newer members of the department joined the project and we want to thank them as well: Patricia Dunn, Kathleen LeDuc, Suzanne Ellis, Lisa Shockett, and Amy Kaufman.

To carry out the Clinical Reasoning Study, Maureen and I assembled a larger research team that spent more than two years studying these therapists. In addition to ourselves, this team consisted of one faculty member from Tufts, Ellen Cohn; several graduate students, Cumba Siegler, Cathy Verrier Peirsol, Terry Sperber, and Suzanne Wish-Baratz; and one undergraduate occupational therapy student, Linda Sicard. Team members helped to collect and analyze data. Particularly during the first year, these students, most of whom were experienced therapists themselves, helped in explaining and interpreting occupational therapy practice for the outside researcher (Cheryl Mattingly). They learned to take field notes, conduct ethnographic interviews, videotape sessions, and analyze qualitative data. Several of them wrote their master's theses based on their research work in the project. They were a wonderful group to work with.

Ellen Cohn has played an extremely important role in helping to analyze the data. She has also been essential in efforts to disseminate the results of the research. She has co-presented with us in various workshops and seminars, paying special attention to the educational implications of the research. She has written several articles based on her analysis of the data and, perhaps most important, served as guest editor for a 1991 special issue of the American Journal of Occupational Therapy on clinical reasoning. This special issue provided a place to get some of the analysis of the Clinical Reasoning Study data in print for the first time.

Subsequent to the original Clinical Reasoning Study, several other research efforts have been carried out that have contributed substantially to both the case material and the analysis presented in this book. One group of graduate students in the occupational therapy department at University of Illinois in Chicago played a central role: Laurie Rockwell Dylla, Jaime Munoz, Kathy Baron, Anita Niehaus, Marcelle Salome, Christi Brdecka-Tuleja, and Lisa Richter. This group began as members of a graduate course on clinical reasoning taught by Cheryl Mattingly. Many members of that course became so interested in the topic that they continued to meet, writing papers and presenting workshops on clinical reasoning in the Illinois area. They formed a Clinical Reasoning Study Group that met for 2 years. They collected and analyzed data based on interviews with experienced therapists. Some of the data from their research can be found in chapters of this book. Some of them went on to carry out research for their master's theses that grew out of these discussions. The intellectual excitement of this group helped to stimulate Cheryl Mattingly to finish her own doctoral thesis, also based on the Clinical Reasoning Study. They are gratefully acknowledged for the important role they played.

The reviewers gave invaluable suggestions in the preparation of this manuscript. We did substantial reworking of several chapters based on their comments, and we wish to thank them for their efforts:

Charles H. Christiansen, EdD, OTR, OT(C), FAOTA
Dean
School of Allied Health Sciences
University of Texas Medical Branch at Galveston

Maureen E. Neistadt, ScD, OTR
Professor
Department of Occupational Therapy
University of New Hampshire

Betty R. Hasselkus, PhD, OTR
Program Director and Assistant Professor
Department of Occupational Therapy
University of Wisconsin–Madison

Maralynne D. Mitcham, PhD, OTRL, FAOTA
Assistant Dean for Research and Graduate
    Studies
Medical University of South Carolina

Alexis Henry, ScD, OTR
Instructor and Academic Fieldwork Coordinator
Department of Occupational Therapy
Worcester State College

Christine R. Berg, MS, OTR
Instructor
Department of Occupational Therapy
Washington University Medical School

M. Carolyn Baum, MA, OTR, FAOTA
Elias Michal Director
Department of Occupational Therapy
Washington University School of Medicine

Jerry A. Johnson, MBA, EdD, OTR, FAOTA
Professor and Graduate Coordinator
Department of Occupational Therapy
Thomas Jefferson University

Kathleen Barker Schwartz, EdD, OTR, FAOTA
Associate Professor
Department of Occupational Therapy
San Jose State University

Lydia Wingate, PhD
Dean
School of Allied Health Sciences
Kansas University Medical Center

Special thanks goes to Charles Christiansen, who cheerfully consented to write the foreword.

Thanks also must be given to the people who have helped in the preparation of this manuscript: Tim Davies, Colleen Gillman, Sonya Bradburn, Lauri Cherbodian, Carol Crotty, Ellen Germeinder, Susan Hamlon, Susan Laborski, Barbara Platt, Michael Roberts, and Mary Beth Schneider.

Maureen would also like to thank Alyson Fleming, Michael Fleming, and Ethel and Vincent Hayes for their constant assistance and support. Lorraine Hendersen and Ann Bonner also deserve special thanks for their unending patience.

Contents

Part I   **Introduction**   I

    Chapter 1   **Giving Language to Practice**   3
           Maureen Hayes Fleming
           Cheryl Mattingly
    Chapter 2   **The Search for Tacit Knowledge**   22
           Maureen Hayes Fleming

Part II   **Occupational Therapy: A Profession Between
Two Cultures**   35

    Chapter 3   **Occupational Therapy as a Two-Body
              Practice: The Body as Machine**   37
           Cheryl Mattingly
    Chapter 4   **Occupational Therapy as a Two-Body
              Practice: The Lived Body**   64
           Cheryl Mattingly
    Chapter 5   **A Commonsense Practice in an Uncommon
              World**   94
           Maureen Hayes Fleming

Part III   **Clinical Reasoning: Taking the Client from Structural
Limitation to New Formulations**   117

    Chapter 6   **The Therapist with the Three-Track Mind**   119
           Maureen Hayes Fleming
    Chapter 7   **Procedural Reasoning: Addressing
              Functional Limitations**   137
           Maureen Hayes Fleming
    Chapter 8   **Interactive Reasoning: Collaborating with
              the Person**   178
           Cheryl Mattingly
           Maureen Hayes Fleming
    Chapter 9   **Conditional Reasoning: Creating
              Meaningful Experiences**   197
           Maureen Hayes Fleming

Part IV Narrative Reasoning: Negotiating the Future   237

    **Chapter 10 The Narrative Nature of Clinical
               Reasoning**   239
               Cheryl Mattingly
    **Chapter 11 Clinical Revision: Changing the
               Therapeutic Story in Midstream**   270
               Cheryl Mattingly

Part V Implications for Practice   293

    Chapter 12 The Underground Practice   295
               Maureen Hayes Fleming
               Cheryl Mattingly
    **Chapter 13 Action and Inquiry: Reasoned Action and
               Active Reasoning**   316
               Maureen Hayes Fleming
               Cheryl Mattingly

Appendix of Clinical Stories   343

Bibliography   361

Index   367

■ P A R T ■

I

Introduction

■

Giving Language to Practice

■ MAUREEN HAYES FLEMING
■ CHERYL MATTINGLY

Introduction

In 1986 the American Occupational Therapy Association (AOTA) and the American Occupational Therapy Foundation (AOTF) funded a large research project which was called the Clinical Reasoning Study. Nedra Gillette, an occupational therapist (OT) and coordinator of research services of the AOTF, was the administrator of the project. Cheryl Mattingly, an anthropologist, and at that time a doctoral candidate at the Massachusetts Institute of Technology, was the principle investigator. In 1987, Maureen Fleming, an occupational therapy educator at Tufts University, joined Mattingly as coinvestigator. The formal part of the study took place from 1986 to 1990. The study continues formally and informally in many ways, both through projects of our own and through those of many occupational therapists working in clinics and studying in graduate schools. Conducting the Clinical Reasoning Study and the subsequent studies and projects has been an intriguing and rewarding process for us and for many colleagues and students. However, one problem has plagued us. People always asked, "When are you going to publish the results of your study?" This question has irked us, not only because we always seemed too busy to devote the long blocks of time to writing that we mistakenly assumed was a writer's privilege, but also because we had a conceptual difficulty. Ethnographic research and action research projects do not yield "results" that can be neatly packaged in columns of numbers to lend a seemly higher order of credibility to the author's pronouncements about the object of study. All research is interpretation, and in ethnography this is especially so. The onus on us was to observe and listen to the therapists as attentively as possible and interpret for you, the reader, how occupational therapists reason in the midst of practice. While this book is based on our research, it is not a report of "findings" such as those reported by investigators conducting quantitative studies. Rather, we present a conception of clinical reasoning developed in the course of carrying out the study. Outlining this conception comprises the major portion of the book.

The conception of clinical reasoning we developed concerns not only *how* therapists think when treating patients, but also something about *what* therapists think about their practice *as* a practice. Together with the therapists we studied, we developed a language for understanding and describing practice. Thus this research project was not confined to the study of isolated cognitive processes that could be called problem solving. It was a project that encompassed the study of real people in their everyday actions, including their language and values. As a result of studying these reasoning processes we learned much about the culture of occupational therapy as well.

A critical aspect of the research design was that clinical reasoning was studied as part of the whole therapeutic process from initial assessment to discharge. Because we looked at the entire process rather than focusing only on assessment, we developed an understanding of thinking in occupational therapy that is very different from that traditionally described in the medical decision-making literature. We assumed from the start that clinical reasoning is a thinking process that happens over time, as therapists interact with patients, and that we needed, therefore, to understand and describe it is an unfolding process. Therapists' reasoning was examined in the context of their intervention and response to clients. This produced a less systematized, though to our minds far more intricate, conception of the reasoning process. The therapist's mental process was always placed within the social context that triggered it—namely, work with patients in particular clinical settings.

This chapter is, in some ways, an overview of the chapters to follow. We briefly discuss the design of the study and examine the role of the language we created to understand the practice. We introduce some concepts that will be elaborated in later chapters. We summarize characteristics of therapists' thinking processes and look particularly at how they are different from thinking processes described in the problem-solving literature. We raise an issue that plagues most practicing therapists, the problem of an "underground practice" created by the conflict between certain OT values and the values of the biomedical culture within which occupational therapists frequently practice.

Not all the things we have to say about clinical reasoning are unique to occupational therapy. While we focus on the practice of occupational therapy, other professionals may find this conception of clinical reasoning relevant to their own practice. This has been the case when we have presented our work to other health professionals, including physical therapists, speech and language therapists, psychotherapists, nurses, psychiatrists, family practice physicians, and pediatricians.

An Ethnographic Study of Clinical Reasoning in Occupational Therapy

THE STUDY

There were two innovative features of the AOTA/AOTF Clinical Reasoning Study. One was the reliance on an ethnographic approach in the study of clinical reasoning. The vast majority of studies of clinical reasoning in the health professions rely on quantitative methods rather than on the extended naturalistic investigation of the practice that characterizes ethnographic research. A second innovation was that ethnography was combined with action research. The boundaries between outside researcher and the research subject were blurred in our study of clinical reasoning, because clinicians who volunteered to be studied also agreed to participate in studying their own practice.

The action research component of this study developed almost (but not quite) by accident. Originally, the primary intent was to do a 1- to 2-year ethnographic study focused on discovering and describing clinical reasoning as manifest in concrete situations of practice. Data collection was to consist of the usual anthropological techniques of participant observation and in-depth interviewing, and videotaping of treatment sessions in which therapists and their clients participated. This study of clinical reasoning did not initially address any concrete practical problems. However, as the therapists who participated in the study became increasingly involved and committed to it as research partners, they discovered that they could take aspects of the research design or findings emerging from the research and apply them to certain practical questions. This study's action research bent grew out of an initial desire on the researchers' part to make the study as collaborative as possible, so that we invited the therapists we were studying to examine their own practice with us. It was an experiment in collaboration. It crossed both disciplinary boundaries and traditional boundaries between academics and practice, and it combined the research interests of the investigators with the practical interests in self-examination and staff development of the therapists. This served as a method whereby clinicians could reflect on their own practice and build into their work schedule a systematic opportunity to examine their own clinical work and that of their colleagues. This resulted in a much more extensive and practical action research project than we initially anticipated.

SEQUENCE OF EVENTS

The site selected was a 900-bed acute care hospital with some rehabilitation wards, including a regional spinal cord unit. The occupational therapy department consisted of 14 therapists working across a wide variety of specializations: acute neurology and cardiology, spinal cord injury, oncology, psychiatry, an outpatient hand clinic, and an outpatient pediatric clinic. Senior therapists from each of these departments became involved in the study. Initially four experienced therapists volunteered to take part. This number gradually expanded to the seven senior therapists, and finally, as the project grew into its second year, it included the entire staff. All of the therapists in this initial study were women.

Data were collected in three ways: through participant observation, through in-depth interviewing of therapists and sometimes patients, and through videotaping clinical sessions between therapists and patients. The research was phased in three segments and moved from open-ended field observations, which relied heavily on naturalistic observation; to more focused interviewing and videotaping of therapists and clients; and finally to the thematic analysis of the data.

The first 4 months of the research were largely spent observing therapists by sitting in on assessment and treatment sessions, staff meetings, lunch hours, and the like. Observations were recorded in field notes. This "hanging around" phase allowed the research team to become familiar with the setting, the pace and schedule of therapists, the range of clinical problems, and with the therapists' interactions with clients. In short, it allowed the team to begin to understand the world within which these therapists lived, and the professional and institutional contexts in which they made their clinical judgments.

The second research stage was much more focused. Therapists were videotaped treating their clients. They were also interviewed before and after clinical sessions. Sometimes patients were interviewed as well. In addition to these highly detailed interviews about particular sessions, therapists were asked to provide larger histories of their work with the clients being videotaped. We asked therapists to describe their reasoning and to tell stories about their work with patients. They were asked to tell, in rich detail, the story of the session and the whole process of working with that particular client. They were also asked to identify what they saw as key decision points, dilemmas, and surprises. Their stories and their experiences of frustration or surprise all served as cues to the underlying assumptions and theories that fueled their reasoning. Finally, they were asked to talk directly about their rationale and their theoretical assumptions in making particular choices and decisions.

The final research stage involved analysis of the data. By the time the data were finally collected, there were approximately 2,000 pages of field notes and written transcripts taken from videotapes of sessions and audiotapes of the accompanying interviews. There were also approximately 30 videotapes of clinical sessions. The research shifted from a purely ethnographic study to an action research study in the process of data analysis. The therapists whose practice we were studying were asked to analyze videotapes of their work with clients and transcripts of their own interviews. However, analysis by the investigators began earlier in the research process. The first group session in which the therapists met together with the research team to begin collective analysis of the data occurred in December 1986, just a month after data collection had begun. These meetings continued throughout the study. As the research project moved into its second year and the emphasis on analysis increased, we held regular meetings with participating therapists at the hospital, where we engaged them in structured analyses of their own videotapes. During the group sessions, therapists were asked to "tell the story" they saw in a videotaped session of a therapist treating a client.

SOME STRATEGIES FOR ANALYSIS

We used storytelling and narrative modes of analysis as a way to help therapists reflect on their practice. One strategy was to have a segment of the videotapes viewed by all members of our group. Therapists were asked to think of the events observed as an unfolding story. Then each was asked to tell their version of the story. Each therapist told a somewhat different story about what they had seen. There were, however, many thematic similarities to the stories. This interpretive strategy highlighted the differences in the overall meaning each participant assigned to what was going on in the session. We asked therapists to view a videotaped session and to divide it into parts as if they were chapters of the story. These chapter titles contributed to the general themes therapists had identified in their stories. We generally followed up with other interpretive exercises that emphasized clinical work as action among multiple actors. These actors could be therapist, client, other medical staff, family members, and even the disease or disability. Sometimes we asked therapists to title the story from the perspective they imagined the therapist in the videotape to have, and then to watch the same slice of videotape again and rename it from the perspective of the patient. At other times, we asked therapists to identify what story they thought the therapist in the tape was trying to enact, and then to pick out what strategies or decisions the therapist appeared to be making in order to try to bring that particular clinical story about. Or we might ask them to examine a videotaped session as a drama and try to describe the nature of the dialogue.

An especially fruitful exercise was to ask the group to find places in a videotape where they saw the therapist getting "stuck" in trying to carry out some therapeutic activity, and then to pick out the strategies they saw the therapist using to extricate herself from the situation.

Looking at their practice as the playing out of stories provided a quite different vantage point for reflection and analysis for these therapists. While they were frequent storytellers about their clinical work in a casual "lunch talk" kind of way, they had never tried to look carefully at their own work using a narrative mode of analysis. This helped them to shift away from thinking of their practice as the employment of technical skills (ranging arms, assessing trunk stability, and the like) to a view of their practice skills and problem solving as an interaction between themselves and their clients. They became much more attentive to how they were implicitly viewing the client in a broader way, how they were constantly developing a picture of therapy as a story that was just a piece of a broader life story of that client.

This narrative reflection also encouraged them to see practice as unfolding and necessarily responsive to unexpected contingencies—a process that was not altogether preordained in the initial treatment plan and that was only partially shaped by their original assessment and planning. Many were initially uncomfortable about thinking of themselves as clinicians who continually, in small and large ways, ran into trouble with clients, so the "getting stuck" analyses were often highly charged. A year later when they reported on how this research had influenced them, nearly everyone mentioned their relief at being able to speak of their practice as a place where things often did not run smoothly and where they and their patients often did not seem to agree about what should happen in therapy. Many appreciated the recognition that part of their clinical skill involved the capacity to continually improvise in order to best respond to what was happening in the immediate setting, and they all grew intrigued with how this capacity to improvise could be better taught to new therapists.

Perhaps the most important outcome of the study was that the therapists became much more conscious of the immense assumptions they were making (had to make, in fact) about the lives of their patients, about what mattered to them. Occupational therapists help clients improve their self-care and their ability to live as independently as possible. Therefore the judgments they make about what constitutes independence and what competencies their clients ought to have are extremely important to therapists' effectiveness. The more we did these narrative analyses of clinical sessions, the more vivid the patients became. Clinical work looked less like carrying out a plan created by the therapist and more like carrying out an interaction in which there were at least two actors—therapist and client.

What Is Clinical Reasoning?

In a sense, the whole purpose of our study was to answer this question as it pertains to occupational therapy. But the more we studied therapy practice, the more complex our notions of clinical reasoning became. There is no one-sentence definition that captures the subtlety of how therapists think in the midst of practice. In fact, we will argue in this book that clinical reasoning involves not one, but several, forms of thinking. Therapists, in other words, think in more than one way. To add to this complexity, clinical reasoning is not reducible to a method (or even several methods) of thinking; it is also a way of perceiving. To talk about how therapists think is necessarily to consider what therapists think about, what they perceive in the way they view their clients, what they focus on as the central problem, what they ignore, how they describe what is physiologically problematic for the client, and even their view of who the client is as a person.

One way to understand clinical reasoning is to differentiate it from theoretical reasoning. While occupational therapists sometimes speak of clinical reasoning as the application of theory to practice, this is a deceptive statement. A grounding in theory is essential for expert practice but does not guarantee such practice. One cannot do without such a grounding, but it, alone, will not yield good clinical interventions, because theoretical reasoning differs from practical reasoning.

Theoretical reasoning is concerned with the general, with what one can reliably predict will hold true in any specific case, or with what will give useful insight into a broad range of particular situations. At the far end, scientific reasoning is the paradigmatic case of theoretical reasoning, because it is concerned with the discovery of universal relationships, especially universal or probabilistic laws. A good theory is useful because it gives us insights into a myriad of situations, allowing us to see a particular situation as an instance of some general category or as caused by some general condition that the theory explains. Solid theoretical knowledge of neuroanatomy and physiology, for example, tells us in quite accurate empirical detail what kind of physical damage we can expect to see when someone has sustained an injury to the spinal column and what part of that damage is likely to be permanent. Because this is general knowledge that holds true regardless of the particular patient, it allows us to speak in great detail about a situation we know little about in terms of contextual specifics. This is the kind of knowledge that can be gained effectively from textbooks.

And yet, theory is not enough. Seasoned clinicians are quick to point this out, though they often find that "knowing more than they can tell" is a very troublesome feature of everyday practice. Occupational therapists often worry that they cannot explain and justify what they do to others outside the profession. They also worry when they cannot explain to students and novice therapists why a particular therapeutic intervention made the most sense with Ms. Jackson but was all wrong for Mr. Green, or how they knew they had to abandon the treatment plan 5 minutes into a session with 2-year-old Joey. Therapists use a certain set of phrases to capture this elusive practical wisdom. They speak of the "art of therapy" or of "getting a feel for what works." What makes it so difficult to translate good clinical judgment into words? And why is knowledge of occupational therapy theories, the biological sciences, and therapeutic techniques a necessary, but insufficient, guide to guarantee good practice? Why does the exasperated supervisor often still exhort the student to "trust me" or "watch me" rather than reciting the relevant technique, rule, or theoretical concept to explain his or her action? (And, for all the imperfection of this exhortation, we know that clinicians believe the most significant educational factor in shaping their own practice was a mentoring clinician.) What, in other words, makes practical knowledge different from textbook knowledge or school-learned technical skill? While clinical reasoning is a kind of practical know-how that deploys theoretical knowledge, it is far more than a simple application of theory. Theory is not enough because clinical reasoning results in *action*. The nature of action compels the actor to do more than apply general theories or techniques.

Clinical reasoning in occupational therapy is quite close to Aristotle's ancient concept of practical reasoning. Practical reasoning, in the Aristotelian sense, results in action. But figuring out how to act, or what course of action to take, is more than an instrumental skill. It involves deliberation about what an appropriate action *is* in this particular case, with this particular patient, at this particular time. This is no mere technical question. Aristotle associates the expert practical actor with a virtuous actor, one who is able to see rightly how to act in a given situation. Aristotle gave the example of the simple practical action of getting angry at someone, or giving money to someone. Even these apparently simple actions require an expertise that is more like wisdom than mere competence, for they require the actor to ascertain what is the right action in a given case. In *Nicomachean Ethics* Aristotle wrote of this:

> So . . . getting angry, or giving and spending money, is easy and anyone can do it; but doing it to the right person, in the right amount, at the right time, for the right end, and in the right way is no longer easy, nor can

everyone do it. Hence [doing these things] well is rare, praiseworthy, and fine. (1985, p. 51)

If this is true of lending money, how much more is it the case for assessing whether helping this recently disabled stroke patient learn to dress himself is the right thing to be doing, what amount of skill is necessary, whether it is the right time, what is the right way of doing it—even whether this is the right person to be teaching dressing skills? While theory directs us to what is generally the case, action always occurs in a very individual context. The very power of theory is that it is general; but this is also its drawback. Any particular situation is always more subtle, and in some way different, from the complexities of the general case. Any theoretical knowledge is bound to be crude and approximate, giving a starting place for action but not giving a rule book. When therapists speak of "individualizing treatment" they are recognizing the same point Aristotle noticed about good practical action: the need to improvise from general heuristics, theoretical constructs, and rules-of-thumb to the specific requirements of a particular situation.

There is, however, an even more fundamental feature of clinical reasoning in occupational therapy that distinguishes it from applied science. Aristotle argued that a major part of practical reasoning includes reasoning about what the nature of "the good" is in a particular case. It required moving from general considerations about the good, to a judgment about what the best good for a given situation was. For Aristotle, the good is not fixed in the way that our scientific knowledge is: "what is good and healthy for human beings . . . is not the same, but what is white or straight is always the same" (1985, p. 157).

The model of professional reasoning treated as applied science presumes that the work of the practitioner is simply to identify which means (including techniques) will best get one to the ends required; hence, such thinking is often referred to as *means-ends rationality* or *technical rationality*. The end, the final goal, what Aristotle calls "the good" is not what scientific reasoning is designed to consider. The diagnostic reasoning of medical science nicely fits the scientific model in the sense that it is presumed that the physician need not consider the end or the good—inducing better health by treating a disease—but only the best techniques and procedures for arriving at the good, means which certainly include diagnosing the disease to be treated. When this good comes into question (e.g., should a dying patient be kept on life-support systems?), this is marginalized in the medical profession as a problem of ethics, which is distinguished from a problem of clinical decision making.

However, Aristotle (1985) made no such distinction. He linked expertise in rational calculation (assessing the best means to achieve the good) with intelligence at discerning what the best good in a situation might be. He connects the need to assess the particular situation, the ability to calculate, the need to discover the best good in a particular context, and the critical role of experience, as well as general knowledge, in doing so. In a brilliantly succinct passage he states:

> The unconditionally good deliberator is the one whose aim expresses rational calculation in pursuit of the best good for a human being that is achievable in action. Nor is intelligence about universals only. It must also come to know particulars, since it is concerned with action and action is about particulars. Hence . . . some people who lack knowledge but have experience are better in action than others who have knowledge. (1985, p. 158)

If one examines the range of professions, it is clear that all professionals sometimes can simply engage in a process of technical reasoning because the ends are not being questioned. The airline pilot, for example, need not reconsider whether he really ought to fly to Washington National after all, because many of his passengers would much prefer Rio as their final destination, nor need he face the additional problem of calculating where he can get the extra gas because he had initially been planning a much shorter trip. Depending on your perspective, occupational therapists are either more or less lucky. They do, very often, have the problem of reassessment while en route. Theirs is a complex practice in which they do have to reconsider and recalculate, often while in the midst of a treatment session. This sort of clinical judgment is almost invisible to the practicing therapist. It simply becomes part of a largely tacit thought process, a habituated expertise that allows the therapist to pay attention to relevant cues and unconsciously shift therapeutic interventions in response to them.

Occupational therapists have to pay so much attention to "the good" in an individualized way because occupational therapy is directed not only to the patient's physical problems but also to the meaning of the disability for the person in his or her life. Clinical reasoning in occupational therapy is directed not only to a biological world of disease but to the human world of motives and values and beliefs—a world of human meaning. Occupational therapists' fundamental task is in treating what medical anthropologists call the *illness experience* (Good & Delvecchio Good, 1980; Kleinman, 1988). The illness experience refers to the meaning that a disability takes on for a particular patient, that is, how disease and disability enter the phenomenological world of each person. Clinical reasoning, taken in this sense, becomes a form of phenomenological thinking.

The extent to which occupational therapists consider issues of meaning quickly became evident in the Clinical Reasoning Study. The therapists that we studied often became involved in a host of problems surrounding chronic illness and disability that their patients viewed as profound. The most ordinary and simple of tasks—eating lunch with an adaptive fork, moving a checker piece with a mouth stick, navigating a wheelchair down a hospital corridor—often triggered deep reactions from patients as they confronted bodies that would never be the same as they once were. As every practicing therapist knows, designing a successful treatment process for a patient goes far beyond grading tasks to increase motor and cognitive skills. It involves creating therapeutic experiences in which patients must deal with very imperfect bodies, often with dying bodies, and still find some reason to struggle for a meaningful life. This is an important clinical task, one that therapists sometimes hoped to avoid but seldom could. Even the therapists who had hoped to treat a hand or a memory deficit often found themselves treating much more because the patient had not just injured a hand or suffered a brain lesion but, in the process, had permanently disrupted an entire life. Even when it was not written into the treatment plan, therapists found themselves having to help patients find some reason to continue doing their hand exercises or to bother to get up in the morning and dress themselves. It appeared that this level of clinical problem was both commonplace and fundamental in occupational therapy practice. This meant that activities like toilet transfer were seen by therapists not just in terms of skill building, but also in light of the patients' experiences of losing old capacities and orientations in the world, and the meaning of their learning new ways of orienting themselves. So clinical reasoning for occupational therapists was not simply scientific reasoning, matching condition to therapy of choice; it went beyond that to a complex practical reasoning aimed at determining "the good" for each particular client.

Giving Unfamiliar Names to Familiar Practices

EXCAVATING THE TACIT DIMENSION

In retrospect, it is clear that the most important outcome of this research was articulating a range of tacit and unexamined features of occupational therapy practice. Sometimes therapists did not express what they knew or were thinking because their practical wisdom was not formulated in words. They knew by doing. While not all that an experienced therapist knows can be put in words, many aspects of occupational therapy practice have been unnecessarily fuzzy, particularly those phenomenological aspects that are not well articulated in biomedicine as a whole. As part of the research process, we began devising a language for features of clinical reasoning that were previously nameless, or viewed as peripheral. The value of helping to give language to practice, especially to the more phenomenological aspects of practice, has become increasingly evident to us.

We did not know when we began this research study that one thing we had to offer therapists was a foreign language that they could use to examine their own practice, seeing familiar things in a new way. Part of the foreignness of the language was simply the result of the multi-disciplinary nature of the research team, especially the collaboration of an anthropologist, an obvious outsider to the field, and an occupational therapist whose graduate education was in phenomenology. The presence of an outsider forced therapists to articulate their thinking in unusual ways. One therapist interviewed as part of a follow-up study by Nedra Gillette explained what this was like. "The external viewer forces people to talk in a different language. Thus they have to think about it [practice] differently, reformulate their notions to explain them in language that the observer can understand." Developing language is a common part of the ethnographic enterprise. It is the result of ethnographic analysis itself, which involves creating taxonomies and finding themes in our observations. In our analytical work of generating codes to "clump" our data, we sometimes borrowed from the language (especially the informal language) therapists themselves used to describe their practice. We used familiar terms such as: "individualizing treatment," "treating the whole patient," "using common sense," "telling stories," "putting it all together," in new ways. Sometimes we drew upon constructs from other disciplines—including phenomenology, literary theory, anthropology, and cognitive psychology—which provided us with a more elaborate, theoretically dense language for analyzing what we were observing and hearing. We introduced exotic constructs (the "lived body," "procedural reasoning," "emplotment," "intentionality," and the like) from a variety of sources. Initially, we introduced new words for pragmatic reasons, as needed, just in the course of sharing with the therapists whom we studied what we were finding, or in asking them to critique our ways of naming what we were seeing in the data. But we quickly recognized that the therapists got intrigued with this "language game," as they helped us learn how to use concepts we were just beginning to formulate, like "creating a future story," or thinking with a "three-track mind."

Given their adeptness, even their thirst, for a language that drifted so far from biomedical discourse, it is not surprising that several years later they identified this as the greatest contribution we made to their practice. One psychiatric therapist said, "Now we have a language to share what we have always been thinking about." They spoke of finally being able to verbalize what they were doing. Another therapist remarked, "Clinical reasoning helps create a language, a framework for thinking about practice that truly makes sense."

They linked this language development to a growing sense of validation as a profession. "When we present to others," a physical disabilities therapist said, "we present ourselves as one who knows what she's talking about and where she stands on the team." One noted that "having a language to share reasoning gives us a feeling of professional identity. In a setting where OTs are definitely outnumbered, the uniqueness of the profession is strengthened." Their sense of validation also came because in the creation of language, we were examining many parts of practice that were usually relegated to the underground as serious and legitimate aspects of practice. Several therapists we interviewed mentioned the importance of speaking of the underground practice, especially since, ironically, many aspects of their professional work that they politically felt they had to hide were precisely those which reflected some of the deepest values of the profession. One said, "We now feel we have been given permission to practice OT, not some sort of PT [physical therapy] for the arms." Another mentioned that her "first impression was that the clinical reasoning study legitimized underground practice." This was an important step for her, she said, because it changed what she felt she could legitimately claim as part of her work. Previously she had felt constrained about what she could include in documentation.

The development of a common language, which helped them first to recognize and then to articulate the large body of tacit knowledge they had in common, was seen as an extraordinary asset, not only to their practice per se, but to their recognition as professionals in their work settings. While confirming a fundamental insecurity of the profession (the assumption that the work of the field is not accorded great respect within the medical model), it also confirmed for these therapists the true value of what they did and allowed them to recognize why OT may not be so highly regarded: it derives from a set of socially relevant assumptions about people and their need to function successfully in their day-to-day lives. Occupational therapy does not address, as its primary concern, matters of curing disease and preventing death. The field, instead, is concerned with life: its quality, its potential, and how it may be enhanced through normal occupations. Language has many values embedded in it. The respondents seemed to imply that this new language was rooted in the fundamental values of the profession, and that it gave them confidence and security in incorporating those values into their practice.

MEANING-MAKING

Many of the terms we created were intended to illuminate those aspects of practice especially concerned with meaning. Occupational therapists use the term "occupation" to imply that occupation involves both action and meaning. Action taking and meaning-making are the central therapeutic processes that comprise occupational therapy. Occupation, as therapists use it, is similar to the concept of action that phenomenologists hold: action embodies meaning. We also noted that action gives form to meaning. Occupational therapists help people whose ability to take action has been limited to forge new relationships between their action taking and meaning-making; and they value the ability to take action in order to participate in the social world. They eschew the more common notion that individuals with limited ability to take action should be excluded from everyday society. They feel that personal worth and meaning should not be reduced along with a reduction in the person's action-taking capacities.

Occupational therapy is focused on quality of life. Activity, OTs assume, is a central force in achieving quality of life. Therapists talk about the value of "engagement" in activity. Engagement means an involvement, a sense of connection with the activity, an investment in the activity. We introduced the concept of intentionality (Schutz, 1970) to connect OTs' implicit understanding of engagement to the more formal concept of intentionality and allow for further explication of the concept. Occupational therapists value self-expression or self-fulfillment and believe these can be achieved through engagement in meaningful activity. Therapists value being engaged in one's life and in one's physical and social contexts and hope that their patients can continue that social engagement when they leave the clinic. As Engelhardt summed up the central concept of occupational therapy very well, "The value of occupational therapy is engagement in the world" (1977, p. 672).

COMMON SENSE

One concept we introduced was the notion of OT as a common-sense practice. Occupational therapy enables patients to engage in the occupations of everyday life: to reenter their commonsense world after they have incurred a disability that has profoundly altered their usual ways of experiencing the life-world. Occupational therapists, as workers in the clinic, in many ways represent the everyday world, because they reteach those very habits and actions which anchor us to the life-world, and the personal and cultural meanings which comprise it. They have patients take action in the hospital in order to return to a meaningful life in the community.

Occupational therapists often say that much of what they do is just common sense. Often, at the same time, they express an element of surprise at the seeming lack of common sense on the part of other members of the hospital staff. We linked their high degree of common sense to both their professional culture, following on Geertz's notion of common sense as culture (1983), and a particular, complex kind of intelligence as proposed by Gardner (1983). Thus, common sense became a term that expressed a particular kind of personal-cultural insight linked to a practical know-how that they saw as characteristic of OT.

INTEGRATING DISPARATE MODES OF REASONING

We also introduced language to differentiate the several kinds of reasoning therapists use in their daily practice. Observing therapists in practice and conversing with them about the way they solved clinical problems made us realize that therapists use a variety of reasoning strategies. Different modes of thinking are employed for different purposes and in response to particular features of the clinical problem complex. Three of these forms of reasoning we called procedural reasoning, interactive reasoning, and conditional reasoning (Fleming, 1989). Another form was narrative reasoning (Mattingly, 1989, 1991). The first three will be briefly introduced in this section and narrative reasoning will be discussed next.

Each type of reasoning is employed to address different aspects of the whole problem. Procedural reasoning is used when therapists think about the person's physical ailments and what procedures might possibly alleviate them or remediate the person's functional performance problems. In this mode, the therapist's dual search is for problem definition and treatment selection. In situations where problem identification and treatment selection are seen as the central task, the therapist's thinking strategies demonstrate many parallels to the patterns identified by other researchers interested in problem solving in general, and in clinical problem solving in particular.

Interactive reasoning is used to help the therapists to interact with and better understand the person. Interactive reasoning takes place during face-to-face encounters between therapist and patient. It is the form of reasoning that therapists employ when they want to better understand the patient as a person. There are many reasons why a therapist might want to know the person better. The therapist might want to know how the person feels about the treatment at the moment; or what the patient is like as a person, either out of sheer interest or in order to more finely tailor the treatment to his or her specific needs or preferences. Further, the therapist may be interested in this person, in order to better understand the experience of the disability from the person's own point of view. Conditional reasoning, a complex form of social reasoning, is used to help the patient in the difficult process of reconstructing a life that is now permanently changed by injury or disease.

The concept of conditional reasoning is perhaps the most elusive notion in our proposed theory of multiple modes of thinking. Yet we are firmly, if intuitively, convinced that there is a third form of reasoning that many experienced therapists used. This reasoning style moves beyond specific concerns about the person and the physical problems and places them in broader social and temporal contexts. The term "conditional" was used because therapists think about the whole condition, including the person, the illness, the meanings the illness has for the person, the family, and the social and physical contexts in which the person lives. Therapists needed to imagine how the condition could change and become a revised condition. The imagined new state may or may not be achieved. The success or failure was very much contingent upon the patient's participation. The client must participate, not only in the therapeutic activities themselves, but also in the construction of the image of the possible outcome, the revised condition.

These reasoning strategies are distinctly different in both form and process; yet therapists shift rapidly from one type of reasoning to another. The reasoning style employed changes as the therapist's attention is drawn from one aspect of the problem to another. Therapists process or analyze different aspects of the problem, almost simultaneously, using different thinking styles but do not lose track of their thoughts about other aspects of a problem as those components are temporarily shifted to the background and another aspect is dealt with immediately in the foreground.

NARRATIVE REASONING: MAKING SENSE OF THE ILLNESS EXPERIENCE

Sometimes we did not give new terms to practice so much as elevate ordinary OT terms and jargon so that they took on greater significance. This was particularly the case in our focus on the narrative aspects of clinical reasoning in occupational therapy. We took seriously a part of practice that therapists generally did not notice—their own everyday storytelling. Therapists we studied often traded stories about patients in the lunch room. This was not gossip. Rather, it turned out to serve two very important functions. It was a method of puzzling out a problem. A therapist might be perplexed about a patient, and perhaps have difficulty engaging the person in treatment or figuring out just what activity might work. The therapist might mention the problem in an offhanded way, and soon one or more therapists would join in the conversation. Often someone would begin with a comment like, "I had a patient like that once. Let me tell you about him." Stories or bits of stories would be shared in an attempt to offer suggestions for possible strategies to try. The storytelling elicited suggestions from the other therapists and these suggestions offered support for the therapist in a "stuck spot."

The other function that these lunchroom stories seemed to serve was a way to enlarge each therapist's fund of practical knowledge through vicariously sharing other therapists' experience. Our hypothesis that storytelling enlarges the practical knowledge of the group is in concert with the concept that many theorists hold: that storytelling is a central way of building and enlarging meanings that comprise the culture. The culture of OT seems to be comprised of a rich fabric of stories. These stories form a bond between therapists and also *teach* them much more than they could learn in a classroom or through their own personal experience. The clinical experience of one therapist becomes part of the collective experience of the group through storytelling. Storytelling was not the only way therapists thought about their patients, but it is a very fundamental one.

When therapists think with stories they are trying to understand the particular problem, to understand the particularity of some person's experience. Narrative thinking is intimately tied to our way of making sense of human experience, especially through an investigation of human motives. The narrative nature of clinical reasoning manifests itself in two ways. First, in the work therapists must do to try to understand the effect of a disability on the life story of a particular patient. Second, in the therapist's need to structure therapy in a narrative way—as an unfolding story—to make the story come true. This is perhaps the most interesting and subtle use of narrative reasoning in occupational therapy practice. Therapy can be seen as a kind of "short story" within the longer life story a client is living. The therapist enters and exits a client's life, playing a part for only a small period. Often this part occurs at a critical juncture in a patient's life, a turning point triggered by the onset of a significant downturn in the progress of an illness. Sometimes it occurs at a critical juncture in an entire family's life, as when a family is just learning to adjust to the entrance of a disabled infant into their midst, or when the head of an extended family loses that role through illness or injury. If we consider disability in narrative terms, as something that interrupts and irreversibly changes a client's life story, then work with a client can be seen as one chapter in that life story.

Therapists were quite accustomed to telling stories, but not to thinking about their stories as evincing a narrative reasoning process. The language of narrative theory was unfamiliar as an analytical category. We introduced concepts from literary theory such as emplotment, narrative desire, dramatic conflict with identified protagonists and antagonists, and suspenseful endings. We asked therapists to think about their work by describing what sort of "story" they thought they were in with a particular client. This introduction of concepts highlighted how intensely therapists cared to make therapy itself an occasion for patients to remake life stories that could no longer continue as they once had when a disability was absent or less serious. The notion of the therapeutic short story threw into high relief the therapeutic task of negotiating what meaningful role therapy was going to play within the unfolding illness and rehabilitation the patient was living through.

It also allowed therapists to be more explicit about the process of treatment as an end in itself. In interviews, it became clear that therapists were not simply concerned with reading a set of treatment objects, but with the whole process of therapy unfolding in such a way that patients were given powerful experiences of successfully met challenges. Often, from their personal point of view, it was not reaching the final goal per se that measured the success of therapy, but the therapeutic experience along the way, where patients developed increasing confidence and commitment to take on challenges, even with their disabilities. This personal perspective on effective practice, however, was lost in the formal language of the clinic. When therapists documented their work in the medical charts or in medical rounds and the like, there was little place to discuss the process of therapy. Official biomedical language invoked a language of instrumental rationality where therapeutic events were represented as isolated, specific techniques (the means) for achieving a series of isolated, measurable treatment goals. The language of narrative allowed therapists to recapture and reflect upon the holistic nature of practice and the importance of the therapeutic experience.

In interviews where therapists were asked to identify how their participation in this research study (or subsequent studies) influenced their practice, they often named the focus on narrative. It helped them consider the patient's future outside therapy, for we had often talked about the imaginative reasoning therapists engage in when trying to construct in their minds the patient's "future story." One said, "In the acute care settings, with the time 'crunch,' narrative is especially useful in helping think about the patient's future, and integrating the patient's past and future." A pediatric therapist mentioned that with her patients, she really had two clients, the child and the family. She used the narrative notion of a therapeutic story to consider two separate stories, the family story and the child's story. A third therapist, who is currently manager of a large rehabilitation unit, described her efforts to encourage therapists in her unit to think in a more self-conscious narrative fashion. She said "therapists can adapt the environment to allow more attention to story building. This is seen as a form of validation." She mentioned that therapists also felt freer to engage in a "greater exchange of their own stories amongst the patients." During analysis of the data, we noticed how often therapists spoke of having "future images" of their patients, and how often the future stories they imagined were created from vivid images they had about what they saw the patient doing when they returned home from the hospital. Several therapists mentioned the value of focusing on the image-making aspects of clinical reasoning.

A highly experienced therapist who works in acute neurology and had been clinical supervisor of students for several years said, "Without a mental image, cues will not be recognized." She helped students notice and develop their image-making capacities. She felt that the sooner students noticed the complex images they were creating from cues they were receiving, the sooner they could become aware of a need to modify those images as further cues warranted. She described this process: "The student forms a hypothesis ahead of time. Then he can compare his reasoning as it enlarges the image, identify recognizable cues, and more easily change the image on the spot." Another therapist who also teaches clinical reasoning to young therapists and affiliating students said that she had begun to have them start building mental libraries of their own stories. She asked them to analyze their clinical experiences as stories by asking themselves, "Who are the characters? Where are you in the story? What is your hypothesis about what is going to happen in the story? What is the moral of this story?"

The remainder of this book considers these constructs in more detail. We consider the tacit nature of clinical reasoning in the following chapter. Part II of the book concerns the nature of occupational therapy as a professional culture in the context of the dominant biomedical culture of the clinic. Because clinical thinking does not happen in a vacuum but in a specific context, we consider the profesional context of occupational therapy and its influence on how therapists decide what clinical problems are theirs to solve. Part II, then, to use the language of Donald Schön (1983, 1987), is about how therapists *set* problems. We sketch those central values and beliefs within this professional culture that influence the judgments therapists make about such basic issues as how to approach a patient, what counts as an "appropriate" goal, and what is "real OT." Parts III and IV take a closer look at the multiple forms of reasoning therapists employ in treating clients. The final section, Part V, raises a series of problems or dilemmas therapists typically face because they often perceive clinical problems. While the practice is often deeply appreciated by both clients and colleagues, therapists can find themselves "misfits" in the clinical setting as defined by the medical model. How they define clinical problems, how they involve their clients, the tools they use, and the ways they reason often put therapists at odds with the dominant professional cultures in which they practice. We hope this book will help therapists articulate their perspectives more clearly and become reflective (rather than apologetic) about what they do and how they think.

■

The Search for Tacit Knowledge

■ MAUREEN HAYES FLEMING

Introduction

One of the purposes of the AOTA/AOTF Clinical Reasoning Study was to discover how occupational therapists think in day-to-day practice situations. Some of the early considerations about the design of the study were based on the work of Donald Schön (1983), who studies how practitioners think in action. He proposed that much of what professionals do is guided by an implicit fund of knowledge gained largely through experience. He further proposed that such knowledge is brought to bear on situations by employing practical theories that organize and make sense of situations so that the practitioner can act in an economical and fruitful way. Some of these practical theories, Schön maintains, are communicated to peers and apprentices and thus become part of the shared repertoire of the group. Schön's intellectual stance that theory can arise from practice challenges the popular scientific notion that practice is simply the application of theory. We agree with the concept that theory can arise from practice. Nedra Gillette, one of the original designers of the study, envisioned that the discovery of these practical theories was one of the central purposes of the study.

Explicating Practical Theories

THE LEGITIMACY OF PRACTICAL THEORIES

The concept that practical theory is a legitimate form of theory is central to the American Pragmatist philosophy of such scholars as William James, John Dewey, and Charles Sanders Pierce. These philoso-phers theorized about practice, but Schön actually studied the day-to-day work of a variety of practitioners. Schön proposed that much prac-tical knowledge is tacit knowledge, shared directly from practitioner to apprentice in real-life situations. The notion of tacit knowledge was proposed by Polanyi (1966) to refer to the knowledge that practitioners have that is known in a direct practical way but is not stated as a formal theory. Polanyi proposed that this practical knowledge or theory is essential to the proficient execution of the acts that comprise expert practice. Polanyi emphasizes "practical wisdom is more truly embodied in action than expressed in rules of action" (1974, p. 54). Such practical wisdom, gained through experience, Polanyi says, resides in the tacit dimension (1966). Schön proposed that this implicit knowledge de-velops as a result of the person's ability to think about or "reflect" upon an event as it is taking place. Thus, through action and reflection the practitioner builds a fund of "implicit" (Koestler, 1948), or "tacit" (Po-lanyi, 1963), knowledge, which is incorporated into and guides the future action (Dewey, 1915; Pierce, 1931–35) comprising daily practice. This practical theory that guides action is sometimes referred to as "praxis," or knowing how to guide one's actions without specifically thinking about them (Bernstein, 1971).

We used the term "theory" in a particular way. We made an as-sumption that therapists' work may be guided by some of the overall or "grand" theories of the profession or other disciplines upon which their academic education is based. However, we also thought it was more probable that therapists would use the personal, practical theories they had developed as a result of their experience. Argyris and Schön (1981) call these two types of theory "espoused theories" and "theories-in-use." "Theories-in-use," they claim, are what actually guide practice and make up for the deficiencies of "espoused theories"—theories that practitioners say they are using—to inform practice. Our search was a search for both the tacit knowledge that therapists have and the theories-in-use that they employed to bring that knowledge to bear on the daily practical problems of the therapeutic situation.

PRACTICAL THEORIES AND PROFESSIONAL EXPERTISE

A problem with any profession is that a large part of expert knowl-edge is tacit. A further problem is that such knowledge often remains tacit. Tacit knowledge is an essential part of what makes a person expert or proficient. Often, however, a practitioner can execute moves that he cannot describe, or make selections she cannot articulate reasons for, even though these were expert performances based on the best ration-ales. While tacit knowledge contributes to the expertise of the individual, it does not contribute to the collective knowledge of the profession. Much of the expertise of a profession develops as a result of the experience and insight of individual practitioners. Practitioners share their accrued knowledge and their implicit "theories-in-use" with their apprentices and colleagues through their daily interactions and through clinical stories; an individual may formulate practical wisdom into a "grand" theory and communicate it to others so that it becomes part of the "espoused theory" of the group. On the other hand, much practical knowledge is not formulated verbally, nor structured as theory or as formal procedures with the accompanying principles of practice.

Practitioners often understand one another and what they are doing but lack a language to describe aspects of the practice or explicate the reasons for it. Although it is essential to recognize the limits of explication and generalized theory to fully comprehend the subleties of a practice, we decided that part of our task was to begin to develop a language to describe therapists' reasoning strategies and processes. This explication would, in turn, yield some other information, such as tacit knowledge about the rules-of-thumb (heuristics) that therapists employed in various treatment situations. Further, this explication would provide a language with which therapists could more clearly communicate with one another about their practice. Fortunately, during the course of our research we discovered several types of tacit knowledge among experienced practitioners, along with many theories-in-use, and, surprisingly, a deeply held philosophy as well. We did not so much discover a set of particular problem-solving strategies as explore the culture of occupational therapy practice, complete with language, values, and even, in some sense, ceremony.

Knowing and Saying

WE KNOW MORE THAN WE CAN TELL

Perhaps Polanyi's most well-known comment is, "We can know more than we can tell" (1966, p. 4). This needs no further embellishment. It is a direct and understandable statement. All of us go about our daily activities acting successfully in situations that defy description. We trust our "sixth sense" to get us through many simple and complex tasks. But practicing professionals are often called upon to say what it is that they know—to "tell" or give reasons for what they are doing. For both political and professional motives it is important that practitioners learn to *say* what they *know*. This is a particular problem for occupational therapists because, although what they do looks simple, what they know is quite complex. To be able to say what one knows can in some way make up for the rift between the surface simplicity and the conceptual complexity of the practice.

Schön (1983) has demonstrated that practitioners of various sorts have a "stock of knowledge" (Polanyi, 1966), which is largely tacit. A simple reason that "we know more than we can tell" is that people can think and act much more quickly than they can verbally describe or explain. So we develop a whole discourse of knowledge that is based more in action than in language. Another reason is that practice is *doing*. A profession develops a practical knowledge of doing that is seldom discussed or explicitly described. Practitioners spend much more time and energy doing than they spend talking about what they do and why. This of course contributes to the elegance of practice. But it does not serve to develop the language of practice. Nevertheless, people learn by doing and learn quite well. The experienced practitioner is thus able to act quickly and do the right thing as demanded by the situation. Buchler (1955) refers to this as making "active judgments" of practice. Finally, there are not enough words to describe everything that people can know and do. As a practice becomes more complex, the available vocabulary to describe it falters.

It is easy to discount tacit knowledge because it is mostly nonlinguistic and appears inferior to more abstract language-based knowledge. Tacit knowledge may be partly articulated but always comprehends more than can be stated. Polanyi stresses:

> Although the expert diagnostician, taxonomist and cotton-classer can indicate their clues and formulate their maxims, they know many more things than they can tell, knowing them only in practice, as instrumental particulars, and not explicitly as object. . . . This applies to . . . the art of knowing and to . . . the art of doing, wherefore both can be taught only by the aid of practical example and never solely by precept. (1958, p. 88)

This tacit understanding of knowing and doing is something that experienced practitioners implicitly trust. They know that they "know what they are doing." They have confidence that they can assess a situation quickly and accurately and quickly "come up with the right answer" or "do the right thing." This implicit confidence in their own ability is probably another factor that contributes to the apparent ease with which experts perform. Yet, they tell us, "It's not easy." Therapists in the Clinical Reasoning Study described themselves as always having to think, always ready to be "on the lookout" for cues that would indicate how the patient was feeling and how the session was going. Good practice was not by any means automatic practice. Therapists thought often and thought hard, and were continually accessing and reassessing their tacit knowledge. Interestingly, therapists often did not realize that they were thinking, unless interviewers asked them to describe their thinking. They envisioned themselves as doing their job and trying to do their best for the patient. It was not that therapists did not think; it was that therapists did not think about thinking. They thought about the patients' problems and how to solve them and how to, as they say, "make the session work." Therapists were often surprised to find how much they knew and how many "bits" of knowledge they included in any one problem-solving task. When they made their tacit knowledge explicit they were surprised at how much tacit knowledge they had.

ACCESS TO TACIT KNOWLEDGE

Tacit knowledge forms the base of all other thoughts and actions that comprise practice. If "we can know more than we can tell," then it is implied that there is something to be known that is not language based. A practitioner often knows how to do things well but cannot describe all the qualities of that performance. While teaching a student, a practitioner often not only gives directions on how a procedure should be executed, but says "watch me" and demonstrates the most complex aspects of the task.

Conversely, one often hears practitioners say, "I learn so much from teaching students." Very often the person is not learning something new. The therapist may be explicitly expressing for the first time knowledge that was once implicit. The clinician may have acquired this knowledge in school and employed it frequently in practice, but may not have verbalized it until the student required that information. In other cases it may be that being forced to explain actions, a practitioner may organize heretofore nonlinguistic experiential knowledge into a verbal description.

The common term "stock of knowledge" refers to the professional's whole collection of knowledge. Much of that collection, or stock, of knowledge seems to be tacit. It seemed to us that therapists had two types of tacit knowledge. One type was specific knowledge that they had once learned in a fairly conscious and sometimes concrete way, and that had subsequently settled in the tacit domain. Examples of such knowledge might be knowledge of anatomy, gained through lecture, study, demonstration, and dissection—knowledge which was once difficult to learn but which eventually became part of the background, working knowledge of the experienced therapist. One could say that knowledge which was once in the forefront of consciousness had "sunk" to the tacit dimension. The other type was knowledge which had never been verbal but was always in the tacit dimension. Such knowledge was acquired through experience and became incorporated in the person's stock of practical knowledge. This knowledge therapists sometimes refer to by using expressions such as: "the look in her eye," "the quality of his gait," or the "tone of the muscle," "just didn't seem right." Here, therapists are expressing an experience-based knowledge that they have acquired but do not have specific words to describe. This tacit knowledge guides the therapists' selection and execution of the repertoire of evaluation and treatment procedures in very significant ways; but sometimes the lack of ability to express just why the therapist thinks the patient has poor judgment or an unstable gait presents a serious problem for therapists and how they are perceived by other professionals.

The Efficient Elegance of Practice

When we have shown videotaped sessions of expert practitioners and their patients, a very common response is often something like: "The way the therapist acted with the patient looked so elegant and effortless. It almost looked like a dance." It is a well-known phenomenon that expert athletes and artists appear to be giving an effortless performance. This is a result of ability, and long years and grueling hours of practice. But even those elegant performances are difficult and require skill, energy, and concentration. It soon became clear that effortless-looking performance is a daily occurrence among experienced practitioners. Experienced therapists informed us that the practice "isn't as easy as it looks." As one experienced therapist put it, "Each new patient or treatment is always a struggle. There is always something new and different that you have to figure out to get the session to go just right." Why are expert practitioners able to perform gracefully and adjust rapidly to complex clinical situations? Why do they do so many things seemingly automatically? Why are many of their day-to-day performances, which were once so difficult to learn, "second nature" (Hayes, 1978) to them now?

One reason for this effortless appearance is that experts are efficient. There is an economy of motions and words. They "get it right" in very few tries. Benner noted this in her study of nurses (1984). This efficiency and economy clearly has something to do with experience. But what? Koestler commented, "The true essence of economy is implicitness" (1948). Experts have an implicit understanding of a whole range of minute details of the phenomena that they understand. They recognize small details and nuances and interpret them with impressive speed and accuracy. Therapists, for example, can feel small changes in muscle tone or see subtle variations in the quality of a person's movement patterns; and they adjust their own tone of voice or body position almost instantaneously in response to subtle cues indicating the emotional status of the patient.

Through constant awareness and processing of their own experience the practitioners can gain a vast repertoire of tacit knowledge that is complex and very accurate. This complex knowledge is based in experience. Often it can be articulated in some form, but the understanding of the phenomenon that is of interest comes to the experienced practitioner in a direct way, not through the lengthy corridors of explanation. An example from Robert Murphy's (1987) account of his experiences as a patient with a tumor in his spinal column may serve to describe this. Murphy describes his encounters with the neurologists who used him as a teaching device for residents:

> A recently retired clinical neurologist asked if he could use my body to demonstrate a standard workup to a young resident. He went through the entire process for an hour, explaining to his student the purpose of each test and the meaning of each of my responses, both verbal and reflexive. By the end, I knew a lot more about my malady, and I also knew that he could have diagnosed my illness without a CAT [computer-assisted tomography] scan or even a myelogram. (p. 37)

Here Murphy recognizes the elegant simplicity of the work of an experienced practitioner with a vast fund of tacit knowledge.

Types of Tacit Knowledge

TACIT KNOWLEDGE: LANGUAGE AND OTHER SYMBOLS

Polanyi (1974, p. 87) refers to three types of tacit knowledge that I will only paraphrase here:

1. Ineffable. This is "knowledge whereby something is known but has not been expressed in spoken language."
2. Intelligible. This is knowledge "where the tacit component is the information conveyed by easily intelligible speech."
3. Symbolic. "Symbolic operations that outrun our understanding." Examples might include a therapist's implicit understanding of subtle aspects of patients' physiognomy or behavior, and a tacit understanding of "what works" in particular situations.

The limited ability to explain all that one knows has been considered a deficit. Looked at from another point of view, it seems wonderful that people can have such extensive and useful knowledge even though language cannot capture it all. However, it does create something of a problem for some professions. When a practice is clearly a complex one, for example, flying airplanes, or being a concert violinist, the outsider assumes that the tacit knowledge is complex and substantial. However, when the practice is thought to be an ordinary task, for example, mothering or driving a car, then there is a tendency to assume that tacit knowledge is neither complex nor extensive. Ordinary tasks are not necessarily either physically easy or intellectually simple. Mothering, for example, is very ordinary but quite complex. And good mothering is considerably more complex than poor mothering. Whether or not tacit knowledge is considered real or sophisticated depends upon individual and cultural stances toward what one considers legitimate knowledge. Our American culture values scientific knowledge and verbal explanation. Knowledge that is implicit and dependant on sensory-motor experience is often considered inferior.

PROXIMAL AND DISTAL TACIT KNOWLEDGE

Polanyi refers to proximal and distal tacit knowledge. Distal (1966, p. 10) tacit knowledge is easiest to understand. It is the knowledge that directly underlies what we are doing. It is that knowledge that we can express, if pressed, in intelligible speech. It is fairly easily accessible to the performer and it is also amenable to verbal explanation: for example; "I am fixing the door knob. I am setting this screw back in its socket so that the shaft will be tight on the knob and it will turn properly." The person can explain *what* they are doing and at least give a surface explanation of the *whys* of the performance.

Proximal tacit knowledge is less accessible, but more essential to what we are ultimately "up to." Proximal knowledge is all the underlying principles, assumptions, values, rules-of-thumb, and "gut" feeling about what we are doing, and why we are doing that. To continue the above example, I know how to hold the screwdriver, angle it precisely to fit the angle of the slot on the head of the screw, know how to exert pressure on the driver through the screw to force it slightly, while simultaneously turning the driver and thus the screw in a clockwise direction. This sort of knowledge perhaps comes from some long-ago instructions from my father, but mostly from the experience that tells me how much pressure is enough, how much torque is necessary, and how fast I can turn the implement in my hand and not cause the screw to bounce out of the door knob mechanism.

Proximal knowledge is "second nature" (Hayes, 1978) to the experienced therapist and generally a mystery to the outsider. The proximal knowledge is the "deeper" understanding but it is more difficult to probe. It is harder for the practitioner to explain or describe verbally. It guides the subtle and complex aspects of practice. Proximal tacit knowledge probably has a great influence on the development of expertise. The neurologist in Murphy's example knew so much about the nervous system and had seen so many patients with various conditions that he immediately knew what Murphy's condition was without the other diagnostic procedures and equipment. This is a good example of the phenomenon of tacit knowledge making expert practice possible.

Learning by Doing: Acquiring Tacit Knowledge

Tacit knowledge is primarily acquired through experience. It is often the case that a person has professional education but does not feel comfortable with his or her ability to perform until he or she has "real" experience in the field. Experience does not serve as simply a vehicle for applying abstract knowledge. It is a way of gaining a more immediate and perhaps far richer sort of knowledge. Most of the perceptions, cues, and templates that various authors refer to as part of a professional stock of knowledge exist in the tacit dimension.

Experience is not simply doing something. It is doing something combined with reflecting on, or making meaning of, the event. Experience is useful, not because one has lived through it, but because one has made meaning of it. The essence of experience is meaning making. Experience, according to Dewey (1929), is "had" or "lived." Experience involves intending to do something, doing it, and reflecting on that experience. Tacit knowledge then is acquired through doing but made useful through reflection. Tacit knowledge is acquired through "having" experiences. This would account for two phenomena that many researchers who study professional expertise have observed. One, people with more "time on the job" tend to be better performers. Two, not all individuals with the same amount of time on the job are equally expert. The number of times that an individual had encountered a particular phenomenon or participated in an event would account for the finding that persons with more time on the job have more expertise than those with less time. Dewey, Polanyi, and Schön all theorize that the capacity to make meaning, or reflect on the phenomenon or event, accounts for the differences in practitioners with the same amount of time on the job having varying levels of expertise. We observed that some therapists appeared to be better or more competent than others. We soon found that the more reflective therapists were the ones who seemed to us to be more competent, in both technical skills required of the practice and, more importantly, in their interactions with patients.

Practice in the Tacit Dimension
TACIT TEACHING

A particular problem with occupational therapy is the ordinary or everday nature of the practice. This is part of the "elegant simplicity"

(West, 1989) of the practice. This everyday quality, however, also obscures the operational and intellectual complexity of the practice and the thinking that guides it. Aside from the general problem that practice of any sort is largely tacit, and the particular problem of the everyday nature of occupational therapy, there are two other aspects of the practice that make understanding the tacit dimension (Polanyi, 1966) important. These two aspects are that much of what the therapists teach patients is tacit and that many activities are structured as implicit meaning-making processes. Teaching patient skills in occupational therapy often occurs in the tacit dimension. Much of the patient's learning in occupational therapy is purposefully structured as tacit learning. "Learning by doing" is a common occupational therapy motto. Learning to do one thing by ostensibly doing another is also a common practice in occupational therapy. It is quite typical for a therapist to have several purposes for engaging in a given treatment activity, but to articulate only one or two. This can make OT activities appear much more simple than they actually are, to patients, non-OT colleagues, or affiliating students. Typically patients think therapists are helping them to *do a particular* task, whereas therapists think they are improving the persons *skill* or overall ability in a *general* area. For example, the therapist may be playing checkers with a person in order to improve fine motor coordination. The therapist may say, "Would you like to play checkers? It's good for your fine motor coordination." The therapist might also be thinking that the game would be good to develop attention and concentration skills, problem solving, social skills, and figure-ground discrimination. Finally, when engaged in the game, the therapist may be mentally assessing the person's sitting balance, attention span, and frustration tolerance. While all professions rely upon tacit know-how, occupational therapy appears to be almost purposefully structured as a practice conducted in the tacit dimension.

In a sense, a treatment activity is almost guaranteed to be not what it seems, especially when carried out by an experienced therapist. For example, an occupational therapist, Mary, was working with a 35-year-old man who had been in a motorbike accident while vacationing on an island in the Caribbean. He sustained a head injury and also some oxygen deprivation due to the length of time it took to get him to the hospital. At the point in his recovery when the videotaped therapy session took place, he had regained fairly good motor function. However, it was quite clear that he was probably not going to regain enough cognitive ability to return to his job as an engineer working with elaborate computer systems. A central question for the OT to address was whether he could learn enough skills and have enough memory and judgment to live by himself, or whether he would need a supervised living situation. In the videotape of a session, Mary simply seems to be helping Walt finish constructing a small paper towel holder and, in fact, she is doing that. But her major interest is not in the towel holder itself, but in what practical living skills he can learn or relearn, and how doing this particular activity can promote learning those skills. She also uses her observations of his behavior while performing this task to determine whether or not he has sufficient problem-solving skills, self-awareness, and judgment to live independently in the community. The simple activity becomes a skill-building activity for the patient. It is also a vehicle by which the therapist's observations are transformed into speculation about current and future functioning.

IMPLICIT MEANING-MAKING

A second feature of the practice that makes it important to examine tacit knowledge is that therapists are often trying to understand, and in some cases influence, patients' tacit understandings of themselves, their disability, and their world. Therapists seem to offer activities that can be interpreted at several levels of depth of meaning. In the above example, Mary had reasons for using the particular task of constructing a towel holder. These were related to both the physical-motor aspects of Walt's rehabilitation and also to the perceptual-cognitive aspects. In addition, Walt had been a civil engineer, so the notion of constructing an object could certainly hold important symbolic meaning for him. Mary offered a construction task to offer some potential for development of a symbolic understanding of himself and his potential future.

Some patients and some therapists do not seem to engage in symbolic meaning-making. Other patients seem to understand these symbolic meanings but choose to keep the understanding of those meanings between themselves and the therapist at the tacit level. Still others are more ready to be explicit about the significance of these symbolic interchanges. In the above example, Mary and Walt did not explicitly discuss, and perhaps did not notice, any deep significance in the construction task or find any parallels in his own reconstruction of his body and his life. Conversely, Aaron, a very young enlisted man in the Army seemed to be struggling with the importance of reconstructive surgery on his hand and his future life. He very much saw the symbolic relationship between the reconstruction of the hand and the reconstruction of his life. He sometimes talked to his OT, "Mit," about whether or not he should have additional surgery and what he was going to do in the future, "probably go to college." At other times, he was quiet and compliant in therapy and referred to his injured hand as "it" or "this thing." Aaron struggled with developing an understanding of both the functional and symbolic role of his injured hand, and vacillated between discussing and ignoring the problems that the injury had created in his life.

It was not clear to us whether the use of symbolic meanings on the part of occupational therapists, in general, was conscious or unconscious. We do not know whether or not they intended to conduct this part of their practice at a tacit level. The literature in the field contains theory about symbolic interaction (Mosey, 1970; Fidler & Fidler, 1978; Llorenz & Rubin, 1967) but most therapists did not seem to explicitly discuss this facet of their practice very much. Some therapists did discuss both the tacit aspects of therapy and the importance of the symbolic level of meaning-making and were quite articulate about those aspects of practice. However, when we have shown videotapes or given case stories to therapists and have asked them to discuss the activity as it relates to the patient's life, therapists are extremely quick to note a whole range of symbolic meanings to which the therapist in the story is directing the patient's attention. Interestingly, therapists in our workshops often find it much easier to assess an activity in symbolic, rather than sheerly biomechanical or technical, terms. This quickness and depth of perception about the symbolic domain strongly suggests that experienced clinicians do, in fact, reason about symbolic as well as skill-building features of activities. It seems that, unless explicitly asked, therapists seldom talk about this part of the reasoning process. Uncovering the tacit knowledge of expert therapists is an exciting task in the archeology of professional knowledge (Foucault, 1972), which is far from complete. Symbolic meaning seems to be more easily captured in clinical stories than in the analysis of single treatment sessions.

Summary

One of the aims of the Clinical Reasoning Study was to make the implicit, tacit knowledge of experienced clinicians explicit. In order to do this we studied both *what* therapists thought about and *how* they conducted their thinking. We were interested to know what sorts of practical "theories-in-use" (Argyris & Schön, 1981) therapists employed to guide their daily practice. We found that professional expertise was enhanced by the use of a myriad of personally constructed practical theories.

Another aim of the study was to identify practical theories that were common to many experienced therapists and to develop a language to articulate those theories. The purpose of this book, in part, is to begin to explicate those theories, to begin to develop a language by which occupational therapists may express and refine both their tacit practical theories and the clinical reasoning strategies they employ, and to explore the tacit values that drive the practice.

Expert practice is difficult to study because experts make complex action look simple. Two factors seem to contribute greatly to the development of expertise: breadth of experience, and depth of reflection on that experience. Because repetition and reflection are both conducted by the individual and are often not raised to the level of spoken language, much professional expertise remains in the tacit dimension. However, we contend that, in order to improve the expertise of a profession as a whole, the individual expertise of practitioners needs to be excavated and expressed in the shared language of the group.

Occupational therapists have a great deal of tacit knowledge. But OTs also employ the tacit dimension in rather unusual ways as a part of their therapeutic strategies. One strategy is the use of tacit teaching. Therapists frequently appear to be teaching one activity while, in fact, they are teaching many skills simultaneously. We were fond of saying that "therapists never do only one thing at a time." Another strategy is to use a concrete activity to allow for the development or expression of symbolic meaning. Therapists often chose particular activities to simultaneously teach a skill and convey a deeper meaning. Another of our favorite sayings was, "therapists never do anything for just one reason."

We were particularly interested in the reasoning processes that therapists used to bring their tacit knowledge to bear on the clinical situations that they encountered and resolved. We found that occupational therapists used many types of reasoning processes to employ their many practical theories. Clinical reasoning, we found, is much more than the identification of a problem and the application of propositional logic to select a solution. Rather, it is the observation and interpretation of a myriad of factors in the problem complex, the generation and integration of multiple practical hypotheses, and the selection and combination from a broad range of potential actions the best resolution of this particular situation. All of this complexity was guided by practical theories that resided largely in the tacit dimension.

Occupational Therapy: A Profession Between Two Cultures

■

Occupational Therapy as a Two-Body Practice

The Body as Machine

■ **CHERYL MATTINGLY**

Introduction

Occupational therapy is a practice that occurs in the cultural domain of biomedicine. Even when therapists are not working directly within a hospital setting, occupational therapy, like all health professions, is strongly influenced by medicine. One of the most interesting features of occupational therapy practice is that it tends to deal with functional problems that fall nicely within biomedicine (treating physical injuries with specific treatment techniques), as well as problems going far beyond the physical body, encompassing social, cultural, and psychological issues that concern the *meaning* of illness or injury to a person's life. This makes occupational therapy rather unusual among health professions. The next three chapters address some of the complexities of a practice that attempts to function within two cultural contexts, the biomedical culture and the professional culture of occupational therapy.

Disease and Illness Experience

Medical anthropologists have made an extremely useful distinction in looking at health care, by separating *disease* from *illness experience* (Good, 1977; Good and Delvecchio Good, 1980, 1985; Kleinman, 1989; Kleinman, Eisenberg & Good, 1978). Although, traditionally, medicine has focused on the diagnosis and treatment of disease, anthropologists argue that much more attention needs to be given to treatment of the illness experience, which involves the way in which disease affects the person's life. Physiologically, the same *disease* can result in a very different *illness experience*, depending on the patient's particular life history and life possibilities. The quadriplegic who is a lawyer with a wife and three children may have the same level of injury as another quadriplegic who is an auto mechanic living on his own. From the perspective of disease, these may be two "C-5 quads," one much like the other. But from the perspective of illness experience—the meaning of the injury in the lives of these persons and how they cope with it— these two people are likely to have very different injuries. A disease focus is concerned with injury to the physical body. An illness focus is concerned with injury to a life.

The medical world does not, as a whole, pay a tremendous amount of attention to the illness experience, which is often viewed as beyond the purview of the health professional. And those who are assigned the task of considering the illness experience rarely pay attention to disease. The medical world tends to be strictly divided between those health professionals who deal with the physical body and with "disease"— physicians being the paradigmatic example—and those, like social workers, psychologists, and pastoral counselors, who are more likely to deal with emotional and social issues surrounding long-term illness. But occupational therapists are concerned with both disease and illness experience. Therapists very often interweave interventions that address both the disease and the illness experience into the same treatment activity. They work toward goals that relate to the physiological prob- lems of dysfunction (thus being disease- or injury-focused) and goals that relate to helping the patient cope with the illness experience, for example, with the fear of returning home, or of never being able to return to work. They have an operating "double vision," in which they perceive and understand their client's disability from both these per- spectives.

This encompassing nature of the practice quickly became apparent in the Clinical Reasoning Study. As an outside anthropologist unac- quainted with occupational therapists, I was almost immediately struck by the fact that the therapists I observed shifted between two quite distinct ways of approaching patients, approaches that appeared to coexist uneasily. During a single session, therapists talked to the patient, got accounts of the patient's problem as the patient was experiencing it, found out about how the patient lived and the patient's family and friends, heard about the patient's worries at changing jobs or having to retire as a result of the illness or accident. At other times in the same session the therapist ignored, or tried to ignore, the patient's stories and complaints and began attending to the patient's body as a purely physical entity. Patients sometimes resisted the move from an experience-focused discussion of the pathology to a treatment of their body as a malfunctioning object. They often grew more childlike in the transition, more passive. In fact, passivity was often required in order for patients to follow the therapist's instructions about how to attend to their bodies, to notice if they could feel the prick of a pin or if moving an injured wrist hurt.

During early observations, occupational therapy looked like a loose confederation of two different practices, each involving distinct conceptions of the body. When listening to patients tell their stories, therapists were treating patients' experiences of the disability and the meanings it carried for their lives. When pricking fingers or ranging arms, they were treating the biomedical body, the body as machine or organism, an entity quite separate from the person because it is treated as distinct from the meaning the body has for a person's life. These two conceptions of the body do not spring from the various practice theories internal to occupational therapy, but from a deeper stratum. They are rooted in underlying conceptions of the relationship between mind and body that have become embedded in Western thought.

Several years of observing, listening to, consulting, and teaching occupational therapists have modified my early perception that it consists of two distinct practices. It is true that occupational therapists often express a sense of tension and unease in their practice as they try to treat both the physical body and the body which a person lives with and experiences his or her life with. In this sense, my early observations reflected a genuine dilemma in their practice, discussed in more detail in the final section of this book. But therapists also are able, at times, to flow quite easily and naturally from one framework to the next, to borrow from both conceptions of the body in framing the problems of patient treatment, and to use either biomechanical means for achieving phenomenological ends or the reverse. Thus, sometimes therapists are able to synthesize these two ways of understanding disability in an effective way, and sometimes they have trouble integrating the two perspectives.

Later chapters of this book, particularly those addressing the multiple "tracks" in which therapists reason, address how these perspectives are synthesized in practice. This chapter and the following one separate these two very different orientations to disability, examining the dramatic differences in treatment that result from seeing disability within predominantly biomechanical terms—as an injury to the physical body—or in terms of the illness experience—as an injury to a life. This chapter considers occupational therapy as treatment of a biomedical body, looking at the centrality of this framework for occupational therapy and for the culture of the health professions as a whole. The following chapter considers occupational therapy as treatment of the "lived body."

THE CASE OF DORIS

The following story of Doris, written by a hand therapist, concerns a time when the therapist got "stuck" in a narrow biomechanical framing of a hand injury—partly because the patient herself appeared to prefer this narrow framing. But, in this case, a focus only on the biomechanical aspects of the injury may have exacerbated the ineffectiveness of treatment in helping the patient regain function of her hand.

Doris

by Mary Black

Doris F. is a 38-year-old black female who was referred to OT at 5 days after repair of her right flexor pollicis longus tendon. On evaluation, she reported that she had sustained the injury while slicing potatoes. She was employed with the State Department of Mental Health as an LPN and reported that although she was financially burdened by this accident, her physician insisted that she not return to work for 8 to 10 weeks after surgery. She was instructed that therapy was recommended 2 to 3 times per week and she voiced difficulty in complying with this due to lack of transportation, finances, and childcare, since she was the single parent of three small children.

Doris's treatment over the next 6 weeks consisted of fabricating a dorsal hand-thumb blocking splint with intermittent dynamic Kleinert traction, edema control, and passive range of motion for the significant edema and joint contractures developing throughout her right hand. Several phone discussions took place between the surgeon and therapist as a result of the patient's declining functional status, despite consistent therapy attendance and seeming compliance with her home exercise program. Rapport was developing between therapist and patient, though Doris rarely made direct eye contact during conversations.

When the therapist went on annual leave, a contract OT carried out treatment for one session. Upon the therapist's return, the following conversation ensued between the contract therapist and the staff OT in charge of Doris's program.

Contract OT:	How's Doris doing now? Have you heard any news on her husband?
Staff OT:	What do you mean?
Contract OT:	You mean you don't know about this?
Staff OT:	About what?
Contract OT:	Doris told me all about how this happened.
Staff OT:	Peeling potatoes?

The contract therapist then went on to relay that Doris's husband was an apparent drug abuser who had threatened to kill her and her children several times. Apparently, he acted on his threats one night, and Doris sustained the laceration while resisting a knife attack; subsequently, he sustained a superficial wound from her and was now in jail without bond.

After a long discussion with Doris's referring physician, the therapist's mixed feelings of anger toward her for not telling the truth appeared, as well as an understanding of her general affect, the realization of her failure as a treating therapist; eventually, an attitude of "Aha!" toward her whole situation surfaced. All this explained her situation and the extreme emotional reaction that caused her eventual diagnosis of reflex sympathetic dystrophy.

The surgeon and therapist continue to struggle with the lack of function in Doris's hand, but have made extra efforts to help her resolve some issues such as returning to work—both for financial and psychological reasons. She continues to struggle with opening up about the situation to those working with her, but allows touch easier and is making eye contact more frequently with her caregivers. Both the surgeon and therapist feel that had this accurate medical history been known prior to 8 weeks after surgery, both Doris's hand function and the treatment approach used would have been different.

Case Discussion

Doris's problem first appears to be a simple physical injury (repair of a right flexor pollicis longus tendon) requiring straightforward treatment techniques (make a dorsal hand-thumb blocking splint, do some passive range of motion, some edema control and traction). But Doris does not get better, despite weeks of treatment. When a contract occupational therapist happens to work with Doris, she later reports to the treating therapist (Mary) what Doris has told her about how the injury occurred. Suddenly the physical decline of hand function makes more sense to Mary. A simple physical problem takes on a new dramatic meaning, when the cause is not a mishap while peeling potatoes but an attack from a husband with a knife.

This case illustrates two important features of occupational therapy practice. One is the tremendous influence and importance of a biomedical way of understanding a clinical problem: here pathology is treated as an injury to the physical body, and healing involves a focus on the physical body. A second lesson from this case concerns the limitations of that biomedical orientation for both understanding and addressing the patient's response to treatment. When the real cause of the injury is discovered by Doris's treating therapist and physicians, and when steps are taken to address Doris's broader life difficulties in preparing to return to work, she responds in ways that directly affect the physical outcome. We find, as the case story ends, that the patient "allows touch easier." As hand therapists are quick to point out, effective treatment of an injury often depends upon patients coming to trust their therapists, allowing themselves to endure treatment that ranges from merely uncomfortable to significantly painful. Trust of the therapist is also required if patients are to use their hands at home in ways recommended in therapy. With such injuries, doing too little too late can prevent maximal healing. Certainly in Doris's situation, Mary Black and the doctor felt that had they understood the real cause of injury, greater improvement in regaining hand function would have been possible. So, while the therapist's biomedical knowledge and skills at addressing the hand as a physical injury were *essential* in treating the client, they were not *sufficient.*

The biomedical way of seeing injury was so powerful in this case that it was only brought into question when the treatment did not work and when it became clear that personal, family, and economic issues were influencing the patient's response to therapy. This case raises several questions to be addressed in this chapter. One, what are the primary values and assumptions of biomedicine and how do they influence the way occupational therapists treat patients? Two, what are the strengths and what are the limitations of a biomedical approach to chronic illness and disability? This case also provides an excellent example of a therapist's ability to see her patient with a "double vision," once the cause of the patient's injury is revealed.

The Biomedical Orientation

A CULTURAL AND HISTORICAL PERSPECTIVE

Biomedicine is organized around several potent metaphors. The philosopher Susan Sontag, in her essay *Illness as Metaphor*, gives a compelling argument about the power of metaphor in shaping a biomedical picture of illness. Sontag uses cancer as her primary example, but her discussion reveals many of the fundamental metaphors which govern the biomedical approach to disease. Cancer cells, Sontag notices, are said to "invade," they "colonize," breaking down the body's "defenses" (1977, p. 66). Cancer is even a kind of alien invasion (1977, p. 68). This is an image-rich language borrowed from the terminology of warfare. (Physicians wage war, even chemical war, on the invaders.) Such metaphors serve to heighten the notion that pathology is a foreign invader with which the physician must go to battle. Oncologists often speak of their personal battles with the cancer cells of their patients (Hunt, in press; DelVecchio-Good et al, in press). These metaphors help to emphasize the separation of pathology from the patient, giving life to the disease entity and drama to a battle between doctor and disease in which the patient is merely the unfortunate bystander, the innocent victim.

The most significant biomedical metaphor, however, is the one that is least obvious, buried in the notion of the "biomechanical" body. This is the metaphor of body as machine. This biomechanical framing (or way of seeing) dominates all of biomedicine, and encompasses a far broader domain than a particular frame of reference within occupational therapy. The conception of the body as machine is based on a powerful Western notion of the body as distinct from mind. In this dualistic view, mind is the seat of intentions, intelligence, and will; the body is a material object, a passive container for the mind. The mechanistic view of the body is particularly appropriate to a practice of medicine that understands the patient as the assemblage of mechanistic processes that are malfunctioning. The body can be conceived mechanistically once separated from the mind. This separation is native to the Judeo-Christian tradition and was articulated and emphasized for science by seventeenth-century philosophers, Descartes in particular (Leder, 1984).

With the rise of modern medicine, the body came to be seen as "merely a machine driven by mechanical causality and susceptible to mathematical analysis" (Leder, 1984, pp. 29, 30). The twentieth-century philosopher-sociologist Michel Foucault (1979) gives a powerful cultural reading of this dualism, painting a seventeenth-century French society initiating bureaucratizing practices in a wide variety of domains—school, prison, the workplace, the army, the hospital—which were based on, and in turn promoted, an increasingly biomechanical conception of body. This vision of body-as-machine was largely motivated, Foucault contends, by an increasingly sophisticated "disciplinary gaze." Training, in many domains, was connected to "strict discipline" of the body, Foucault notes (1979, p. 170). The problem of surveillance of large masses of people became of primary concern. Foucault notices the use of uniforms in many settings, where bodies were dressed in an indistinguishable way. He argues that people were being trained, in effect, to see themselves as objects, possessing biomechanical bodies whose special feature was that they were all the same. Describing the eighteenth-century organization of school, as one example, he speaks of the "disciplinary gaze" as a "normalizing gaze" exerting pressure on individuals to "conform to the same model so that they might all be subjected to subordination, docility, attention in studies and exercises, and to the correct practice of duties. . . . So that they might all be like one another" (1979, p. 182). He singles out the growth of the "examination," used in schools, hospitals, the military, at work, and the like, as exemplary of a whole social world moving toward a normalizing, objectifying perception of the person (1979, pp. 184–185).

THE BIOMECHANICAL VIEW IN MEDICINE

The biomechanical view in medicine is constructed on the realization that, as a machine, the body is susceptible to mechanical interventions. This assumption is basic to the explosion of medical discovery that began in the seventeenth and eighteenth centuries and still continues.

> The scope of clinical possibilities thus widens commensurate with that of expanding research and technologies. As machine-like, the body can be divided into organ systems and parts to be repaired, surgically removed, or technologically supplemented in relative isolation. (Leder, 1984, p. 30)

In making medical diagnoses, modern physicians of the eighteenth century sought to free themselves from phenomenology, that is, from linking the diagnosis to the patient's experience of the illness. The history of medicine since the eighteenth century is a history in which medical professionals have come to depend less and less on the patient's perceptions and understandings of their illnesses. Diagnostic practice has come to rely, in part, on ignoring or passing quickly from the less reliable data of patient reports to more precise information gleaned from diagnostic instruments and laboratory tests.

Foucault argues that this process began with a revolutionary shift in the basic categorization of disease. "The doctors of the eighteenth century," he says, "identified (disease) with 'historical,' as opposed to philosophical, 'knowledge'" (1975, p. 5). Disease was reclassified as an *object* that had an *observable* history. The task of the modern doctor as he emerged in the 1700s was to carefully observe and track that history and, in this way, to come to an understanding of the nature of particular types of illness. Medical case histories were developed to record that process.

A critical consequence of this new understanding of disease was that the patient and the disease were separated. Prior to the advent of modern medicine, doctors thought each sick person as having his own ailment. The radical shift of the eighteenth century was that instead of seeing ailments as belonging to the patient, diseases were believed to "have their own identity" (Feinstein, 1973a, p. 215). Diseases were seen as completely distinguishable from the patient and his or her personal history. They had their own "natural history" that could be observed from the clinical course the disease took in patients in general. A new form of medical case study recorded that natural history and carefully separated it from the way the disease held meaning for the patient, and for those involved with the patient as a person, and from the way in which its history was involved with the personal life of the patient.

The notion that diseases had their own natural history was not completely new. The Greeks as far back as Hippocrates held such a view (Sacks, 1987). The new conception may have been reintroduced as part of a new form of institutionalization of treatment, the "birth of the clinic" (Foucault, 1975). Increasingly, the ill went to hospitals to be treated rather than staying at home, and this allowed the comparative observation of the same disease processes across numerous cases.

The separation of patients from their disease was also strengthened by the new study of corpses. As doctors began doing autopsies, they could look beneath the surface manifestations that ill patients presented to them and trace effects that could not be seen by the naked eye. Through examination of corpses, doctors developed a "medical gaze" into the basic anatomical structures of the body. This allowed them to know more about the nature of diseases and their routes through the body than the patient could reveal or directly sense.

The development of new diagnostic instruments in the nineteenth century further separated patient from an experienced body and patient from physician. The medical sociologist Starr (1982) describes the impact of new technical tools, like the stethoscope, which allowed the physician to extend his medical gaze. Such instruments encouraged and sometimes even required the physician to "move away from involvement with the patient's experiences and sensations, to a more detached relation, less with the patient but more with the sounds (and sights) of the patient's body" (p. 136). These instruments allowed doctors to see and hear the body in ways the patient could not, and gave the medical professional access to cues that the patient could not interpret. In an important sense, medical professionals came to know their patients' bodies much better than did the patients themselves.

The biomedical mode of conducting medical practice and clinical reasoning are now a familiar part of chart notes, reimbursement procedures, and medical rounds. They are institutionalized in myriad forms throughout the medical system and they underlie the way most medical professionals see their patients and their patients' ailments. Treating disease as an entity apart from the patient and the patient's experience of it was a critical turning point in the development of Western medicine.

Because the biomedical model has focused on the diagnosis of disease, within medicine, the essential clinical skill for the professional has been the ability to investigate the particular symptoms evinced by a patient (which may be felt and experienced in unique ways by different patients)—signs that physicians can discover from their own investigation and treat as cues to a deeper, more hidden level of reality, the pathology. This identification allows the professional to extract from his or her repertoire of treatment interventions those scientifically proven to be effective in treating this disease state.

Through this process, the physician moves from the particular symptoms a patient may complain about; to the particular ways that patient's body looks, sounds, and feels; to a general disease category. This movement from the particular patient's body to a general pathological condition is essential in helping the physician or other health professional know what kind of treatment is appropriate. The biomedical concern to link the idiosyncratic particular with a general law or state of affairs (such as a disease category) is related to a concern for effective intervention. If professionals can come to recognize general processes underlying particular cases, then general techniques can be designed to change those processes in predictable ways.

Certainly some medical interventions work in this way. For instance, if the physician learns to recognize a unique set of aches and pains as a fractured femur, she can perform a standardized procedure with predictable success. This procedure can be learned and applied in Hong Kong to a 60-year-old man or in Cincinnati to a 15-year-old girl with similar results.

Analogously, certain aspects of occupational therapy practice can be standardized because certain aspects of occupational dysfunction can be predicted to follow from certain pathological conditions. Occupational therapists draw continually upon a biomedical approach to their patients, particularly in their focus on the disease or medical condition of the patient. To return to Doris, the therapist clearly oriented her treatment approach to Doris' medical condition, which she describes in some detail in her written case. Also, therapists often take a biomedical approach in treating deficiencies in the body, a focus that is also evident in the case of Doris. Both of these biomechanical emphases will be discussed further below.

The Biomedical Orientation in Occupational Therapy

SHIFTING CONCEPTIONS OF OCCUPATIONAL THERAPY

Occupational therapy is a profession that has had a shifting relationship to medicine. During some historical moments it has been more at odds with biomedicine than at others. When I first began observations of therapists, I knew almost nothing about the history of the profession. In retrospect, it seems remarkable that my first impression of witnessing two professions that treated two different bodies was reflected in the literature on the history of how the profession has developed.

In giving a brief sketch of occupational therapy's role vis-à-vis biomedicine, I rely heavily upon several scholars within occupational therapy, most notably: Rogers (1982a,b), Kielhofner & Burke (1977), Bing (1981), Levine (1987), Kielhofner (1983), and Reilly (1962). These scholars have, by and large, depicted this profession as having undergone a major paradigm shift. They describe the profession as having an early orientation which dramatically shifted after World War II. During the first half of its life, occupational therapy was grounded in a philosophy that was an outgrowth of Moral Treatment, a movement that bears some resemblance to a phenomenological conception of the body, especially as it evolved in the occupational therapy movement. The second half brought with it a powerful biomedical framing of what was to count as appropriate clinical problems for occupational therapy, what one prominent theorist in the field called a "scaling down" of the profession to "match kinesiological, neurological, or intrapsychic view(s) of human nature" (Rogers, 1982b, p. 714). What is described historically as a paradigm shift of the entire profession looks rather messier in practice, where it appears that both paradigms live simultaneously. The Clinical Reasoning Study research team observed a sometimes difficult, sometimes creative and fluid, synthesis of two perspectives about how to understand and treat clients with disabilities. In a historical light, this may be the result of an ongoing attempt by individual therapists to integrate two distinct streams of practice and belief to which they became socialized as members of the profession.

The early paradigm, with its emphasis on appropriate adaptation to life roles, on meaningful work, on creativity and play, and its explicit critique of the medical model, began to lose its persuasive force by the 1940s. Most theorists document a shift toward a much more biomedically based paradigm of practice, which began to take place in the postwar era. During this time, many external pressures, especially pressures from physicians questioning the efficacy and scientific basis of occupational therapy, exerted themselves on therapists and initiated a reaction in the profession that involved a move to a more physiologically based practice. A profession that had a strong grounding in moral treatment theory and the arts and crafts movement through the 1930s thus shifted into one where there was a strong division in the field, as many therapists became concerned to ground their practice in a more medically acceptable way. The traditional crafts approach to treatment as well as the broad, holistic conception of the nature of chronic illness, fell into increasing disfavor. Those famous looms which often dominated the occupational therapy treatment room were moved to attics and basements.

Rogers describes this shift toward a more medically directed way of thinking:

> Like many health care professions, we embraced the prevailing philosophy of reductionism to build our scientific development. Reductionism had the net effect of limiting our view of the client, the environment, and occupation. Instead of conceptualizing independent behavior as a molar event, involving a client and a broad contextual milieu, it became a molecular event, involving fragmented responses and equally discrete external stimuli. (1982b, p. 714)

According to theorists within the field, there were two primary reasons for the effectiveness of the pressure to shift toward a biomedical approach to occupational therapy, with its emphasis on exercises and strength building, rather than occupations in the richer sense intended by the early founders. One was the Depression and the question of financial survival. Scientifically demonstrable treatment effectiveness became much more important to ensure job security. The other was the rising power of physicians across health professions. The American

Medical Association became the accrediting body for the profession. Occupational therapy became increasingly specialized, a process that still continues. Much, though not all, of the specialization was related to diagnostic category.

Three approaches to occupational practice arose which better fit a biomedical framework. These are still extremely powerful within occupational therapy. One is based on a kinesiological model. Here musculoskeletal integrity is emphasized and treatment approaches address the problems of increasing range of motion, strengthening muscles and improving coordination (Rogers, 1982b, p. 714). The principle of this practice is to "mobilize, coordinate, and strengthen bodily segments; to develop physical skills and endurance for necessary bodily improvements; to test the physical components of occupational fitness; and to promote psychological stability through intelligent adjustment to unalterable physical limitations" (Kielhofner & Burke, 1977, p. 683). A second practice model is neurological. Functional independence is treated as it relates to capacities to integrate sensory input. This model focuses primarily on perception and its relation to cognitive, motor, and emotional development. The physiological focus is the neuromuscular system and the relation between sensory input and motor output. A third key practice model (though one which is now waning) is based on a psychoanalytic treatment of occupation where "primary importance was placed on the unconscious phenomena, with exploration of here and now feelings and behavior as a means to arrive at an awareness and understanding of intrapsychic conflict" (Kielhofner & Burke, 1977, p. 683). While a psychoanalytic model deals with mental rather than purely physical disabilities, it is still very much a disease-focused model, and in that sense quite congruent with biomedicine.

CURRENT CONCEPTS OF PRACTICE

In response to a perceived reductionism in the profession, many occupational therapists in the 1960s began writing articles in the national journal advocating a return to the original, holistic beliefs that the profession had begun with. During the 1960s and 1970s yet another frame of reference, called *occupational behavior*, began to emerge from the work of Reilly and her students, who attempted to ground occupational therapy in the early conception of the occupation cure. This has been developed by one of her students, Kielhofner, under the designation "Model of Human Occupation." It also continues to be explored, in a somewhat different vein, at the University of Southern California under the leadership of Florence Clark. This group is in the process of developing an "occupation science" to undergird the practice of occupational therapy.

Both biomedical and occupational behavior frameworks are currently powerful in the field. The biomedical influence in occupational therapy is alive and well. Speaking from the study of actual practice, things look far from unified. And yet, in interesting ways, therapists appear able to integrate in practice what is highly disparate in theory. On the whole, the therapists who were part of the original Clinical Reasoning Study or our subsequent studies tend not to slot their practice within any particular practice theory or overall paradigm. Our discovery of a "two-body" practice within occupational therapy may simply be the result of two systems of values which, by now, are deeply embedded within the professional culture. Certainly, the values and beliefs that belonged to the early occupational therapy movement can still be clearly heard, even in the most reductionist of therapists. It is more common than not, for instance, for even those therapists most wedded to biomechanical treatment modalities to give their patients strength-building exercises while simultaneously exhorting them to become more self-reliant, and explaining that increases in muscular strength will allow increased autonomy by allowing them to move, and hence live, more independently.

The biomedical influence in occupational therapy is probably most pervasive in two ways, despite differences in specialization, practice settings, or ostensible adherence to a practice theory. First, there is a continued emphasis on medical diagnosis and dysfunction as a key which orients therapists in practice. Second, there is a strong emphasis on "fixing" discrete deficits (physical, cognitive, even emotional) and heavy dependence upon accompanying treatment modalities designed to improve skills for those targeted physiologically based functional deficiencies. This atomistic "check-list" approach to treatment is supported by reimbursement and chart documentation procedures. These procedures, at least as conceived by most practicing therapists, promote long lists of discrete problems and accompanying lists of treatment modalities and goals targeted to address them. The diagnostic focus, and the atomistic check-list focus, better fit a biomedical approach to disability than the holistic approach advocated in the early days of the profession.

THE DIAGNOSTIC EMPHASIS

Rogers and Masagatani (1982) found, in their research on clinical reasoning in occupational therapy, that the medical diagnosis was the most critical factor influencing how therapists assessed their clients. The therapists who were studied in the AOTA/AOTF Clinical Reasoning Study also used the medical diagnosis as an important organizer in developing their treatment plans. They linked medical diagnoses with generally expected dysfunctions, and these dysfunctions, in turn, pointed them toward certain treatment activities and procedures. To know a person's pathology was to be able to predict with high probability what physiological difficulties one would encounter. To be able to predict dysfunctions meant the therapist could also predict what interventions would improve the body.

The dominance of medical diagnosis in orienting therapists is clear from the many stories we have asked therapists to write about clinical cases, as well as from interviewing therapists. Almost invariably, therapists begin their stories by giving the diagnosis. Here are some representative examples from the first sentences of various written cases where the patient is introduced to the reader. These are quoted verbatim:

> "Anthony is an 8 y.o. (dx: spastic quad c.p.) who will be entering the 2nd grade in the fall."
> "I received a telephone call from a woman I knew from the local community. She was a pediatric nurse at the local hospital. Her two children, Brian, 3.5 yrs. old with severe cerebral palsy-quadriplegia, ? m.r., seizure disorder and Antony, an 19 month old, who seemed to be developing in a typical fashion."
> "Ann was a 26-year-old woman who had given birth and subsequently had a stroke. She was admitted to a N>C> rehab hospital with right hemiparesis."

As is obvious from these examples, the medical diagnosis and associated probable dysfunctions give therapists a familiar starting point, a general guide to help them anticipate what kinds of treatment interventions are likely to be most appropriate. Sometimes it has seemed as though the therapeutic process begins in a biomedical mode and gradually shifts to a more phenomenological one, as therapist and patient begin to develop a relationship with one another, and the therapist comes to see the patient as a particular individual. Certainly when therapists tell and write stories about their work with patients, this shift often occurs. At the start of the case example, we are given the diagnosis, but as the story proceeds, we begin to be confronted with the person who has the disability.

One reason the biomedical framing figures so large in the therapist's attention is that disease categories are not individualized, not tailored to the particular patient. The therapist can view a new patient as just another example of a general diagnostic category, another "spastic quad c.p." Therapists often do not have much time to treat patients; there may be little time initially for exploring a patient's particular life situation or the personal, family, and cultural factors influencing how the physiological difficulties are being experienced or handled by the patient. The medical diagnosis provides a certain initial shortcut.

Sometimes, therapists also get involved in puzzling about the diagnostic status of their patients. There can be tremendous drama around the process of diagnosis when symptoms and signs are unclear or inconsistent. Often a great deal is at stake in discovering the correct diagnosis. The power of the biomedical model, of course, is that, in many cases, if a diagnosis can be made accurately, there are known methods of treatment that can cure or alleviate the illness. Even if outright cure is not possible, accurate diagnosis may allow significant healing. It is not surprising that therapists also occasionally get involved in this essential medical drama.

A favorite genre of clinical story that therapists like to tell concerns times when they recognize a misdiagnosis that their colleagues have made, or when they discover a critical feature about a patient that can make a diagnostic difference. Since patients are asked to be active in therapy, therapists often have a chance to observe their patients and their bodies in ways not possible when the patient is undergoing a passive examination by the physician. This activity-based assessment and treatment process can thus sometimes give therapists valuable information about a patient's pathological condition.

The following case, which is quite dramatic, revolves around diagnostic puzzles as a therapist begins to see a patient, Sue, who presents an "unusual configuration of cognitive and perceptual deficits." The therapist wonders how much of this patient's symptoms are caused by pathology and how much (if any) are "put on" as the neuropsychologist suspects. The diagnostic puzzle is essential in giving the therapist an initial question that she asks during her home visits. The unusual nature of the patient's symptoms provides subsequent puzzles for the therapist, puzzles the therapist must solve in order to offer Sue the most effective adaptations for her home.

THE CASE OF SUE

Sue

by Anonymous

This patient was a 28-year-old white female who was seen 1 month after a car accident in which she suffered a "bang" to the head but was not hospitalized. Upon returning home, her friends noticed she had memory difficulties and an inability to organize herself, but she did not seek medical treatment until 3 weeks after the accident, when she began to have temporal lobe seizures. Neuropsychology testing was done on an outpatient basis, and the results revealed multiple deficit areas with no consistent pattern. The neurophysiologist expressed an opinion that many of her deficits were "put on." A referral was made to OT to evaluate her ability to function in the home.

My impression of the patient before meeting her was mixed—either the patient was faking disability for insurance purposes (certainly a plausible scenario) or the nature of the head injury was very diffuse (possibility that

I felt was plausible as I could remember one particular 18-year-old learning-disabled patient who had a very unusual configuration of cognitive and perceptual deficits).

Out first treatment session was at Sue's home. Sue was a large woman, about 225 pounds, who greeted me graciously and was extremely verbal and articulate. I was struck by her verbal intelligence and felt she exuded a capable, competent air unlike that of any head-injured patient I'd seen. She invited me in, through the living room and into the kitchen, and I was astonished at the contrast between this socially adept woman and the disheveled and chaotic living environment. The house was a mess. There was cat hair covering the furniture, tons of clutter, and five cats jumping off chairs and rubbing against my legs as I proceeded to the kitchen.

Therapist:	I've come to talk with you about the difficulties you've been experiencing since your car accident. I'd like to work with you on some solutions to these difficulties. Can you tell me about some problems we ought to work on together?
Sue:	I'm having trouble finding things in my cupboards and I can't remember whether or not I've fed my cats. I love my cats, I don't want to mistreat them, and I'm afraid I forget to feed them. I used to be so good to my animals.
Therapist:	It seems like one goal we could work on might be finding ways we can help you remember things. Feeding your cats is one of these things. Are there other things you have difficulty remembering? What about feeding yourself? Do you prepare balanced meals for yourself?
Sue:	I make myself TV dinners in the oven. I always cook them the same but sometimes they aren't cooked well. I eat them anyway.

Her mother had marked the 30-minute print on the timer with a red dot. She always cooked her TV dinners for 30 minutes.

Therapist:	Can I look in your freezer?

She nodded yes. I open the freezer and pull out some TV dinners. Some had 30-minute cooking times, others 45 or 55 minutes. I deduce we can simplify her meal preparation by finding kinds of TV dinners she both likes and can cook at the temperature. On a hunch, I opened the refrigerator. It was empty except for cat food.

Therapist:	When did you last go to the grocery store?
Sue:	I tried to [tears]. The cart doesn't look like it fit through the door. I could see it wouldn't fit. Anyway, the carts and all the people made me confused. I had a seizure. I had to come home. My mother will bring me some food.
Therapist:	Did you try to push the cart through the door?
Sue:	No, it didn't appear to fit.

I thought that there would be therapy for perceptual problems that revolve around activities that say, "Try it—I know it does appear not to fit but go ahead and try the activity." I am convinced her head injury symptoms are very real. I am sure her memory difficulties extend to difficulties taking her medications appropriately, and she may have more seizures on the days she forgets to take her meds.

I open her cupboards. There is no organization. Foil wraps, saran wraps, wax papers, and so forth are in all different drawers

Therapist:	Maybe one thing we could do or try is to organize your drawers so that like things are together?
Sue:	Yes, please. [She smiles.] Let's label them when we're done organizing. I have one more problem I want to address. I can't use my vacuum cleaner. It makes me nauseous. [She opened the closet and pulled out a new Royal canister vacuum cleaner.] I start out okay and then I get sick. I need to vacuum the cat hair.

I'm puzzled.

Therapist:	I have no good idea about why vacuuming makes you sick. Did it make you sick before your accident?

She shook her head no. I'd have to think on this one. We begin to organize her cupboards and agree to meet again to continue in a few days.

I'm sitting in a graduate school class taught by Shirley Stockmeyer. The topic is peripheral vision. She gives an example of motion sickness and nausea as a result of visual distraction in the peripheral visual field. My mind wanders back to Sue. Could her nausea be related to peripheral visual distortion when vacuuming? I call her up: "I have an idea—can I try your vacuum cleaner?" I travel to her home with my upright vacuum cleaner in my car. I try her canister. The hose and motor trail in the peripheral visual field. "Try my upright, Sue." Sue vacuumed with the upright and did just fine. She was happy. I was thrilled. This $3,000 tuition finally proved to be practical!

Biomedical Treatment Approaches: Fixing the Deficits

When occupational therapists operate within a biomechanical frame, they focus especially on the development of the patient's skills and strength; activities are conceived as exercises in skill building. This may involve exercises in the usual sense (e.g., lifting weights) or functional exercises, such as learning how to guide a wheelchair after a stroke, or learning to do a bed transfer as a paraplegic. It may mean focusing in on discrete skills, memory retraining and the like, which assess, in a check-list kind of way, a series of deficits. What gives these tactics their biomedical orientation is not simply what gets treated (body impairments), but rather a way of understanding a client's problems as a series of discrete difficulties related to diagnostic category rather than to the context of the individual patient's particular life history.

Occupational therapists observed in the Clinical Reasoning Study almost always asked patients to work with them during treatment. Even when they attended to the body in a strictly mechanistic way, the patient was rarely as passive a partner as in other medical encounters. Patients were never as separate from their disability as they are when, for instance, a surgeon operates, or a nurse listens to a pulse. Even initial assessments by occupational therapists generally required some level of participation by patients, because occupational therapists gather so much of their information about the extent of functional disability through asking the patient to perform tasks, rather than through examination of the patient's passive body with specialized instruments. Thus, in occupational therapy, passivity and detachment of the patient are not the best indicators that therapists are operating within a biomedical mode.

When therapists worked within a mechanistic frame, this was most evident by the way they defined the problem they were treating. In addressing the biomechanical body, problems were defined as deficiencies in strength or skill, as in the following example of a therapist working with a patient with a spinal cord injury. This example records an interchange between therapist and patient which occurred at the beginning of a treatment session. As the scene opens, the patient and the research assistant sit in a corner of the large spinal cord treatment room together. They are waiting for the occupational therapist who has left to get some adaptive equipment for the session. The patient asks the research assistant what she is doing there. The researcher says, "I'm here to watch the therapists to try to learn what makes good therapy." The patient replies, "It's in getting stronger." The therapist returns to the patient and they have the following conversation:

Therapist:	What did we talk about that we are going to do today?
Patient:	[No response.]
Therapist:	[Unclear] and the stick?!
Patient:	I'm tired.
Therapist:	You've already had your PT today?
Patient:	Yes. We're going to use the deltoid aid?
Therapist:	You need more power. The deltoid aid will help and the weight class too. . . . [Some discussion between them about schedule changes as the therapist begins to range the patient's hand.]
Patient:	Could I use the deltoid aid to get my arms to come up?

Therapist: Let's see. It pulls you up, right? In order to get your arms strong enough to lift them up you must hold them up as long as you can once they are up there. We can later rig up weights and attach them to your arms so that you pull them up as you lift. Did you want to use the deltoid aid to help pull your arms up or down? [Therapist begins to have patient actively exercise his left arm. Counts to ten.] Now hold it. Let's try to do four sets. Maybe on the other side we'll be able to do five sets. You are stronger over there, aren't you? [She repeats exercise three more times.] That was the fourth set. Can you do another?

Patient: Yes.

Therapist: OK, let's go for it! Could you really feel it?

Patient: Yeah.

Therapist: I could see the muscle popping away. [She moves to the other side and starts the exercise. The patient lifts his arm and tries to hold it for the count of ten. Exercising continues.]

Here the therapist defines the patient's problem as lack of strength. "You need more power," she tells him when he asks if they are going to use the deltoid aid. The entire session is devoted to exercises with the deltoid aid, which are intended, as the therapist tells him, to build his strength. The patient shares the therapist's perception of his problem, at least as it relates to occupational therapy, for he tells the researcher before the session begins that what makes good therapy is "getting stronger." And although he appears reluctant at first to begin work, he is soon actively considering the possibilities of the deltoid aid for strengthening his body, as when he asks the therapist if he could use it to get his arms "to come up." He not only appears to work his body hard in the session (evidenced toward the end of the session when the therapist asks him twice if he wants to quit and he tells her he wants to finish), but he participates at another level when he hypothesizes additional possible uses of the adaptive equipment for arm strengthening. Here he defines a problem he wants to work on. The patient comes to attend to his body, much as the therapist does.

Therapists provide ways for patients to attend to the mechanical aspect of their bodies more carefully and precisely than they otherwise might, so that they learn to recognize the healing process in terms of subtle measurements of bodily change. They train patients to read their bodies for signs of biomechanical progress and to interpret these signs as markers along a successful therapeutic path.

In the following example, a hand therapist is using a goniometer to measure the range of motion a patient has in his injured hand. She tells the patient to lift his hand off the table as far as he can, bending at the wrist. With effort he lifts his wrist. They then have the following conversation.

Therapist: I think it's right now where it's going to be.

Patient: Yeah, there's only so much you can do for it.

Therapist: Yeah, actively you can move it about 20 degrees, which isn't a lot, but it's still better than zero. And you can bend it down about 50 percent, which only gives you a motion of 30 degrees, you know, the actual amount of motion you can do back and forth, which isn't much. So anything we, this (upcoming surgery on his hand) will do, will obviously be better. . . . [Continues measuring in other positions.]

Therapist: Just for a lark, let's look at your improvements. Good, you gained 40 degrees of motion going up and you gained 30 degrees of motion going down. That's a lot and that's a big, that's what I was most concerned about because if you can't do this [she rotates her forearm—supination and pronation], if you can't do it, there's not much you can do.

Patient: Yeah.

Therapist: You can't turn a key.

Patient: You can't turn anything. . . . [Therapist continues asking the patient to position his hand in different ways and taking measurements.]

Therapist: Bring your thumb down toward your little finger and hold it. [Patient does so. Therapist measures his thumb motion.]

Therapist: Thumb's better, you can bend this part.

Patient: I can bend the whole thing more.

Therapist: It's loosening up. Hopefully your thumb won't be that tied up. I don't know. [Patient agrees in low tone. Words were unclear.]

The therapist mentions later in the interview that she measures the progress of her patients partly for her own records and partly for them, to help them see improvements. Hand therapy is very painful and tedious and gains are often difficult to observe. Measuring becomes a way to show that the pain and frustration is worth the effort. The therapist uses a special measuring device, the goniometer, and interprets the numbers to help the patient see improvement. She tacitly asks the patient to see his problem—and hence his progress—through the subtle increasing ranges in hand motion that have taken place.

By the end of the interchange recorded above, the patient is also noting the improvement in his thumb range. He echoes the therapist twice in this exchange. Once it is to amplify her statement of his problem; her "You can't turn a key" becomes his, "You can't turn anything." The second time it is to amplify her statement of his progress; "You can bend this part" becomes "I can bend the thing more." In his repetitions and amplifications, he is aggressively taking up her way of seeing his body.

The extent to which the two examples above stay within a mechanistic way of seeing the body is more strongly evident by what is omitted than by the conversation and focus of activity itself. Very likely, in both these cases where the patients are invested in regaining strength and mobility in their body, that regaining strength carries immense meaning in terms of self-image, as well as quite practically, in terms of what they can do in the world. A few degrees of mobility or a few pounds more weight lifted can mean all the difference in what these patients, both working-class men in their twenties, can make of their lives.

Such focus on the biomechanical body has direct, well-understood implications at the phenomenological level for the patient. In the above examples, neither patient nor therapist voices a translation of their explicit focus on biomechanical improvements into the implicit meanings that the patient's injury and recovery carry for them. The treatment activity in both these examples carries strong cultural meaning, as an exercise entailing significant pain, which requires them to make a "manly" effort. What is omitted is any explicit focus, either through activity or conversation, of the broader phenomenological world the patient inhabits. The hand patient who comes to echo the therapist in her statements of his problem and his improvement leaves unspoken a more experientially and semantically dense way of seeing his problem.

As is the case with all the therapists in this study, however, this therapist does not always treat his injury purely as a hand injury. On other occasions this patient has talked to the therapist about what this hand injury has meant in his life, including increased depression, increased drinking, and increasingly serious marital problems. Prior to the injury, which was sustained at work, he was a construction worker, the major wage earner in his family. After the injury, his wife went to work while he stayed home with the two children. Biomechanically speaking, the injury was to his hand. From the perspective of the illness experience, the injury was to his life.

When therapists and patients frame problems biomechanically, there is a personal and meaning-centered resonance that is bracketed, as if by tacit common consent, but rarely disappears. Patients, however, do not always consent to this biomechanical framing, and in such instances the therapist may choose to reassert a biomechanical reading of the problem, as in the following instance.

A therapist who treats acute neurological patients is seeing a patient who has suffered a second stroke. She is focusing on certain motoric and perceptual problems that the strokes have caused, especially the patient's inability to attend to his left side. During the following interchange, the therapist has placed his arm in a transparent air cushion, a plastic wrap that she then blows up. A nurse has come in the room and is curious about the use of the air cushion. The therapist and nurse have a short conversation about it, in which the therapist explains, "I'm using it for isolated motor control." The patient, who has been almost silent throughout the whole session, then suddenly says, "I wish God could do a miracle on me. I can't use my arm as I should." The therapist then turns to him and replies,

> "Well, you are doing much better. You can give yourself a lot of credit. You and others have been working hard. What keeps you in the hospital is not so much weaknesses as a lack of attention on your left side. You don't need a wheelchair. It's safety. It's attending to the left side. So that's the most serious thing. That's what you need to work on."

The patient frames his problem in religious and existential terms, in the language of despair. His drastically weakened arm is not a biomechanical condition but one of life's cruel tricks. His statement follows on the "medical talk" between therapist and nurse, and stands in jarring contrast to it. The therapist's quick response is to reject his interpretation of his problem and to reframe it in biomechanical terms. She does this in three successive moves.

Her initial response is to simply deny the existential meaning he has assigned to his disability, declaring "You are doing much better." Next, she then reframes the problem, telling him his difficulty "is not so much weaknesses as a lack of attention on your left side." She might be telling him that he is mistaken about the problem giving him the most trouble, believing it is his motoric weakness when it is actually a perceptual problem. But given the statement he has made, "weaknesses" seems to refer to the way he projected himself as weak, as needing a "miracle" in order to improve. Finally, she moves without pause from her reframing of the problem to an attempt to direct his attention to his hand in a biomechanical way. She directs how he should think about his problem, and she asks him to participate with her in careful attention to his biomechanical body:

> *Therapist:* Now on this one, just use your wrist to come up gently. I don't want you to stiffen your body. So look at your wrist and make your wrist stay up. You're doing it without working too hard. Mr. _____, you are not looking at your hand. Are you looking at your hand?

Patient:	Trying to.
Therapist:	Don't look at me, look at your hand. Make it come up to my hand. You are learning how to move all over again. You are telling yourself how to move. That's why you have to look at your hand. I cannot make it work on my own. We both have to do it together.
Patient:	Yes, yes.

In shifting the patient away from his way of seeing to her own, the therapist is also asking the patient to see how he can improve his condition. She tells him that what he is doing with her is "learning how to move all over again." The foregrounding of the biomechanical gaze is interesting, in this example, because it provides the more optimistic view. Enclosing the disability within a biomechanical problem opens the possibility to see successes that might be invisible from a phenomenological point of view. The two different ways of seeing operate at different depths of suffering and despair. But there are other times when an overreliance on the biomechanical framing of a problem can prevent even biomechanical healing. The case story of Doris told at the beginning of this chapter provides a good illustration of this.

Describing the Disability: "Chart Talk"

THE IMPORTANCE OF TALK

Describing clinical cases to colleagues plays a substantial role in a therapist's work day. Therapists in the Clinical Reasoning Study spent approximately one-third to one-half of their time in meetings with colleagues or in writing chart notes. This time was spent discussing patients, describing clinical problems, outlining and justifying treatment approaches, citing treatment goals. There was a weekly departmental meeting among the occupational therapy staff, weekly interdisciplinary meetings with medical staff in particular diagnostic wards (neurology, psychiatry, etc.), and supervision meetings between senior occupational therapists who were supervisors for staff therapists.

The main topic in all of these meetings, except perhaps the weekly departmental staff meeting, concerned the presentation and review of case loads. The status of each patient would be reviewed, with discussions around the efficacy of particular treatment approaches, problems the patient was presenting to staff, any new medical complications, or possible discharge dates. Therapists were continually called upon by colleagues to provide descriptions of their work with patients and to evaluate the patients' status. Therapists also talked to one another casually, over lunch, in the hall or in their offices, about the patients they were seeing. And, in the everyday course of treatment, they talked to the patients themselves about how the therapeutic process was going or about the nature of the patient's disability.

CHART TALK AND STORY TALK

A biomechanical way of understanding disability and of framing clinical problems shows up, not only in what therapists do in treatment, but in how they describe what they do. When a disability is presented biomechanically, therapists typically outline a list of general problems that have clustered around a particular patient. The tendency toward an atomistic portrayal of clinical problems is also characteristic of the way treatment modalities are described. Treatment is often pictured as a serial collection of isolated actions, a linear sequence of events. General problems are connected, one by one, to treatment interventions, with outcomes of interventions matched against the initially identified problem categories. When a history is given, either of onset of disability or of treatment process, that history is of the pathology and its course through treatment, not of the person who possesses it. The particular experience of the patient is downplayed or left out altogether.

Alternately, when therapists consider the meaning of the disability for the patient's life, their discourse moves into a narrative mode. They begin to tell stories. Clinical problems and treatment activities are organized in terms of some unfolding drama the narrator sees in the work with a patient. A cast of characters emerges. Motives are inferred or examined. Feelings often dominate the drama, where the narrator intersperses descriptions of what happened with interpretations of how the patient felt or her own emotions when certain events transpired. Both the patient's illness experiences and therapist's experience of treating the patient take center stage. Idiosyncratic events occur in many of these stories: unexpected difficulties, or a great success that couldn't have been predicted, though the therapist might have hoped for it. Therapists and patients often get surprised in the story. Usually there is some suspense surrounding the telling, except in the briefest tales.

The dual practice of occupational therapy is visible in the dualistic way therapists describe their work and their clinical reasoning to one another, to their patients, and to outside researchers. Therapists talk about their work, drawing upon two distinct language. One is a biomedical discourse, a language of "chart talk." The other was a narrative discourse, a language of personal experience.

These two modes of description—"chart talk" and "story talk"— play a powerful role in giving therapists two languages for making sense of patients, two ways of envisioning clinical work. The same patient can be described through both forms of talk. This chapter and the following one examine the relation between the "body" therapists treat and the form of discourse they use to describe what they are seeing.

These two frameworks for making sense of human experience have been discussed in detail because, obviously, they help to illuminate differences between a biomedical way of understanding disability and a phenomenological one. A good example of the significant difference between these two frameworks emerged out of an exercise we asked therapists to carry out at the very start of the research project. We asked therapists participating in the study to write out a description of a patient that had presented them with problems, one where they had gotten "stuck." They were to define the problems and write up the case in any way they chose.

Therapists presented their cases in two distinctly different ways. Some wrote stories about the therapeutic process and especially about the experience of treating the disability from the point of both therapist and patient. These were accounts that centered on the meaning of the disability from the patient's and therapist's perspectives. Other therapists described their problem case primarily in biomechanical terms; experiential aspects were minimized. A nice illustration is the quite different way two therapists presented cases that concerned hand injuries. One confined her description primarily to the biomechanical body, referring only briefly, and as a kind of postscript, to the disability and its treatment in an experiential way. The second described her problem in such a way that the biomechanical was buried within a narrative description of how the disability was affecting the patient and herself. The first account is given below. The second account is given at the beginning of the following chapter.

FIRST THERAPIST: THE BIOMECHANICAL MODE

The Man with the Amputated Hand

by Deborah Slater

The experience I've had most often as a hand therapist is a result of the natural cycle of recuperation after injury: that is, maintaining motivation, and creativity in dealing with the inevitable frustration, both in myself and the patient, over a long haul of rapid, then slow improvement, with many plateaus in between.

This was especially true in the case of a young man who received therapy over a period of a year and a half. He had amputated his right dominant hand in a hydraulic log splitter. The hand was replanted, with fractures pinned and soft tissue repaired, after which he started on an aggressive rehabilitation program. The long-term problems that required multiple attempts at solution (some effective, some not) were:

- Lack of metacarpal phalangeal [MP] flexion.
- Lack of thumb rotation and subsequent functional opposition.
- No active motion in the interphalangeal (IP) joints of the little finger.

What I tried for each problem was:

Problem I: MP flexion.
- Wrist splint with rubber bands and finger slings for dynamic flexion.
- Discontinued night resting extension splint since patient was in extension and active extension had improved.
- Joint mobilization.
- Coband wrapping in flexion and active assistive range of motion.
- Ultimately, 11 months after the injury, surgical capsulotomy to MP joints and extensor tendon release.
- Alumafoam splints to concentrate flexor power at MP joints.
- Flexion assist wrist splint with betapile strap to flex IP joints.

Problem II: Lack of thumb rotation.
- Wrist cuff with dynamic thumb sling to pull into palmar abduction and opposition.
- Functional "opposition" activities with decreasing object size.
- Aquaplast web spacer.
- Resistive prehension for strengthening.
- Dynamic thumb sling attached to wrist splint to stretch web and position thumb in palmar abduction.

Problem III: Little finger limitation of motion and limited flexion, all fingers.
- Massage to break up adhesions.
- Resistive exercise for same.
- Flexor tenolysis 14 months after the injury (significant improvement.)
- Splint with finger nail loops for rubber band traction.

Reviewing this case pointed out a few things to me. One was the need to work closely with the physician because well-times surgery moved the program along significantly, and therapy maintained and built on these improvements. I also had to come to grips with the fact that we cannot control all outcomes: for example, sensory return, which has important implications for ultimate functional usage, is generally poor in adults, and there is no way to change that. This patient saw good improvement from all the modalities tried, but some were more effective than others. There were long periods of time with little or no improvement and patient attendance also lagged—the end is sometimes never in sight for them, too. Therapists and patients alike get bored. It is hard to maintain creativity and motivation. And sometimes you just cannot find a solution as good as you want!

Case Discussion

Deborah describes a situation of extreme frustration, a familiar, difficult scenario for hand therapists. What is interesting about this case, in the context of this chapter, is how Deborah frames the clinical problem and how she describes her treatment task.

She lists three problems for therapy.

1. Lack of metacarpo-phalangeal flexion.
2. Lack of thumb rotation and subsequent functional opposition.
3. No active motion in interphalangeal joints of the little finger.

She then takes each problem in turn and describes the therapeutic approaches used to treat that physiological difficulty.

Interestingly, these specific physiological problems are framed by problems that hint at the phenomenological domain, but these are not taken up as target issues to which her therapy is directed. The therapist mentions at the beginning and end of her case that a major difficulty was the frustration of the patient at the plateaus in therapy. She also hints at her own frustration at lacking control over the progress of treatment and her recognition that there is often more to physical healing than "fixing" a hand. An important feature of "chart talk" is that while in actual practice, therapists are likely to confront and have to reason through problems in domains that fall well outside the biomedical one, there is often no official place in the institutional world of clinic (or even, perhaps school) to address these broader issues. Thus the talk of therapists, especially what is written into chart notes or offered in formal staff presentations, often sounds much more biomedical than what has actually occurred. It is unlikely that Deborah simply ignored her patient's frustrations at the lack of progress in therapy. But often therapists do not feel that this is a part of their practice or that it is "reportable." The final chapters of this book look at the problem of the "underground" nature of many of the clinical problems therapists actually deal with, such as those hinted at in this case.

Summary

Biomedicine plays a powerful role in occupational therapy. There are good reasons why therapists are trained in the language and tools of biomedicine, in anatomy and physiology, in kinesiology and neurology, but the limitations of biomedicine are also clear to practicing therapists, as the case of Doris shows. If therapists want to be effective, they invariably find themselves addressing concerns that are not strictly biomedical, ones in which they must remember the patient as person, not as "another quad down the hall."

Therapists do seem to need a "double vision" in order to do their job. That is, they need to view their patients as diagnostic categories and collections of physiological or mental dysfunctions on the one hand, and as quite particular people with quite particular lives on the other. Seeing the person behind the disability is the subject of the following chapter.

■

Occupational Therapy as a Two-Body Practice
The Lived Body
■ CHERYL MATTINGLY

Introduction

In the previous chapter, we made a distinction between a biomedical orientation toward disease, and the anthropological concern with illness experience. Occupational therapy, as we mentioned, pays attention to both of these in rather equal measure. The last chapter looked at how occupational therapists address the disease in their practical focus on medical diagnosis and on treating disease-related dysfunctions. This chapter looks at the second orientation, examining how therapists treat the illness experience.

When therapists direct their treatment interventions to the illness experience of their patients, they are treating disability in a phenomenological mode. "Phenomenology" is a philosophical term that has come to be used in a variety of ways. We use it in this book in two primary senses. In the first sense, it offers an alternative conception of the body to that recognized in biomedicine. The underlying metaphors of biomedicine treat the body as a container or machine, both a physical container for the mind and, in the case of pathology, as a physical container of foreign pathogens. But a phenomenological conception of the body is very different. From this perspective, the body is no mere machine, nor a mere container for the mind (as reservoir of meaning) but is an indissoluble part of a person's experience of the world. This different view of the body provides a different view of disability. If our experience of our body is inseparable from, even constitutive of, our experience of our world, disability is an interruption or injury to a whole life.

In the second sense, phenomenology looks at persons, not as isolated individuals with internal physiologies and intrapsychic structures (though they possess these), but in the context of how they live their lives. Particularly, this phenomenological approach involves understanding people in terms of their daily practices, life histories, social relationships, and long-term projects, all of which give them a sense of meaning and a sense of personal identity.

The centrality of *action* in constituting the world we live in is crucial to this phenomenological tradition. The place of action in helping to create and recreate our world is examined by a number of phenomenological philosophers whose writings have influenced our interpretation of the place of phenomenology in occupational therapy. In this book, the most central of these philosophers are Alfred Schutz, Martin Heidegger, and Maurice Merleau-Ponty. The role of the person as actor in constituting his or her "life-world" is of particular importance to a profession like occupational therapy. This is both because of the importance of activity as a treatment intervention and because of the frequent recognition by therapists of how disabled patients, who have become limited in their actions, experience their world in a very different way.

A second tenet of phenomenology is central to this book: the continual nature of the human effort for *understanding*. The phenomenologists we draw upon also emphasize the continual effort required to understand one another, and the centrality of this effort in living our everyday lives. Not only action, but also the capacity to understand one another, is necessary to inhabit a (comparatively) commonly shared world. As one philosopher writes, "The fact that the life-world exists shows that men somehow cope, in their common-sense, routine way, with the need to understand each other" (Bauman, 1978, p. 176).

The problem of understanding is important to the practice of occupational therapy. Therapists have the problem of understanding their patients. While, from a biomedical point of view (that is, from the perspective of the medical diagnosis), therapists may understand what is going on physiologically, this still leaves the puzzle of how a particular patient with that disability is making sense of it, is coping with it, is grieving over it. And patients and their families often have the problem of understanding themselves. When a person becomes afflicted with a sudden stroke, or must be hospitalized for another manic depressive episode, or becomes progressively more paralyzed by the growth of a spinal cord tumor, life changes. This change is not only a change in action, in capacity for doing. It also involves changes in recognition and understanding of oneself. Persons can no longer recognize themselves, can become lost in trying to reconstruct a life history that gives them any place from which to continue. When an active athlete has a head injury, or a factory worker permanently injures his hand, these do not merely require new job training. They also require the quite painful process of helping patients to see themselves in new ways, to return to lives that will never be the same.

CASE EXAMPLE IN THE PHENOMENOLOGICAL MODE

The following case provides an interesting contrast to two of the cases related in the previous chapter. In the case of Doris, the story is told by the treating occupational therapist, and it is the contract occupational therapist who discovers how her hand was injured. But in the following case, the storyteller, rather like that contract therapist, is "just visiting." She is not the "real" occupational therapist, and, she too is the one who discovers the deeper meaning of the hand injury because the patient reveals the story behind it, as she has not done to her treating therapist.

What is most important, in both these cases, is how an injury, which from a purely physical standpoint may not be that serious, can, from a phenomenological point of view, be immense.

The Visiting Therapist

by Kay Schwartz

I was visiting a colleague at her clinic. She invited me to join her as she was treating one of her patients—we'll call her Ms. Anna Anderson. I introduced myself as an occupational therapist and a friend of her therapist, and sat down beside Anna.

Anna started to ask me questions about my work and my studies, and we found that we had some common interests. I asked her about the injury for which she was receiving treatment and how her treatment was progressing. She explained that she had injured her middle finger when a window sash fell on it, that there had been a lot of blood, and that her two children had been frightened by the accident and the trip to the emergency room of the local hospital. (I observed to myself that the injury looked to be a relatively minor one and was responding nicely to therapy.)

Then Anna remarked that her husband had recently been killed in an automobile accident and that there had been a lot of blood. After she had made the remark, I felt as though time stood still while myriad thoughts raced through my mind. I sensed this was an important revelation. Who else knew this? I wanted to look at my colleague, but I felt that eye contact might deflect the focus of attention away from Anna's statement. But why would she share it with me, a relative stranger? How did she see me? What did she expect from me? I became aware of my own discomfort. I could feel her pain and horror at having her recent injury be a catalyst for reliving her husband's death. The intensity of feelings was hard for me to endure, and part of me wanted to ignore the remark and go on as though it had never been spoken. But I sensed this moment was an important one and I knew I must acknowledge it.

After what was probably a 30-second pause, I responded to Anna's remark by saying that her injury must have been a horrible time for her if it reminded her of her husband's death, and she said it was not. She said that it was a very hard and lonely time for her, and a frightening one for her children. I asked whether her surgeon knew about her husband's death and she said no. She criticized her doctor for treating her as though she were just a finger and not caring about the rest of her.

I was tempted to lecture her, and tell her that if the doctor had known her situation his approach may have been different. I did not lecture her, however, because by this time I had concluded that the role Anna cast me in was one of a sympathetic outsider—a professional, but not one she was responsible to—and that the best thing I could do was to acknowledge that her feelings were legitimate and natural and to hope that this discussion would lead her to separate her injury from her husband's death.

Anna then began talking in generalities about her disappointment with some health care providers. I asked her whether occupational therapy had been beneficial, and she said that she had enjoyed that part of her treatment the most.

While we had been talking, Anna had been exercising. At this point her therapist intervened to bring her back to her therapy and to discuss her progress and her home exercise program. Then Anna said goodbye and that she had enjoyed talking with me. I said the same and that I wished her continued progress.

When she had gone, I asked my colleague if she knew about the husband's accident. She said no, but that it explained a good deal about Anna's worry over her injury.

When I reflect back on why I behaved as I did, I would say that my behavior was, in part, shaped by my clinical experience in treating patients with physical disabilities, where I had learned the importance of helping them deal with their feelings as a way to come to grips with the implications of their physical problems. I had learned in graduate school to check out my assumptions, to make sure that the conclusions I drew were, in fact, what people meant. Finally, I had learned during my own therapy to endure that uncomfortable feeling that comes to me when I, or someone else, is sharing a revelation that is filled with strong emotion.

Case Discussion

Because there can be such disparity between the meaning of the disability from a biomedical and physiological point of view, on the one hand, and from the point of the view of what it means to the patient, on the other, medical anthropologists have come up with an extremely useful distinction. They have distinguished the category "disease" from the meaning of the condition for the patient, which they call the "illness experience" (Good and Delvecchio Good, 1980; Kleinman et al., 1978; Kleinman, 1988). In the case just recounted, it becomes markedly apparent that Kay pays almost exclusive attention to the patient's illness experience, with only a cursory glance at the physical injury, which tells her that at the level of body injury, nothing serious is going on. Of course, Kay is in the unusual position of being the visiting therapist, with no responsibility for this person. Anna is not her patient. If she were, it is much more likely that this concern with the patient's illness experience would be intertwined with attention to the biomedical condition, with the physical injury.

Phenomenological Roots within Occupational Therapy

The term phenomenology is a recent addition to the language of occupational therapy, but certain tenets of phenomenology are shared by the early tradition within the field, with its special amalgam of values and beliefs based on both the moral treatment movement and the arts and crafts movement early in this century. The emphasis both on purposeful activity and on understanding the person are core values in the profession, and connect the profession to phenomenological concerns developed in philosophy. Before turning to current practice, this section offers a cursory sketch of that history. Again, there is heavy reliance on a small number of theorists in piecing together this history, most notably Rogers, Kielhofner, Burke, Levine, and Bing.

At least some of the phenomenological emphasis currently visible in occupational therapy probably stems from its origins within the moral treatment movement, and perhaps even more from its connection to the arts and crafts movement. The first years of the profession were highly influenced by the Moral Treatment movement in the United States, a movement rooted in eighteenth-century reforms in the treatment of the mentally ill in England and France. Moral Treatment was directed at creating new methods of caring for the mentally ill, in which occupation in purposeful activity was central (Bing, 1981, p. 502). Activities were viewed as both diversions from morbid thoughts and an avenue for altering patients' emotional excesses. Activities were especially perspicacious, so the theory went, when they became part of regular employment that would organize daily life and offer a real social role (p. 504).

The Moral Treatment movement spread in the 1800s, and occupation was considered an integral part of the approach. The movement adhered to a strongly optimistic view that mental illness was curable, if the insane were treated correctly. Insanity occurred when people, through an excess of emotion and faulty habits, lost their connection with the mainstream of social life (Kielhofner & Burke, 1977, p. 678).

Moral Treatment had embedded in it an assumption that mental illness stemmed in part from maladaptive responses by individuals to their social world and that health could be regained through "accommodating or adapting individuals to the general mores of values of their culture" (Engelhardt, 1977, p. 668).

The Moral Treatment movement essentially died in the United States by the mid-1900s, but it was revived, in a rather different form, in the twentieth-century occupational therapy movement, which was an amalgam of the older Moral Treatment philosophy and the arts and crafts movement. The most clearly "humanist" streak in occupational therapy has its roots in this arts and crafts heritage, with its emphasis on creativity, on the need to create objects that are both useful and beautiful, artifacts of which one can be proud. The arts and crafts movement was an upper-class rebellion against the "machine age" and a pastoral call to an earlier time when craftsmen rather than machines produced society's goods. Levine quotes Ruskin (a key proponent of this movement) as arguing that one needed a society where "humans, not machines, completed objects" and thus where "work was not abstracted from life but had a place at its very core. The manufactured goods of his [Ruskin's] own time he found to be both aesthetically and morally unsatisfying because the worker was treated like an extension of the machine, completing only part of the finished product" (Levine, 1987, p. 248). It is interesting, in looking at contemporary occupational therapy practice, to see it as an integration of biomedicine, with its central metaphor of body as machine, and an arts and crafts tradition, with its view of the machine as "morally unsatisfying."

The idea of using craft making as a medically therapeutic approach to the mentally ill is credited largely to two people: Susan Tracy, a nurse who, in 1906, ran a craft-based "occupations training course" for nurses working at Adams Nervine Hospital in Boston, and physician William Dunton, who was convinced that an "occupations cure" was highly therapeutic to the mentally ill. In addition to the efforts of these two, there were several other early attempts in the first decade of the twentieth century to run what were called "sheltered workshops" for patients to produce well-made crafts that could be sold (Levine, 1987, p. 250). The occupational therapy movement was based on the idea that "the 'scientific' prescription of arts and crafts could cure a variety of chronic problems generally considered outside the domain of medicine" (p. 250).

The occupational therapy movement was in part a response to the rising prestige of medicine, and particularly a physiologically centered approach to medicine, which was taking place in the first decades of this century (Starr, 1982; Kielhofner and Burke, 1977; Levine, 1987). Occupational therapy grew, in part, out of dissatisfaction among some physicians with this narrowing of the medical perspective. Some dissenting physicians, notably Herbert Hall, William Dunton, and Adolf Meyer, were concerned with the development of medical therapies that preserved a sense of the mind-body unity and, even more broadly, of the role played by the larger social and physical environment in influencing mental and physical health (Levine, 1987). Adolf Meyer's address to the Fifth Annual Meeting of the National Society for the Promotion of Occupational Therapy in 1921 illustrates this sense of dissatisfaction. He began his talk by taking direct issue with a diagnostic approach to medicine and advocating a much more holistic and social view of medical problems:

There was a time when physicians and the public thought the art of medicine consisted mainly in diagnosing more or less mysterious diseases and "prescribing" for them. Each disease was supposed to have its program of treatment, and to this day the patient and the family expect a set of medicines and a diet, and a change of climate if necessary, or at least a rest-cure so as to fight and conquer "the disease." No branch of medicine has learned as clearly as psychiatry that after all many of these formidable diseases are largely problems of adaptation . . . and psychiatry has been among the first to recognize the need of adaption and the value of *work* as a sovereign help in the problems of adaptation. (1977, p. 639)

Hall, Meyer, and Dunton all turned to the arts and crafts movement as a basis for an "occupation therapy" for the treatment of the mentally ill. The marriage of these two movements is important in its modification of some of the "work cures" that were used in mental asylums. While the new occupational therapy movement firmly believed in work, it was equally adamant about the kind of work it considered therapeutic. There is an interesting parallel between these assumptions and those voiced by a political philosopher schooled in phenomenology, Hannah Arendt. In *The Human Condition*, Arendt makes an interesting separation between labor and fabrication and, in language that closely resembles that of the arts and crafts reformers, speaks of the integrity of fabrication—of a making in which the end product is, in an important sense, the product of that maker. Labor, by contrast, lacks this integrity for Arendt; it is that sort of activity where people cannot have creative ownership of their work or the sense of integrity that comes from a process of making things which are an expression of oneself.

Arendt's distinction between fabrication and labor is useful in expressing the kind of work the original occupational therapists had in mind, a making that allowed an integrity and ownership to the maker, rather than work that was merely useful and demanded no creativity or pride from the worker. The early occupational therapy workshops and clinics stressed solid workmanship and a high-quality product. Pictures taken of the products patients made in those early clinics show beautiful woodworking and weavings. Even today, although the crafts focus of occupational therapy has lost favor, it survives in such things as the traditional auction at the annual national association meeting, where therapists auction their own handicrafts to raise money for the American Occupational Therapy Foundation.

The notion of "occupation," as it developed in the occupational therapy movement, was not confined to a theory about the curative potential of work, not even the comparatively creative work of the craftsperson. There was a more complex notion behind the advocacy of occupation as therapy, and it had to do with a view of human life that consisted of a kind of occupational rhythm, a movement through time, which balanced certain occupations fundamental for human health. Health required not only productive work but recreation—play—and rest. This is still a very fundamental tenet within occupational therapy (Kielhofner, 1983; Rogers, 1982b; Reilly, 1962). The occupation cure was intended to introduce this balance for those who had become un-balanced, and to do so, not through talking, but through doing. "The only way to attain balance in all this is actual doing, actual practice, a program of wholesome living as the basis of wholesome feeling and thinking and fancy and interests" (Meyer, 1977, p. 639). Notably, the kind of work that the early occupation therapists gave to their patients was the sort that is culturally ambiguous in terms of being either work or play, being work for some and play for many others. Occupational therapists had the task of constructing environments, carefully graded to increase the challenge to the patient, where they introduced increas-ingly complex activities that pushed patients to increase their capacities to perform complex, meaningful, and socially appropriate tasks and, in this way, adapt themselves to the "real world" outside the institution. The patients' engagement in these activities was to prepare them to adapt to reality. The emphasis on adaptation and the definition of illness as a maladaptive response to an external environment, rather than an internal process, was one of the most important distinguishing marks that separated occupational therapy from the medical tradition, both in physical medicine and in psychiatry.

There was an early emphasis, not only on the kinds of occupational activities that might be therapeutic, but on the role of the therapist in functioning as a "firm but gentle" guide to patients, carefully struc-turing and adapting activities to the particular needs of the patient at particular points in their recovery process (Bing, 1981; Rogers, 1982b; Meyer, 1977).

Phenomenology in Current Practice: Treating the Lived Body

THE LIVED BODY

Phenomenologically speaking, sickness and disease are not merely a matter of malfunctioning parts but involve the breakdown of the patient's social modes of operating in the world, the ground of expe-rience, that which gives a life-world. The disabled patient is one who suffers a reduction of this ground of being-in-the-world, in the form of a failure of bodily movement, which, as we have seen, can be described at one level in biomechanical terms.

The "lived-body paradigm," as it has come to be called, derives from phenomenology, particularly the work of Maurice Merleau-Ponty. Merleau-Ponty (1962) argued that bodily acts are not merely mechanical, and that many volitional acts are not merely mental, that is, they do not merely arise out of explicit judgments and acts of will. Phenomenologists argue that the body mechanism is intentional in the sense that it is directed outward toward the world, so that one can speak of bodily intelligence, or even of the bodily ground of all intelligence. "The body," Simone de Beauvoir wrote, "is not a thing, it is a situation . . . it is the instrument of our grasp upon the world, a limiting factor for our projects" (quoted in Murphy, 1987). There may be no better description of the phenomenological body.

Merleau-Ponty based his argument on studies of sensory perception. He saw sensory perception as neither a mechanical process nor a type of thought. Working from the findings of Gestalt psychology, he argued that sensing already recognizes a set of meanings, because the perceptual field is always at the outset structured by the observer into foreground and background features. The features that make up the foreground of the scene are then treated as its significant features. He linked the existential work of creating significance through the initial act of seeing—sensing significance so to speak—with the active body.

The sensing of the lived body is tied to its capacity of self-movement. Through movement, new perceptual fields are revealed; movement helps bring some objects more clearly into focus, while neglecting others. Self-movement is an essential aspect of sensory perception, and perception lays what Merleau-Ponty considered the precognitive groundwork for all clearly volitional, purposive, and cognitive acts, for acts of will.

Not only is a person's experience of her body reduced if she is disabled and movement is constricted, she also quite literally loses much of the world around her. She is no longer able to construct the objects of her world in the complex, multiviewed way that she could when her body moved freely. This means that a loss of bodily movement, a constriction, is not purely mechanical. It directly affects body intelligence, body seeing.

This loss of body, of the possibility of movement, directly impacts a person's self. Merleau-Ponty argues that a phantom limb, for instance, is not merely a physiological or psychological problem, but also a problem of being-in-the-world. Our body gives us a "natural momentum that throws us into our tasks, our cares, our situations, our familiar horizons" (1962, p. 81). When our natural way of moving through the world is lost, the world itself, as we have inhabited it, is lost. For if the objects that make up the world are constructed from perceptions, and perceptions depend on our movements, which orient those perceptions, then loss of movement and accompanying loss of ability to perceive in the normal way means loss of objects. We can no longer grasp the world as we did when we could move freely, unimpaired.

It is this loss of our way of being-in-the-world when we are disabled, he argues, that makes it so difficult to accept the bodily losses that come with disablement. Our capacity for movement is directly connected to our sense of self. Merleau-Ponty writes:

> What it is in us which refuses mutilation and disablement is an I committed to a certain physical and inter-human world, who continues to tend towards his world despite handicaps and amputations and who, to this extent, does not recognize them *de jure*. (1962, p. 81)

REHABILITATION OF THE LIVED BODY

In their practice of talking to patients and eliciting stories from them, the occupational therapists in our study were closer to a phenomenologic than to the biomechanical framing of disability. They also addressed the lived body in the course of presenting therapeutic activities as a basis for the patient's reorientation in the world. This understanding of the meaning of therapeutic activity was often recognized by both patient and therapist. In concrete terms, for instance, this meant that activities like dressing were seen not just in terms of skill building, but were also understood by clients and therapists in light of the patients' experiences of losing old capacities and orientations in the world and of the meaning of learning new ways of orienting themselves.

The anthropologist Robert Murphy (1987) wrote an autobiographical account of his own illness experience, a degenerative disease caused by a spinal cord tumor, which left him paralyzed from the neck down at the time he wrote his account. He notes the difference he experienced between his treatment by neurologists and by rehabilitation specialists. He was struck with the irony that neurosurgery and clinical neurology were among the most prestigious medical specialties while rehabilitation medicine ranked among the lowest. The irony was that neurology, as Oliver Sacks (1984) has also noted, "is essentially a passive science" because neurologists can only examine and diagnose. Rehabilitation, on the other hand, is an active science, where both patient and therapist work together to discover the patient's real limitations and to continually try to transcend those limitations. Because of the problems occupational therapists tackle, they deal not only with physical ailments but also with the patients who have them.

Robert Murphy experienced rehabilitation therapy as a kind of game where therapists "urged, cajoled and nagged" him and his fellow patients to push harder than they felt able and where "today's painful overreach may become tomorrow's routine accomplishment" (1987, p. 51). He tells of one day when

> a young paraplegic woman was helped to her feet, given a walker, and told to walk. After about five steps, she told the therapist, who was walking just behind her, that she was tired and wanted to stop. The therapist told her that she was giving up too soon and ordered her to

continue. The other therapists and their patients echoed him, telling her that she could do it, forming a cheering section as she struggled onward. She soon stopped again, this time begging to be put back in the wheelchair, but the therapist was adamant. Finally, after she broke down in tears and shows signs of collapsing, the chair was brought up behind her and she fell into it. Everybody in the gym applauded, and she wiped away the tears and grinned in triumph. (1987, p. 51)

This happens to be a story about physical therapy, but it belongs just as surely to occupational therapy. Rehabilitation medicine in general, and occupational therapy in particular, fit precariously in the medical mold, requiring so much more active and collaborative a relation between clinician and patient than is the norm in biomedicine in general.

In rehabilitation, patients are very much involved in their own recovery. They must claim their disability rather than separate themselves from it. The powerful autobiographic accounts given by vivid and informed writers like Murphy and Sacks about their own experiences of disability, as well as the everyday talk of patients to their therapists, emphasize, over and over again, the assault to one's sense of identity that deep injury to the body causes. To become disabled is to become disembodied, alienated from one's own body. Therapists' efforts are directed, in part, toward a patient's "re-embodiment"—a reclaiming of the body—and this involves helping patients articulate a new sense of self.

The following section looks at how therapists address their therapeutic intervention to help patients place their experience of illness or disability within the broader context of their lives.

Treating the Whole Person

Occupational therapists have always presented themselves as concerned with the patient's relationship with the disease, with the "whole person." They are concerned with disability as a meaningful experience, especially inasmuch as it has affected the patient's capacity to move through the world, and to take up the occupations that have shaped his or her life and given it significance. "We [occupational therapists] are concerned with understanding the occupations of human beings, the ways in which people organize the activities that fill their lives and give their lives meaning" (Parham, 1987, p. 555).

The functional assessment, which is the occupational therapy equivalent of the doctor's diagnosis, generally requires that the therapist go beyond gathering information and assessing the patient's physiological condition. It requires that the therapist pay some attention to the patient's unique life history and to how the patient sees and understands her or his condition. In the course of treating patients, occupational therapists generally address, in some way, the experiences and perceptions patients have of their disabilities, their struggles with these disabilities, and how those activities that have given their life meaning are affected.

This concern with a patient's experience of disability derives in part from deep beliefs that belong to occupational therapy's professional culture, and have been discussed in some detail earlier in this chapter. Yet the phenomenological perspective, from which illness and disability are treated as meaningful experiences, although seemingly fundamental for the problems occupational therapists tackle, is actually quite neglected as an articulating and legitimizing framework for practice. Occupational therapists are trained much more systematically in the biomedically related sciences that provide them with a way of seeing the biomechanical body. They are required to take courses in anatomy and physiology, in biomechanics and neurology. Such courses form the core of their education. There is no such core of courses to equip occupational therapists to treat the phenomenological body. They learn little or no philosophy, sociology, anthropology. The psychology of disability as an illness experience is addressed incidentally, in less pedagogically emphasized, clinically oriented courses designed to teach skills in patient interaction or group leadership.

Yet the phenomenological body is the one therapists encounter just as often as the biomechanical one, in attempting to carry out their practice with real patients. They are drawn into the phenomenological world of these patients, by the way they work with them as much as by the questions that they ask. The meaning that the patient makes of an illness enters directly into the therapeutic process, because this process is built on a practice of "doing with" the patient. This requires therapists to devise treatment goals that are meaningful enough to patients that they are motivated to work hard, as partners in the therapeutic process. The therapists thus find themselves constantly confronted with the interpretive task of translating between their way of seeing and the patient's. If the goals that the therapist pursues are too far afield from the patient's perception of their functional needs, therapy is likely to be stalemated.

Therapists also continually refer to their interpretations of patient meanings, to modify treatment directions or to attempt to persuade patients to see their disability in a different light. They often see possibilities where patients see none, and commonly attempt to help patients fight despair and passive resignation in the face of their disabilities. Robert Murphy, commenting on his own resistance to therapy and his enormous depression as he faced a deteriorating body, notes that "[rehabilitation] therapists must breach imposing psychological barriers to reach their patients and enlist their cooperation in the long tedious process of reconstructing their bodies" (1987, p. 54).

Effective therapy requires that patients be committed to a long path where gains are so slow they are difficult to perceive, or are counteracted by a faster rate of deterioration. This means that therapists must address the problem of motivation. They must tap into commitments and values deep enough within patients to commit them to such a process. No matter what the technical and physiological expertise and orientation of the therapist, or what practice theories he relies on, effective collaboration requires treating the disability as more than a biomechanical matter that can be separated from the experience of the patient.

Therapists were often required by their own interest in involving patients in therapy to create stories and theories about who patients were and how they experienced their disabilities. But therapists' interest in the phenomenological body is not necessarily motivated so directly by strategic concerns. Therapists often revised their planned treatment activities in small ways as the patient voiced concerns that they had not anticipated prior to the session. In fact, they often insist on interrupting their plans to respond to such concerns.

A concern for the patient's experience of disability is revealed when therapists begin an activity that reflects a planned agenda and, in the course of carrying out that activity, they shift the activity to accommodate the patient's concerns. In the following example, taken from field notes, the therapist opens the session by initiating an evaluation of the paraplegic patient she has seen only once or twice before. The evaluation involves a standard set of questions intended to provide information on the patient's cognitive, motoric, and self-care status.

Therapist:	Do you remember what my name is?
Patient:	No.
Therapist:	What letter does it start with?
Patient:	Patty.
Therapist:	What did you have for breakfast? (Patient replies. Therapist asks questions about the tape recorder which he has put on his bed and he replies.)
Therapist:	How is your back doing?
Patient:	It's giving me some pain.
Therapist:	Remember how I was going to ask you some questions? We can do that or we can do some relaxation exercises first.
Patient:	You're the doctor.

| *Therapist:* | Well, I'm not the doctor. Which do you prefer? How about the relaxation first, to help with the pain? |
| *Patient:* | OK. |

In this interchange, the therapist interrupts her evaluation when she asks the patient how his back is doing. He tells her he is in pain, and she stops to teach him how to do a relaxation exercise, an "interruption" that lasts for about 10 minutes, including the exercises, before she returns to her evaluation format. She takes his pain seriously, and seems to expect him to demand that she do so, as when she tells him, "Well, I'm not the doctor. Which do you prefer?" After telling him he is to choose, she chooses what she believes he ought to prefer—relaxation exercises to help relieve his back pain.

She implies that being a good patient for the occupational therapist is not the same as being a good patient for the doctor. Good occupational therapy patients are ones who make choices—albeit choices within a list presented by the therapist. Good patients are also those who take their experiences and the feelings related to their disability seriously. The therapist later tells the patient to "know that when you have pain, it's telling you something. You can separate yourself from the pain, but you also have to take care of it."

Later in this session, they discuss his medications. He tells her, "I don't give a crap about what a medicine's for, but I guess I should." She replies, "You do need to know about your meds' side effects. Suppose you start getting a reaction of some kind, you'll know that it's from the med. You have to be your own pharmacist. Know what to do when you start feeling side effects." This exchange is similar to the one about pain quoted above. The therapist again picks up the theme that being a good patient—or a competent disabled person—involves taking responsibility for one's condition, coming to know your body and what it is telling you, knowing how to treat yourself. But this time she asks the patient to attend to his body as the medical professional might, learning to read his body so that he can recognize the effects of medication. In both instances, but especially the latter, the therapist wants the patient to use his bodily experience as a source of information that will help him to care for himself somewhat like a medical professional might. Competence here means learning to "be your own pharmacist." Here phenomenological and biomechanical frames blur in an effort to "treat the whole person."

Therapists also spend a great deal of time talking to patients. While occupational therapy is very much an action-based intervention, where doing takes priority over talking, therapists work to combine both, and often use the "doing" to raise sensitive issues and to ask patients to communicate their own personal experience of disability and how they are making sense of it. The following section considers the efforts of therapists to communicate with their patients and to let patients know they are willing to listen to their perspective.

Communicating with Patients

The phenomenological frame enters practice in quite another way as the therapist and patient roles become less clearly defined when therapists ask patients to become partners in ordinary conversation. Therapists rarely relinquish control of interchanges. There are many markers that the setting is professional. "We are not equals here" is one indelible message of the hospital setting. And yet there are moments, often initiated by the therapist, when the patient is asked to participate in an activity or coversation as a "whole person," as someone who brings a whole self to the interchange.

Therapists make an extraordinary effort to talk with patients, to find some way of making contact, no matter what their physiological status. The following two examples are situations in which therapists work to engage or include in conversation patients who cannot speak. In the first, the patient is comatose. In the second, much more elaborate and complex conversation, the patient is very alert but is unable to speak aloud because of a tracheotomy and can only mouth words.

The first of these examples is an initial meeting between a therapist and a patient. What is telling about this example is not what gets said, which is very little and strictly medical, but the therapist's sustained efforts to make contact with a comatose patient. This session involves an evaluation of the head-injured patient, a 29-year-old woman who was in a car accident the week before. The therapist begins by approaching the patient and saying, "Hi, I'd like to look at your eyes." After lifting her lids, and touching her chin and the bandages on her head, the therapist tells the patient, "I'm going to look at your arm." She then tells her, "I'm going to move your arm a little bit." After ranging the patient a few minutes she says, "Ginger, see if you can lift up your arm for me." There has been no discernable response by the patient to any of this, but the therapist continues to speak to the patient. The following day the therapist again sees the patient, this time in the company of a physical therapist. She begins her second day's work by saying, "Hi Ginger, it's Susan. We're going to work with you and move you body." She continues to speak directly to the patient as she works with her, though speaking of her in the third person when she discusses her with the physical therapist. After this session , the occupational therapist was interviewed by the researcher and asked about why she talked to the patient.

Interviewer: I noticed that you did a lot of talking with the patient and the physical therapist did almost none. Could you explain that for me?

Therapist: In general the OTs do more talking and interacting with the patient. I am dealing with the cognitive-sensory aspects of the person. OTs do a lot more problem solving with patients. For OTs, technique is secondary. . . . She [patient] responds to tactile stimuli, that is why I touched her when I talked to her."

The therapist "overreads" what the patient can offer as a partner in conversation. She acts on the assumption that the patient may be able to understand her and she continually probes, watching for responses. She does not know, of course, whether this patient can hear her or not, but makes the most positive assumption, on the chance that if the patient can hear, she should be treated as a person and talked to as a person, not as a mere body. The therapist justifies her communicative attempts, in contrast to the physical therapist who speaks directly to the patient only once during the session, by saying that occupational therapists need more mental involvement from their patients. Although the therapist only addresses the patient in what (if the patient were awake) fits narrowly into a biomechanical mode, her persistence in attempting to establish contact with this comatose patient, on however minimal a level, exemplifies the pervasive concern among occupational therapists to bring their patients into the therapeutic process.

The second example is, in one sense, the natural extension of these interests in bringing patients in. Therapists tended to overread the capacities and commitments of their patients as active partners and willing collaborators more often than they tended to underestimate them. This was connected to their constantly emphasizing to patients that, though they were disabled, their personhood was not completely identical with their injury. Although the patient in this second example is also a silent participant, the conversation itself could hardly be more different in tone from the preceding one.

The therapist initiates a three-way conversation involving the patient, herself, and a male nurse. This conversation occurs in the large spinal cord unit when a male nurse happens over to chat with the occupational therapist as she is treating a patient. The patient, who is quadriplegic and has lost both legs, has also had a tracheotomy and cannot be understood except by lip reading. This therapist, like all the therapists I observed, was adept at lip reading, and she functions here as an informal interpreter, ensuring that the two men, patient and nurse, are in a conversation together. The therapist initiates the conversation by introducing the two men and then asking the nurse if he had heard what the patient, whom we will call John, had said to a famous football player, a Boston Patriot, who had come in to visit another patient the day before.

Occupational therapist (to male nurse):	Long day, huh? You love your job.
Nurse:	I like it.
Occupational therapist:	Good. Do you know John?
Nurse:	We have met on occasion.
Occupational therapist (asks John):	Do you know that guy?
Nurse (to both):	The good-looking one.
Occupational therapist:	Yes, dream on. That's what John keeps saying about himself. Do you know what John said to Andre Tippett yesterday?

(John mouths something to the OT that causes her to laugh but which the PT and the researcher cannot understand.)

Nurse:	What is that? (OT laughs)
Nurse:	What did he say?
Occupational therapist:	He didn't say that. He was seeing Mike (another patient) and Andre came in and we were talking for a while. And then I said to him, "Did you meet my friend John?" He says, "Who's John?" So John went to say something to him and he couldn't hear him, so he comes down like this to John's ear to listen. And I said, "You won't get it that way. You can't hear him. You have to read his lips." So the first thing John says to him is, "What happened in Denver?" [The Patriots had just lost the Superbowl in Colorado.] So Andre looks sort of baffled and then John says, "I was very disappointed."
Nurse:	Is that what he meant?
Occupational therapist:	Yes. Right to him. And you should have seen his face. He was like . . .
Nurse:	He knew.

Occupational therapist:	John is like hysterical. So Andre realized John was joking and he started laughing too. We were all laughing.
Nurse:	You know, I know him.
Occupational therapist:	Do you really?
Nurse:	Yes, we both went to the University of Iowa.
Patient:	Is my time up?
Occupational therapist:	No.
Nurse:	We both went to the University of Iowa and he was a senior and I was a freshman and I was on the swim team and he was on the football team and all the athletes in the college were in the same dormitory.
Occupational therapist:	Yes.
Nurse:	So I had friends on the football team, wrestling . . . and one night we went downtown and there aren't that many bars. There was only one or two, so I was where everyone goes dancing to meet people of the opposite sex. And I went down with some of my friends and I saw him and we started hanging out in this bar. And he would go dancing and he was getting every girl he wanted. Probably because he is Andre Tippett, so I didn't have any such luck. I was trying my damnedest.
Occupational therapist:	Ahhh, we feel bad for him, don't we John?
Nurse:	So finally I went up to him, and back then I couldn't handle myself well enough. I put my arm around him and went, "Andre, how did you get all these girls, you have got to tell me." He is like, "What are you doing?" "Well, I just go ask them to dance, and as soon as we start dancing, bam, they are gone. They hate me." And he said to me, he said, "You dance too much like a white man. I'll teach you how to dance." So he brought me out on to the dance floor

and was like, "No matter how fast the dance, be slow, be cool, because girls like that. They see all you white guys jumping around, hopping, raising your hands. Don't do that. Just be cool. It's always like this, no matter how fast you dance."

Occupational therapist: John agrees.

Nurse: It's true.

Occupational therapist: Say this again? (Patient says something which is not audible.)

Occupational therapist: And you, 'cause you dance like that . . .

Nurse: That's true . . .

Occupational therapist: . . . you got all the girls.

Nurse: Next time you go to a bar, watch them dance. No matter whether it is a fast song or a slow song. Same speed, same moves. The white guys were just jumping all around and doing that. I mean, no girls want that. And so, he taught me. Well, anyways, we went out on the dance floor, and he was like, "Show me what you did on this song." And, like, all the football team was looking on. I felt real stupid. And so he is like, "No, no, no, no, no. Like this. Do this and imitate me." He would grab my hands and say, "Put your hands here." So I was dancing with him.

This joking story exchange begins when the therapist introduces the two men, an ironic introduction which already sets the stage for the stories that follow. The nurse reminds the patient that he is "the good-looking one," to which the occupational therapist replies "Yes, dream on. That's what John keeps saying about himself." Her retort defines the two men as being alike and includes the patient in her response. Since John is a quadriplegic who has lost both legs, this is an ironic response; but the irony is ambiguous, for she often compliments John on his "beautiful blue eyes" and by his own account he was always quite vain about his appearance. She follows this up with a story about John. She tells John's story, and in so doing, she conveys something about John. The entire story could be seen as an extended introduction of the two men, mediated by the occupational therapist as she conveys to the nurse, and perhaps more importantly to the patient, a view of John's identity. The story she tells is about John's boldness and wit, about a quadriplegic patient using humor to off-balance a famous football player. The nurse counters with a story about his own encounter with the famous football player. In this story, the storyteller is the one who fumbles, a simple inversion of the first theme. There is also, in both stories, a theme about the off-balancing of culturally typical power hierarchies: a paralyzed man shows up a whole man; a black man shows up a white man. This theme of the fluidity and unpredictability of power is reinforced by the final exchange between occupational therapist and nurse as the nurse leaves. The nurse's name is called over the intercom. He parts with a final joking remark.

> *Nurse:* They probably want me to tell them my Andre Tippett story. So that's how I learned how to dance. He's a football star and I'm . . .
>
> *OT:* . . . making beds.
>
> *Nurse:* Cruel, but true.

This exchange on the ironies and unpredictabilities of power is also an episode of bonding, in which teasing and tricking are cast in a friendly way. Both are friendship stories with happy endings about the possibility that very different sorts of people can find ways to make real contact with one another. In the first story, everyone laughs together at the end. In the second story, an inexperienced white man learns how to attract girls.

The storytelling that the occupational therapist initiates conveys multiple messages about the meaning of this patient's disabilities. One clear message is that while such an experience may be devastating, the patient has not lost all of his force as a social actor. In an encounter with a powerful man, he still has resources to equalize the relationship. He may be disabled but he is not powerless. The public identity that the first story gives to the patient is that he is a strong man, someone who still has some ordinary perspective on the outside world (he can be disappointed that his Boston team lost the Superbowl) and who still has intelligence and social skills that he knows how to use to advantage. Another strong message is that it is still possible for this patient to connect to the world and to other men. This message is given both by the content of the first story, which is about bonding through kidding between a disabled man and an enormously physically able man, and by the placement of that story as part of an introduction between the nurse and the patient, itself an encounter between the able and the disabled. While the occupational therapist's help as a translator and commentator are essential in informing the nurse about John, she also participates in generating an impression that John's powers of kidding exceed in some ways what the nurse may yet be allowed to know, for the joking that precedes the storytelling is initiated in part by a remark that John makes to her and that causes her to laugh, but which she treats as a private joke, refusing to communicate it to the nurse.

Perhaps the most essential and subtle phenomenological task that therapists undertake is the work of helping clients find their way back to the "real world," that is, the world outside the hospital or therapy room. Even therapists who treat outpatients, or go to people's homes, or see children in school, are involved in helping clients make a kind of "return": that is, therapists are deeply invested in helping patients find ways to create meaningful social homes, to find places in the everyday world as far as possible. There is an incredibly strong anti-segregationalist streak in occupational therapy. Disability, therapists would say, is no excuse for isolation or for a useless life. The remnants of the moral treatment movement can be felt in these strong sentiments. The next section of this chapter looks at how therapists address the problem of helping their patients "return," especially when that means that patients can never simply go back to a life they once lived, to social roles they once occupied, or do what the "able-bodied" do in the social world.

Returning Patients to the "Real World"

Occupational therapists are transporters; they help patients make transitions from hospital to home, from sick role to active social member. They contextualize the skills that they teach in terms of patient lives back home, lives which go beyond the "sick role" of the hospital patient. They work at the interstices of the patient's life, treating patients in settings apart from everyday life—like the hospital or an unlikely corner of the grade school—but orienting patients to the everyday life to which they will return. Therapists work to embed the activities they ask patients to carry out within their own life stories. They often ask patients to discover connections between therapeutic activities in the hospital and their personal lives at home. In all of these ways, the therapeutic activities take on a meaning that goes far beyond technical assistance at skill building. Therapy sessions become microcosms of life, which therapists hope patients will build on and expand in their return to the larger life outside the hospital. It is thus that occupational therapists aid their patients in the journey back from the hospital world and the sick role, to the everyday world, and to the more complex and responsible roles of being father, sister, friend, worker, and the like.

A CASE OF RHEUMATOID ARTHRITIS

A quite powerful example of this concern to facilitate return is given in the following story, written by an experienced therapist, about a single session with a patient readmitted to the hospital for a chronic case of rheumatoid arthritis.

Another Surgery

by Mary Evensen

This session is with a woman in her mid-fifties who has been in the rehab hospital approximately a week and a half. Her primary OT approached me the day before I treated the patient and told me that the patient has had rheumatoid arthritis [RA] for a long time and that she has been getting a lot of help at home. Also, the patient is a "VIP" [her husband is on the hospital's board of directors] and she is "very hard to work with" because she doesn't want to do anything for herself. The OT shared with me that she didn't know what to do with the patient besides transfers, and that she probably needs hand splints, so my input would be appreciated.

My initial impression from this discussion was that this seems to be a novice approach to treating persons with chronic RA . . . not knowing and/or understanding the disease, the therapist concludes that it is the patient's fault for not actively participating. Having heard other therapists express this frustration (due to lack of experience), I decided that I would not bias my judgment of the patient based on this description. (I have specialized in arthritis treatment for the past 7 years.)

To initiate the treatment session, I glanced at the primary OT's written treatment plan and then approached the patient to introduce myself. She was sitting in a wheelchair, wearing a cervical collar, accompanied by her private duty nurse.

Therapist:	How is your morning so far?
Patient:	Okay.
Therapist:	Did you sleep well last night?
Patient:	Yes, I guess so; but, I feel so tired.
Therapist:	Did you have a good breakfast?
Nurse:	(Answering for patient) She ate it all.
Therapist:	How about PT? Tell me what you worked on this morning.
Patient:	We just did some walking. . . . We didn't go too far, but I'm exhausted . . . really tired! I don't know why!
Therapist:	What would you like to work on in OT this morning? (pause) What do you think the most important thing is for you? Maybe something that is giving you the most trouble?
Patient:	I can't think of anything special.

I explained that her primary OT felt it was important for us to work on transfers and I asked the patient if she agreed that transfers were important.

> **Patient:** Yes, but I just came from PT where we were working on walking and getting up and down from the wheelchair (with a sigh), I *really* feel exhausted. All I really want to do is lie down and get some rest.

From this, I agreed that the patient seemed tired and that we could work on wheelchair to bed transfers to allow her to rest, and then work on some other things while she was resting.

> **Patient:** (seeming surprised) You really think so! Is that okay!?
>
> **Therapist:** Sure it's okay. Sometimes with arthritis you need to rest so that you don't overdo it.

In agreement, we left the OT clinic in order for the patient to return to her room. As we waited for the elevator I explained that I could teach her some ways to help not getting so tired . . . what we call "energy conservation." This is especially important for RA since it's "in your system" [systemic], not just where the joint is affected.

Upon arriving at the patient's room, I assisted the patient, locking her wheelchair brakes, and asked her what kind of help she needed or wanted.

> **Patient:** I want to try to do it for myself . . . as much as I can anyway!
>
> **Therapist:** That's good. I want you to do it for yourself. . . . I'll just be here for safety and if you need me to help.

This interchange made me reflect on the comments of the primary OT (". . . she's very hard to work with . . .") and I wondered—that description doesn't seem like this woman!

Once comfortably positioned in bed, I asked the patient questions about getting ready for discharge in an effort to focus and prioritize our treatment. At this point, she explained that discharge was uncertain since she needed to have surgery for her neck—a halo—but, it hasn't been done because her lab tests [blood] were not right . . . some anemia. Then, she asked,

> **Patient:** What do you know about this type of surgery? Is a halo really necessary?
>
> **Therapist:** If the spine in the neck is unstable, it can put pressure on the spinal cord and cause further weakness and potentially paralysis in both your arms and legs.

Patient:	That's what the doctor told me too. But, I asked him if I really needed the halo . . . and he said "yes." He even gave me the names and phone numbers of some other people who have had this type of surgery. I talked with one of them and the most aggravating thing he said was that the nurses didn't always take care of his skin . . . especially the scalp where the screws are; and, the most painful thing was when they tighten the screws without any anesthetic! . . . So, I was wondering what I should do with my hair . . . if I should have it cut, or how to style it. I like it long. (The patient's hair is just past shoulder-length.) I've always had it that way. How will I be able to wash it?
Therapist:	That's something we can help you with in OT. We can adapt it by using a reclining wheelchair and a specially shaped basin.
Patient:	Like the beauty salon?
Therapist:	Sort of like that. With one of our other patients, we even taught her family how to do it so that they helped her almost every day.
Patient:	This is very important to me. You may think it's silly.
Therapist:	No, not at all.
Patient:	It's just that I'm very vain. I've always been that way. I like to look "just so." I've been used to putting my makeup on everyday, even when I was home alone.
Therapist:	Have you been wearing any makeup in the hospital?
Patient:	No, not yet.
Therapist:	Do you have any here with you?
Patient:	Some.
Therapist:	Do you want to put a little on now . . . before lunch?
Patient:	No, not now
Therapist:	(reencouraging the patient) This is the rehab part of the hospital where we help people get ready to go home. That's why we wear regular clothes here. So, it would be good idea to start wearing some makeup, like at home.

From this, the patient confessed that she *hadn't* been wearing makeup at home prior to her admission . . . really, she hadn't been able to do anything besides lying in bed! She started describing how terrible it felt to have her family [children and grandchildren] come and visit her—lying in bed.

Patient:	How awful they must feel to see me just lying there! Then I wonder, why me? Why do I have to go through all of this? Why me?

Obviously, the patient was very distressed and not coping well with this illness experience—seemingly the most severe she had experienced. Thinking that she must have had some episodes of successful coping with RA over the years, I asked . . .

Therapist:	How long have you had arthritis?
Patient:	About 15 years.
Therapist:	That's a long time. We know that RA is unpredictable and it has its "ups and downs." How have you dealt with that in the past?
Patient:	You know, it never really seemed bad until I started having my surgeries. The rest of the time I just forgot about it and went on living my life. But, the first surgery was on my wrist . . . about 10 years ago. Look at my hands now! My fingers are getting more and more crooked.
Therapist:	Do you exercise your hands?
Patient:	Some . . . I do this (demonstrating flexlexten) and this one (thumb opposition).
Therapist:	Good, keep that up!
Patient:	Then, after my wrist, it was my ankle . . . then my hip . . . then another ankle surgery. Through all of them, I held myself together. I wore makeup and all of that. I went out to dinner . . . like I did before . . . after I recovered. But now, this one . . . another surgery . . . I don't know how I'll get through it!
Therapist:	That's why your therapy is so important now . . . to help build up your strength and tolerance and your ability to help yourself *before* the surgery so that your recovery will go smoother.
Patient:	Well, I suppose we should try some work now.
Therapist:	How are you feeling?
Patient:	I feel exhausted.
Therapist:	It's okay to rest. Rest is an important part of the treatment for RA.

I went on to describe the principles of energy conservation—planning, prioritizing, pacing, and positioning—and, I encouraged the patient to identify a personal example in order to apply these principles. This lead us to a discussion of how her life-style has changed . . . has been compromised, because of illness.

Patient:	I used to entertain a lot and go out to dinner with my husband and his friends . . . at least once a week. I can't do that now!
Therapist:	Why not?
Patient:	I can't go out in a wheelchair!

Therapist:	Why not?
Patient:	I'm too vain.
Therapist:	How about a walker?
Patient:	I did that once . . . but, I won't do it again. I feel like everyone gawked and stared at me. I'm too vain.
Therapist:	You know, things are changing. More and more physically challenged individuals are getting out there and doing what they want to do. They're not letting their disabilities stop them . . . eating out in restaurants . . . going to shopping malls, museums, the theater, ball games . . .
Patient:	Really?!
Therapist:	Yes. And other people seem to be getting used to seeing them, too. I don't think they stare so much. . . . I know when I see them, I'm happy for them! I know they're doing what they *want* to be doing . . . what's important to them! What do you think the most important thing is to you?
Patient:	Being with my family—my children and grandchildren. Look what they've brought me (room decorated with flowers, cards, drawings by grandchildren, teddy bears, potpourri). There's their picture (on the bedside table). Look at my beautiful grandchildren. I want to be able to be with them . . . to hold them. Some of them came to visit me here in the hospital, and one of them in particular seemed to be afraid—seeing me in the wheelchair. So now when I know they are coming—I'm in bed.
Therapist:	How do you *like* to be when you're around them?
Patient:	Sitting on the couch . . . like in the picture.
Therapist:	Have you tried that since being in the hospital?
Patient:	No, I mostly sit in the wheelchair.
Therapist:	Well, that's something that we can help you with in therapy . . . the transfers like you've been practicing. Also, improving the strength in your arms . . . to hold the children. How does that sound?
Patient:	Good.
Therapist:	So, we talked about a lot of things.
Patient:	Yeah, but we didn't get very much work done.
Therapist:	What do you mean?
Patient:	Well, I rested most of the time.
Therapist:	Was that important?
Patient:	Well, I was tired.
Therapist:	So, is it important to rest when you are tired?

Patient:	I guess.
Therapist:	Remember what we talked about . . . balancing work and rest to save your energy and not to get overtired.
Patient:	But I *do* want to get better.
Therapist:	So you have some priorities to work on this afternoon . . . building up your sitting tolerance and arm strength, along with your transfers, so that you can hold your grandkids.
Patient:	My family is the most important thing to me.
Therapist:	Ready for lunch?
Patient:	Yes, I think so. Thank you so much for letting me rest. I really appreciate it!

Concerned about the extent of the patient's psychological distress, I phoned the psychologist and described the discussion with the patient. The psychologist told me that the patient has major depression and has been referred to a psychiatrist for consult and treatment. She thanked me for sharing this information and stated she would use the goal of being around and holding her grandchildren as a key point of treatment this afternoon . . . to help motivate and activate the patient, since she has been minimally participating in therapy. I also shared this information with the primary OT and asked her to followup with the psychologist.

Case Discussion

This case illustrates many of the themes that have already been raised in this chapter. It also reveals the intense shame many disabled people feel about their own bodies, and about how others will perceive them. In the role of transporters, therapists deal with the problem of stigma, or what the sociologist Erving Goffman (1963) has called "spoiled identity." The disabled suffer not only a dramatic shattering of life stories through accident or disease, not only the imperative to revise their lives to suit those bodies, they also confront a society that views them as a less than normal member, even though they have left the "sick role" of the hospitalized patient. When therapists treat the "whole person" they treat a different person than the outside social world is willing to acknowledge. Goffman notes that the stigmatized person is one who has lost his wholeness in society's eyes. "He is reduced in our minds from a whole and usual person to a tainted, discounted one" (Goffman, 1963). Enabling persons to "live on the outside" and take up active lives in society also means helping them to confront the enormous fears that accompany tackling the social world with a "spoiled identity." Competencies at specific activities of daily living become symbols of how to take on that frightening, dismissive social world. Through these regained competencies, patients can in some ways regain their status as "regular" members of society. Therapists help to transport patients back to that status through everyday activities.

The patients whom occupational therapists treat have had their lives seriously interrupted by a disabling disease or trauma. They must imagine new lives for themselves, "begin a new life story," one might say. The attempt to recover as far as possible their former lives requires a radical reimaging of how to go about the simplest daily tasks. While the therapists in this study generally concentrated on teaching patients such simple skills (simple, that is, from the perspective of the nondisabled), skill building in itself was rarely the ultimate goal. They tried to organize therapeutic activities not simply to build skills or strength, but to provide experiences through which patients might see how they could effect a transition from the hospital and the sick role back to a life of comparative independence. This made it important to listen to patients' stories about their previous "well lives" and to the concerns they had about attempting to reenter those lives.

Blurred Frames: Integrating Treatment of the "Two Bodies"

In theory, the biomechanical and the phenomenological frames oppose one another. And it is easy to choose examples from the practice of occupational therapists in which they function so fully within one frame or the other that this opposition is clear. Therapists themselves feel the tension between these two, as when they discuss the dilemma of needing to both "treat that hand" and "treat the whole person" and the two tasks seem to require different approaches to the patient, or to work against each other.

But often therapists work and talk with their patients in a way that shades one framework into the other. Therapists and patients tack back and forth between these two perspectives, relying now on one, now on the other. Asking a client how a hand feels when ranging it may yield, quite naturally, a broader discussion about how the patient feels about therapy or about difficulties he is facing at home. Sometimes when that occurs the therapist may cut off the patient's exploration of these associations. In most such instances the therapist seems concerned to stay within a biomechanical frame. But often the therapist will allow or even encourage patients to respond to a narrowly posed question with a more wide-ranging discussion of their feelings and experiences.

Sometimes a single therapeutic activity can have meaning within both frames. For example, a therapist may range a patient's hand while listening to her talk about feeling depressed, the physical touch helping to create a context in which the patient can reveal himself.

Some therapeutic activities dwell in the margins of both frames. One example of this comes from a therapeutic interchange described earlier in this chapter, in which a therapist talked to a patient about what to pay attention to in his body and how to manage his care relative to the side effects of medications. Therapists refer to this sort of interchange as "patient education" and identify it as one of their primary therapeutic tasks. Patient education often entails directing attention to the patient's physiological body. When this attention serves the therapists' need to gain better information about patients' physiological status, the interchange is conducted within the biomechanical frame. But attending to the body as a locus of symptoms can also provide the basis for a bit of education designed to help the patient become more adept at interpreting the biomedical meaning of what she feels. In these instances, therapists teach patients some elements of biomedical language to be used in interpreting their own condition, somewhat as a medical professional might. This enables the patient to regain a sense of independence and control over a body which is not only subjective, but has the practical consequence that the patient can tell others what is needed in terms of professional medical help as the condition changes.

Whether an activity or conversation fits within the biomedical or the phenomenological frame is not determinable by any narrow criteria. It very much depends on the context of activity, especially on how the patient responds to the therapist's intervention. This may mean that patients come to learn a subtle interplay of these two discourses, just as therapists do. Consequently, there may be no simple demarcation between the patient's experiential language for the disability as an injury to one's life, and the use of elements of the biomedical interpretation of such symptoms and signs related to the nature of the disease or trauma. In these ways, the patients' mastery of some areas of biomedical thinking can have direct implications for the ways in which they construct the meaning and experience of disability in their lives.

Summary

The phenomenological aspects of occupational therapy practice are essential, and often require subtle and fluid reasoning by therapists, who must ascertain at what level they should ask the patient to consider the *meaning* of the disability as an illness experience. A purely biomedical conception of clinical reasoning that treats the major task of the health professional as the identification of disease (or related dysfunctions) and the planning of disease-specific treatments leaves out too much of importance in the way occupational therapists must think in their work. Their concern to help patients transcend limits is implemented, not only in what Robert Murphy calls the long process of restructuring bodies, but also in their use of therapeutic tasks and conversations to advance a necessary restructuring of the self. Whether tacitly or explicitly, occupational therapists in this study recognized, though perhaps fleetingly, how closely one's sense of body is connected to one's sense of self. They constantly structured experiences in ways calculated to allow particular patients to transcend the physical limits that they thought would now govern their lives. This growth often occurred only through an accumulation of almost imperceptible gains achieved at the price of agonizing effort. The intended effect, however, was not only a compensation for earlier losses in physical ability; it was meant to begin a reconstruction of the self that recognizes and values those possibilities and qualities of life that remained open.

■

A Commonsense Practice in an Uncommon World

■ MAUREEN HAYES FLEMING

Introduction

The work of occupational therapists is focused on the work of other people. The therapist's role is to enable others, who are ill, injured, handicapped, or compromised in some way, to regain the ability to participate in society through occupation. The specific aim of OT practice is to develop or *recreate* a person's ability to *engage* in *occupations* in *everyday life*. The way occupational therapists use the term "occupation" is somewhat different from its usual usage. Definitions of occupation abound in the OT literature. The concept of occupation is not limited to formal employment but is broadened to any work, or as the therapists say, "purposeful activity." An "occupation" may be either a formal job or role, or a day-to-day activity that occupies one, such as gardening. A concept that is included in most definitions, though sometimes implicitly, is that occupation involves both action and meaning. In this chapter we discuss a concept of occupation that underscores the dynamic relationship of action and meaning, as observed in the AOTA/AOTF Clinical Reasoning study and in other studies of, and conversations with, occupational therapists in the United States, Canada, and several European countries. We propose that action taking and meaning-making are the two central processes that comprise occupation as these therapists have constructed that concept.

A Therapeutic Practice Rather than a Medical Profession

Because they often work with individuals who have illness or disabilities, and frequently work in hospitals, occupational therapists are often referred to, as part of the "medical team." However, while occupational therapy is important to rehabilitation, it is not a medical profession.

> Occupational therapy is described as a health discipline rather than a medical discipline. This is because occupational therapy's focus on the effects of disease or injury on everyday living is a uniquely non-medical focus. (Christiansen, 1991, p. 4)

Occupational therapists do not generally treat the disease or the disability per se. Occupational therapists treat the *person* for whom the *consequences* of the disease or injury have been disruptions in the individual's ability to participate in everyday activities. Physicians are concerned with the cause of the disease. Occupational therapists are concerned with the consequences. Some therapists seem to focus primarily on the physical effects, whereas others concern themselves with the emotional and social consequences as well. Occupational therapists like to say that they focus on the person's abilities, not disabilities.

Though occupational therapists often work in hospitals, their role is to prepare people to function when they return to the "real" world of home and community. In a sense the therapists do not so much treat problems as prepare people to address problems once they have returned to the normal world. We found the concept of therapy, which implies that patients work on their own problems under the expert guidance of the professional (therapist), to be very appropriate in characterizing the practice of occupational therapists. Their work is therapy, rather than treatment, that is, it involves the application of a solution.

Occupational therapy is a different practice from medicine, with a different focus. Victor Kestenbaum, a phenomenologist who is interested in how patients make meaning of illness, points out that medical practices and health practice require different "habits of mind" (1982, p. 3). He differentiates medical practice sharply from health practices. He further advocates that *health* professionals adopt the "phenomenological habit of mind" (p. 8) in order to understand their patients' illness experiences. Such habits of mind organize our way of making sense of a situation and become part of our professional culture. We found that, implicitly, occupational therapists do take a phenomenological approach to their clients, even though they do not use the formal language of that branch of philosophy. We discovered early in the project that giving therapists some of the language of phenomenology to express some of the habits of mind they already possessed, but for which they had few words, helped therapists and ourselves in many ways. It made it easier for us to understand the practice, its values, and some of the core habits and meanings that direct the whole culture of the profession.

COMMON SENSE AND CULTURAL VALUES

It may seem strange to the reader that a book whose title includes the rather erudite sounding phrase "clinical reasoning" would have a chapter on common sense. But common sense, we will see, is a valuable form of interpretation (sense making) which allows the person to take necessary action. Because occupational therapy is focused on the ability of individuals to take action and often requires considerable action by the therapists as well, common sense is especially helpful. But there are two more important points to be made here. One is that, as Clifford Geertz (1983) has pointed out, common sense is a particular type of intelligence which is worthy of study, even though it is difficult to study because of its "invisible" nature. Geertz comments:

> When we say someone shows common sense we mean to suggest more than that he is just using his eyes and ears, but is, as we say, keeping them open, using them judiciously, intelligently, perceptively, reflectively, or trying to, and that he is capable of coping with everyday problems in an everyday way with some effectiveness. (p. 76)

Underscoring his respect for common sense, Geertz says "common sense is both a more problematical and a more profound affair than it seems." (p. 77)

Another important point Geertz makes is that common sense is part of a cultural system. As such, common sense is not an automatic process or a given. Rather it is a kind of knowledge that is based in the *values* of the particular culture and the *operations* (sets of actions) that are plausible within the culture. We all know that some values that are important in one culture may be unimportant or nonexistent in another. Similarly, some actions that are permissible or expected in one culture may be seen as offensive in another. In this book we are not going to say much about culture in the usual sense, but we are going to focus to some extent on the culture and values of occupational therapy. In many ways the cultural values of occupational therapy are its strong points. However, there are many times when therapists find themselves in difficult situations, and in conflict with the cultural values of other professional groups with whom they work. Their values are an important influence on their reasoning processes, on the actions they take, and on the activities they help people to learn. In some problematic situations we encountered, however, it was difficult for the therapists to deal with the professional value conflicts that occurred. This led to some clinical reasoning problems that arose from time to time, some of which will be discussed in this book.

IMPLICIT AND EXPLICIT CULTURAL VALUES IN OCCUPATIONAL THERAPY

There are several excellent resources in the OT literature that address the philosophy of OT and the values of the profession. Here, I will rely on Engelhardt (1977) to help make a few points. One is that OT is focused on *quality of life*. Second, "the point of focus [of OT] is the individual capable of activity" (p. 667). Here, there are really two concepts: the focus is on the *individual*, and the aim is to help the person become capable of *activity*. A third point is that activity is a central force in achieving quality of life.

> OT . . . does not seem to be essentially bound to concepts of disease at all. It is instead focused on the success of individuals in finding fulfillment through human activity. (p. 670)

In our study we found that many OTs were strongly committed to the value of self-fulfillment through engaging in everyday activities. However, some therapists did not seem to have a deep commitment to that value and were much more focused on the biomedical aspects of the practice. A fourth concept or value of OT that Engelhardt notes is the value of *engagement*. Occupational therapists talk about "engagement in activity." This is an expression both of an idea and of a value that they hold. The idea is that engagement is an involvement and a sense of connection with the activity, an investment in the activity; the value is that it is important to be engaged in what one does. This is important because it enables the person to find self-expression or self-fulfillment in activity. Occupational therapists also talk about the importance and value of being engaged in one's life and in one's physical and social contexts. Engelhardt expresses this in a simple and elegant statement: "The value of occupational therapy is engagement in the world" (p. 672).

Some of the cultural values of OT that underlie the commonsense aspects of daily practice may be stated as follows:

- To be able to take action is an important aspect of being human.
- Self-expression and self-fulfillment are basic human rights.
- Engagement in activity leads to self-understanding, self-expression, and self-fulfillment.

- Participation in the physical and social world is another basic human right.
- Engagement in everyday activities is an important way of participating in the world.

CASE EXAMPLE: VALUES IN PRACTICE

The following therapist's story will be used as an example to illustrate many of the aspects of OT, its cultural values, and the commonsense aspects of its practice. Values help this therapist select what problems to address, and common sense helps her implement a program that resolves the problems in an uncomplicated but by no means simplistic way.

Ann

by Maureen Freda

Ann was a 26-year-old woman who had given birth, and had subsequently suffered a stroke. She was admitted to a rehab hospital with right hemiparesis. When I first met Ann, she was very depressed about being separated from her new baby and her main fear was that she would not be able to adequately care for the baby on her own. Adding to this fear was the knowledge that her insurance would not cover any in-home services. Her husband was her only family, he worked at construction every day, and they lived in a trailer park. In order to go home with the baby, she would need to be very independent.

The initial therapy sessions were centered around tone normalization, with an emphasis on mat activities, along with traditional ADL [activities of daily living] training in the mornings. Ann's husband visited daily and usually brought the baby with him. At first this was extremely frustrating to Ann, since she could not hold the baby unless she was sitting down with pillows supporting her right arm. She continued to voice anxiety around the issue of going home and being able to care for the baby. Her husband was also very worried about how this transformation would take place—the transformation from Ann as a patient to Ann as wife and mother. I spent a lot of time talking to both Ann and her husband about the necessity of normalizing the tone and improving the movement of the upper extremity as a sort of foundation to the more complex functional skills Ann was so anxious to relearn.

Eventually it was time to spend the majority of the treatment time on functional skills. The two areas we focused on were homemaking and childcare. The homemaking sessions were fairly routine and traditional in nature. However, it proved to be a bit more difficult to simulate some of the childcare activities.

Our first obstacle was to find something that would be like a baby. We settled on borrowing a "recus-a-baby" from the nursing education department. We used this "baby" for the beginning skills such as feeding and diaper changing. Ann had progressed, but she still had slight weakness and incoordination in the right arm and she was walking with a straight cane. The next step was to tackle walking with the baby. We, of course, practiced with a baby carrier. We also had to prepare for the event of carrying the baby without the carrier. I wrapped weights about the "baby" to equal the weight of the now 3-month-old infant at home. Ann would walk down the hall carrying the "baby," and I would be following behind jostling the "baby" to simulate squirming. (We became the talk of the hospital with our daily walks!!) Ann was becoming more and more comfortable and confident with these activities, so it was time to make arrangements to have the real baby spend his days in the rehab with his mother. This was not as easy as it might seem. The administration of the hospital was not used to such requests. But with the right cajoling in the right places this was eventually approved. The real baby now replaced "recus-a-baby" on our daily walks and in the clinic. While these successes were comforting to Ann and her husband, the fact remained that we were still in a very protective environment. The big question was yet unanswered—would these skills hold up under the stresses of everyday life, alone, in a trailer for 8 hours daily?

Never being one to hold to tradition, I decided to go to administration another time with one more request. I wanted to do a full-day "home visit" with Ann and her baby. This too was approved, and a week before Ann's scheduled discharge, she and I set out for a rigorous day at the home front. Once there, all did not go smoothly; Ann fell once and practically dropped the baby. She was very anxious and stressed, but we managed to get through the day. We talked and solved every little real or perceived difficulty. Both Ann and the baby survived the fall and the "almost" dropping. When we got back to the hospital, Ann, her husband, the social worker, and I sat down and realistically discussed and decided what kind of outside help was a necessity and what Ann could really accomplish in a day. Ann's husband adjusted his schedule, a teenage neighbor was brought in for 2 to 3 hours a day, and Ann was able to do the majority of the care for her baby.

Although this was not a story with a lot of pitfalls, I have been 5 years without my own patients; this was and is the most vivid of my clinical stories.

Case Discussion

In Maureen's story we see the elegant simplicity of the practice retold as a series of negotiations between several "actors": the patient's medical condition; Ann and her family, and even neighbors; the therapist and her professional knowledge; a few other workers in the hospital; and Maureen's skill at enlisting their aid or approval. Orchestrating all these factors is no easy task, but she managed it smoothly. Part of the reason for this is that all of these requests, therapeutic designs, and plans made good sense—good common sense. One central way in which all this made sense was that the whole treatment revolved around returning Ann to her home and family— transporting her back to her usual life-world. Who could deny a request for a "recus-a-baby" or a home visit in the face of this eminently sensible goal?

The Life-World

The concept of the "life-world" has not been part of the mainstream of occupational therapy literature; however, it is a concept that therapists seem to implicitly understand. The concept of life-world is the idea that we exist in a day-to-day world that is filled with numerous important, subtle, and complex meanings. These meanings form a substratum or a backdrop for everyday actions and meaning. Often these meanings are tacit or "taken-for-granted" (Schutz, 1975, p. 32). They are so much a part of ourselves that we do not even interpret objects or ideas as either present or questionable. The life-world is our immediate common world. It is the people, objects, contexts, and meanings that make our lives intelligible. Our life-world, though seemingly ordinary, is alive with meaning. The life-world is comprised of the individual, family, and social groups; the physical and cultural contexts in which they exist; and the habits and meanings developed and sustained through their interrelationships.

Schutz defines life-world as:

> Life-World; also: World of everyday life. The total sphere of experiences of an individual which is circumscribed by the objects, persons, and events encountered in the pursuit of the pragmatic objectives of living. It is a world in which a person is wide awake, and which asserts itself as the paramount reality of his life. (1975, p. 320)

When a person is ill or injured, those habits, meanings, and personal and contextual relationships change. The ways in which the individual participates in the life-world changes. Reentering the life-world after an illness or injury is a physically, psychologically, socially, and existentially difficult endeavor. Assisting persons to accomplish this is the task that occupational therapists as a group have taken on. The degree to which individual therapists participate in this endeavor varies. Some are content to train the physical body to perform "activities of daily living." Others engage the patient at a deeper level, at the phenomenological level. They actively help people struggle with the personal and social meanings that accompany the difficult transition back to the life-world, now that one has a changed body and, usually, a changed self-image and social position.

In Maureen's story of Ann we see how she skillfully worked with Ann at both the physical and the phenomenological levels. The work with the simulated and squirming baby is one example of how Maureen used the physical activity to help work at the phenomenological level as well. The coordination and balance practice was important at the physical level, but even the (commonsense) thought to simulate the baby so carefully with weight and wriggles demonstrates work at the phenomenological level. This conveyed meaning to Ann that her therapist thought of her as a person who could be a good mother. The home visit was clearly a way in which Marueen helped Ann with the important and often frightening return to the world of home and to her life-world. Interestingly, this very sensible home visit required special negotiations with the administrator in order to acquire permission to actually go out into the real world of Ann's home so as to best tailor the final aspects of treatment to Ann's new life.

Engagement and Intentionality

In the story of Ann we see that Maureen, the therapist, tries many ways to restore Ann's ability to participate in her everyday life as a woman and a mother. Together they practice taking care of a baby (action taking), while they are also remaking Ann's sense of her self as a mother (meaning-making). Occupational therapists often use the term "engage," as in the "the person is engaged in an activity." This seems to us to imply that therapists place special importance on the person's *willing participation* in action taking and meaning-making. This interest in participation in the world is similar to a concept that phenomenologists refer to as "intentionality" (Schutz, 1970). The concept of intentionality is complex, but worth some discussing here. Part of Schutz's definition of intentionality is that intentionality is "the most basic characteristic of consciousness" (1970, p. 318). But "consciousness" is not used the same way it is used in medicine, as in, "The patient is unconscious"—or in psychology, as in "The thought was unconscious." Consciousness, to phenomenologists, means not simply a biological or psychological mechanism, but encompasses a person's orientation to the world that includes an interest in being in, and aware of, one's world. It includes a sense of awareness, and the possibility of apprehending and participating in aspects of one's world. It is a sense of connectedness to the world, and at the same time to one's self and one's being, that has a certain amount of intensity to it. Schutz goes on to comment that "it is always the consciousness of something; it is directed toward something" (p. 318). This directedness is also a quality that OTs want to see and that they try to encourage in their patients. It makes sense that, if a person is going to regain the ability to function in the physical and social worlds, then he or she needs to be oriented toward it. One's intentional state needs to be oriented to that aim. (Other philosophers such as Merleau-Ponty [1963] define intentionality slightly differently. Schutz's formulation seems to us to be more similar to the OT concept of engagement, so we are using that here.)

The concept of intentionality, consciousness directed toward something seems very like the OT concept of engaging in activity. Occupational therapists have long claimed that "purposeful activity" is more therapeutic than are processes, such as repetitive exercise, that are not directed toward an immediate external objective or, as they say, "a goal." Therapists formerly used examples such as: Weaving a rug is better exercise than simply making the same arm motions against resistive weights, because the person can focus on a purpose, making the rug. Today OTs tend to use more immediate daily tasks such as simple meal preparation, using a telephone, or planning a trip to the store as their therapeutic activities, but the concept of meaningful activity remains.

At least part of the OT idea of meaningful activity must be linked to OTs' recognition that patients "perk up" and participate in activities that are interesting to them. This interest or interaction between the person and the activity, this engagement in activity, is therapeutic. The reason it is therapeutic may be that it has sparked patients' intentionality. Intentionality is a sense that is very much diminished when a person is ill or injured. We are making the claim here that, together, *intentional* action taking and meaning-making are the elements that make the practice therapeutic. When these elements are present, there is therapy, not simply treatment. Intentionality, this engagement with objects and activities of interest, is necessary if the person is to marshal the forces to participate in the difficult process of "rehabilitation," and the even more challenging task of existing in the community, in the everyday world, doing everyday activities, while disabled.

In the story of Ann, Maureen first points out that initially Ann was too depressed to participate in activities that highlighted her separation from her baby. This loss of intentionality, Merleau-Ponty (1963) points out, is common in illness. It is certainly understandable that intentionality would be temporarily lost in situations, such as Ann's, where one has been severely injured or disabled. When Ann's ability to participate in the world has been compromised, it is understandable that her willingness to participate would be diminished or even destroyed. Maureen used less meaningful activities, such as "normalizing tone," until Ann was ready for more meaningful activities, such as taking care of her baby.

Therapy as Reconstruction

Occupational therapy originated with the training of women to assist soldiers who were physically or emotionally injured in World War I so that they could learn skills that would enable them to engage in productive work in the postwar society. These women were called reconstruction aides. They were from upper- and upper middle-class families and had a college education. They were usually 25 to 30 years old and married. Their purpose was the "reconstruction" of the working lives of persons who were forever changed as a result of the physical, psychological, and social insults of war. (See Hopkins & Smith, 1990 and Christensen & Baum, 1991 for overviews of the origins of occupational therapy.) Although the term "reconstruction" is seldom used today, the therapist's concern to help a person reconstruct a life that has been interrupted by illness or injury is still a central theme in OT practice.

Reconstruction aides organized as a profession. The purpose of the profession was to study the effects of occupation in restoring people to a socially meaningful life. Early authors stressed the importance of considering both mental and physical health. They trained individuals with disabilities to do activities, skills, routines, and tasks that were viewed as precursors to work. Examples are self-care, and the broadly defined "activities of daily living" (ADL); or the work-related skills important at the time, such as weaving, woodworking, typing, leather work, and sewing. Later, therapists took on the task of training individuals with emotional or cognitive impairments to participate in some social role activities. Eventually, occupational therapists moved out of hospital environments and worked in the public schools, public health programs, nursing homes, retirement communities, and industrial settings. The concept of occupational roles, tasks, and skills was broadened and refined. Categories of activities such as preschool, perceptual-motor, cognitive, social, and life skills for infants, children, adolescents, adults, and the elderly were developed. Today, occupational therapists work with anyone who encounters difficulty in participating in activities of daily living or social role activities. Therapists view their role as helping a person learn or relearn the essential functional activities of everyday life. Which particular activities of everyday life are important is determined by individual therapists in collaboration with their patients. The person's interests, abilities, goals, family, and social contexts are considered. Therapists want to address a person's particular life goals, tasks, and interests. This method of constructing an understanding of what the problem is and what services are needed based on the interests of the particular person is quite different from the typical view that professionals know what "should be done" to treat the clinical condition. It makes good sense that if the OT is interested in treating the person, it is a good idea to inquire about the person's wishes.

In the story, both Ann and the therapist worked very hard to reconstruct Ann's ability to work as a mother. Ann constructed a statement of the problem and both therapist and patient reconstructed her skills. Maureen carefully orchestrated that reconstruction, both through the actions she and Ann took and the depth of engagement they had with each other. The tasks Maureen chose, and which aspects of the tasks she selected to have Ann engage in, were based on interpreting

Ann's level of intentionality or ability to participate in the life-world at any given time. Tapping into her intentional state and orchestrating purposeful actions, Maureen helped Ann to recreate her skills to participate in the world, but more importantly to reconstruct a sense of self.

CONSTRUCTION OF THE THERAPEUTIC PROBLEM

The idea that OTs help clients reconstruct their lives following an illness or injury is a powerful one, but one that seems to be inconsistently represented in the literature. Patients' lives are certainly influenced, redirected, even misdirected by illness and injury. Occupational therapists help to restore people to a level of function that enables them to engage in everyday activities.

The concept of construction seems to be used implicitly in OT in several ways. One is that the patient and the therapist work together to "construct" the problem. That is, that they collaborate to define what the patient thinks the problem is, and what aspects of the problem the patient wants to work on. A typical example is Dan. Dan is a computer scientist who was in an accident and became a paraplegic. One of the problems that he and the OT could have worked on was dressing and showering. However, these tasks were quite difficult and exhausting for Dan. He decided he would hire a personal care attendant to help him with those activities and save his energy for work. In OT, he decided to work on "transfers" such as transferring himself from bed to wheelchair, and wheelchair to car, and learning to drive a car with hand controls. The therapist and the patient "constructed" Dan's problem as need for energy conservation, transportation, socialization, and employment, and they selected the OT activities accordingly.

Another way the concept of construction is used is in the way some philosophers and social scientists use the term "social construction." This means that cultural, social, and personal meanings are "constructed" or built up as a result of human interaction. In this process, subjective meanings are taken as if they are "knowns" or "givens." Berger and Luckman (1967) claim that all social life, including culture and language, have developed or been constructed as a result of social interactions and the meanings made out of them. Many of the therapists and patients we observed seemed to be engaged in a process of social construction. They shared meanings and special words or routines with patients that built small social systems within the microcosm of the clinic and their relationships with the patient. Patients often learned OT jargon, and OTs often learned specialized words from a patient's job or family life. Little rituals such as items being set up in particular ways, or therapists' comments like, "Well did your roommate snore last night?" were common and were often part of the opening moments of a treatment session. One patient "charged" his therapist a thumb wrestling match at the end of every session as his reward for working hard in therapy. Another "charged" a joke at the beginning of the session as a sort of fee that the therapist had to "pay" to enlist his participation in therapy. These shared meanings and routines helped liven up the sessions, but they often had deeper meaning than that. They helped form bonds between therapists and patients who were working very hard together to construct and find ways of dealing with very difficult problems. They were important building blocks in the social process of reconstructing the patient's life.

An even deeper use of the notion of construction is that individuals who sustain permanent injuries are changed forever; their lives have changed and their sense of self has changed. Occupational therapists help people construct a new life by assisting them to relearn how to do everyday tasks that can reconnect the person to the everyday social and physical world. Some therapists are able to help the person construct a new sense of self as well. This is a complicated idea and an even more complicated practice. Aspects of the idea and the practice will be discussed throughout this book.

It seems implicit in Ann's story that Maureen and Ann found much important meaning and formed a bond that sustained them in their work together. Maureen's comment that "this was one of the most vivid memories of a clinical story" expresses that bond. One can almost see the construction process as Maureen recounts every step of the way in the process of helping Ann construct new meanings, and reconstruct a new self and a new life for herself, her husband, and their baby.

The Meaning of Everyday Activities

Occupational therapists feel that everyday activities are significant and meaningful. They have a firm belief that it is important to be able to perform everyday activities and that those activities are essential to one's sense of self-worth. In a very direct manner, OTs view activities of daily living as essential and important—a concept that most able-bodied people either reject or take for granted. Therapists have an implicit belief akin to Berger and Luckman's notion that "the reality of everyday life maintains itself by being embodied in routines" (1967, p. 149). Berger and Luckman comment that among the multiple realities there is one that

> presents itself as the reality par excellence. This is the reality of everyday life. Its privileged position entitles it to the designation of paramount reality. The tension of consciousness is highest in everyday life, that is, the latter imposes itself upon consciousness in the most massive, urgent

and intense manner. It is impossible to ignore, difficult even to weaken its imperative presence. (p. 21)

Everyday routines or tasks maintain the person in a positive relation with both the objective, and subjective social world. Thus, for better or worse, our performance of socially meaningful tasks—everyday activities—shapes our own and other's views of ourselves. Therapists help a person attain, retain, or regain these social meanings and values by relearning everyday activities. They have a strong belief that the ability to perform everyday activities is inherently linked to a sense of personal dignity and sense of self-worth. This is expressed in many ways. An example from a videotape of a "novice" therapist will illustrate this point.

Karen worked with Ella, a very elderly and ill lady. Karen's tone of voice was quiet, firm, and reassuring. She asked Ella, "What did you do today?" Karen carefully listened to the reply and responded with, "That's good." She then proceeded to do some preliminary range-of-motion activities. Then, Karen asked Ella to sit up on the side of the bed and put her slippers on. This took about 4 minutes to accomplish. Karen watched patiently and made some encouraging and reassuring sounds.

One might ask, "Why would a healthy young woman spend all that time insisting that a frail lady put on her own slippers, when Karen could have easily put them on for her?" The answer is that Karen believes it is important for people to be able to do as much for themselves as they can. She believes that patients understand this and do want to do as much as possible for themselves (when they are physically and emotionally ready for it). Therapists think that performing one's own self-care tasks is so linked to one's human dignity that they assume that patients will feel a profound loss if this ability is lost. This is not simply a loss of a skill, but a loss of a more essential part of oneself, the ability to participate in meaningful activities.

Occupational therapists feel that "performing"—by which they mean "doing something"—is an essential part of human function. They feel participation in life and the world through action makes life meaningful. Phenomenologists refer to "being-in-the-world" as an important aspect of human existence. Occupational therapists refer to this active "being-in-the-world" as "functional performance." This is a rather dull, mechanistic sounding term to express a fairly eloquent idea. The idea is that people find meaning in active participation in being-in-the-world, and that meaningful connection of person and life-world is maintained, at least in part, by action. Action taken in the world forms a persons's physical relation to the environment. The meanings made through that active participation are important social meanings which connect the individual to other human beings.

Occupational therapists sense the significance of helping a person maintain these important physical and social ways of being in the world. An example is Suzanne who works with terminally ill cancer patients. She insisted on maintaining their daily activities even though she could see both physical and cognitive deteriorations that contributed to reductions in their "functional performance." Many people would say this is a waste of time and money. Why "rehabilitate" someone who is going to die soon anyway? But Suzanne believed that someone should live with dignity, not die efficiently. She felt that they should participate in the world, even though there were dire predictions about how long that person would live.

Another assumption OTs make is that the ability to participate in the social world and perform, as they say, "personally desirable social roles" is a basic human right, and an important part of people's perception of their place in the social world. This participation will also influence other people's perceptions of an individual. Therefore, the tasks the OTs take on are to help the person regain the ability to perform critical activities, and thus maintain the social role and sense of social place and self-worth that accompany those activities.

Matthew, a lawyer with a central cord injury, is a good example of this relationship between the individual's ability to perform in the life-world and his sense of personal and social self. Matthew, his therapist Patty said, had not yet "adjusted" to his performance limitations. It was a difficult situation, because with the particular sort of injury he sustained there are no standard predictions regarding the degree of "return" the person will experience. No one could tell him whether he would eventually walk or have a useful amount of hand function. He was very upset about his injury. He referred to himself as "a cripple" and insisted that he would overcome his condition. He was determined to return to his law practice. In fact, he did eventually walk with a cane and have fair hand function and returned to the family law firm. Patty worked with him on writing, both handwriting and computer typing (even though these were inappropriate goals for that time in his rehabilitation process), because he saw writing as a very important part of being a lawyer and insisted that she teach him to write. She also worked on tenodesis movements, shoulder strengthening, opposing digits, and use of the mobile arm support. These activities were more usual ones for this stage, based on consideration of the physical aspects of his treatment process. Patty explained most of these strengthening and range-of-motion exercises to Matthew in terms of their relevance to writing, thus linking the strenuous—but seemingly meaningless—exercise program to the more desirable future task of writing.

The assumption that performing everyday activities and a sense of self-esteem are interrelated seems to be universally held by the occupational therapists. It is an assumption that definitely directs practice.

It is also clear from the videotapes, and even more clear from direct observation of, and conversations with, patients that they feel that these two factors are interrelated and essential to rehabilitation, and to the patient's ability to "adjust" to disability.

We have always had trouble with the notion of "adjusting" to something as awful as a permanent physical injury. Therapists, too, said that they did not think people actually "adjusted" in the sense that the disability was acceptable to the person. "Cope" or "adapt" were not quite right as descriptors of what therapists sensed was a resolution of the personal struggle that their patients experienced. The notion of patients constructing a new self with which to reenter the life-world and form a new life seemed to them to be more reflective of their patients' personal experiences of rehabilitation.

The Uncommon World of the Clinic

CLINIC WORLD VERSUS LIFE-WORLD

The modern hospital operates on the basis of a set of implicit and explicit norms and assumptions that are generally referred to as "the medical model." These assumptions include concepts such as: Medicine is a scientific practice; diseases are objective entities that can be scientifically discerned and treated with a particular process; the person is not to blame for having the disease; and clinicians should maintain an objective perspective on the condition and a professional distance from the person who has the disease.

The world of the clinic is not, for most people, part of their life-world. It is another world, even an otherworldly place. The environment is different. The steel, plastic, tile, electrical signals, and lighted dials immediately convey an unnatural sense of mechanical control and nonhuman power. Not only is the physical environment different; the social environment is different. It runs according to strict, but not necessarily discernable, social rules. Conversations are conducted in specialized languages, or not at all. The social meanings of the hospital staff are often conveyed in gestures, postures, and stylized conversations. One enters a hospital and one enters a different world. One's personal and social meanings and understandings are rendered useless. This is not a change of environment and therefore meaning, like that on entering a church, a school, a library, a restaurant, a beach house, a museum—where one is an outsider who can quickly discern the rules and thus quickly learn to function within the constraints of the context. The hospital is an environment where the person is a patient and therefore an outsider. The language is not one's own. A person enters the clinic world and becomes a patient. An injury or disease has entered the hospital, and one's body accompanied it there. The hospital is a society, a culture unto itself. This culture is a world apart from one's ordinary life-world. People usually do not even wear their own clothes while in the critical stages of care and recovery. They do not have familiar objects, furniture, or pictures around them. Everything belongs to the hospital.

The scientific model has been interpreted by and incorporated into the medical culture of the clinic. In the hospital, as in the lab, science and subjectivity are never supposed to interfere with each other. The assumption is that if science is to thrive, then the subjective reality of the patient should not interfere. The social system of the clinic exists to maintain the scientific treatment of the disease, not to understand the personal experience of the individual and the influence of the disease on one's sense of self. There are definite advantages to the medical model, and certainly to scientific medicine. These are not to be denied. However, the person may suffer the social "side effects" of this view, where the disease is the object of attention and the person is its unwitting container.

TEMPORARY OR TRANSITIONAL WORLD

For most people, entering the hospital is a temporary event. One has an appendix removed, gives birth, or has a bone set. The physical discomfort and inconvenience are indeed minor, especially in light of the relief one finds at having been skillfully rescued from accident or disease. The hospital stay is temporary, and one recovers, goes home, and resumes more or less the same life, in the same life-world. People who stay in a hospital only briefly are usually not tremendously affected by the social norms and other impositions of the culture of the clinic.

But for some individuals and families, the relief that the patient has lived through the long hours of surgery is quickly overshadowed by the knowledge that the person will never be completely whole again. A life was saved, but one realizes that some of the body and its abilities were lost. Often, one's life, in the most true sense, was lost, though one's body, or most of it, was saved. In such cases, the clinic becomes not a temporary world but a transitional world. In this transitional world one learns that you cannot simply get better and go home. This is when one is very much affected by the clinic and its culture.

Typically the patient stays in the "regular" part of the hospital, for example, the postsurgical floor or acute care section for a few days and then is moved to the rehabilitation unit ("rehab") of the hospital or another rehabilitation institution. Rehabilitation units or hospitals are the transitional world. They are a world that is not strictly medical, but they are not a part of the regular community or the usual life-world of the person. Here one engages in activities and procedures that will rehabilitate the body and ready it for a return to the "regular" or commonplace world. A person might reside in this transitional world for a short or a long time, depending upon the injury and other factors. This world is not one in which physicians are central to the patient's future. The time for medical intervention is over (or mostly so), and the fate of the person's physical condition is close to sealed. In this world there are no dramatic rescues, no narrow escapes, no miraculous cures. This world is filled with hard-working therapists of many types, who put patients through paces day after day in an attempt to increase the usefulness of their remaining physical capacity and to maintain the health of their bodies and minds. Therapists have commented that this is the time when the family typically brings in photographs of the person, in better times. It is not uncommon for a high school graduation picture of the person to appear in the room, critically placed so that the staff can see the picture that represents the "real person" to the family, not the "patient" that the staff sees. The families want to maintain an image of the person in the usual world. Often it is not clear to the family whether or not the patient will return to the real world as the person he or she once was. One wonders how closely the person in the bed will resemble the image in the photograph. There is always the hope that this, too, is a temporary world. But for many it is not. It is a transitional world. It is a world in which one practices to return to the usual world in an unusual condition.

In rehabilitation one learns new skills, new ways of doing things, and acquires a new view of oneself and one's future life and life-world. Here is where medicine and nursing start leaving off and rehabilitation or entering one's new life really begins. Here the person encounters therapists almost too numerous to mention. To some extent they are all transition therapists, helping the individual to adjust to, or learn skills for returning to, the community. However, because of their special focus on function, the occupational therapists play an important part in the transitional world. Occupational therapists are central to the process of returning to the community. They teach the functional skills the person needs to be able to perform everyday tasks. They also help the person regain, or acquire, social role activities and skills. Further, some therapists help the person to reconstruct their self-image and life goals. At all three levels, occupational therapists help in the process of reconstruction and return to the community. They are a particularly critical element in the process of making a transition from the other-world of the clinic, back to the usual world of the community, and possibly to at least some meaningful parts of the life-world in which the person once participated.

THE OCCUPATIONAL THERAPIST AS TRANSPORTER

Occupational therapists try to help the person regain both function and meaning. The role of the OT and the task of teaching new ways of engaging in everyday activities has an influence upon clinicians' reasoning. The therapist's task is not to save the person's life, as is the physician's task. Rather, the occupational therapist's task is to help the person remake a life that has been changed by illness or injury. To do this, the therapist teaches new ways of doing everyday tasks that the person will need to be able to do once she or he returns to the community. The therapists also help patients remake their sense of self so that they can make the transition from patient in the hospital to citizen in the community. As such, the therapist's role becomes the symbolic role of "transporter." The physical and social barriers and supports in these two types of settings are considered carefully in the therapists' reasoning. The therapists' role is that of symbolic transporter because they help people imagine what their new life outside the clinic will be like. Many are not actually able to go to the community with their patients the way Maureen did with Ann. However, many engage in community-like activities with their patients in the hospital, much as Maureen did when she made the hospital corridors stand in for a sidewalk that Ann might someday traverse with her actual, squirming baby. Therapists help people imagine themselves in the new environments, roles, relationships, habits, routines, and skills that would comprise their new lives. The transporter role is at the same time vague, complex, and important, and in it therapists employ a considerable amount of imagination, an openness to experience, and a willingness to tolerate uncertainty or ambiguity. This role seemed to be highly valued by the therapists and patients but seems ill-defined by the profession or its literature.

COMMON OBJECTS AND ACTIVITIES IN AN UNCOMMON WORLD

The world of the clinic is full of unusual apparatus, rituals, and language. Occupational therapists, however, use ordinary objects—combs, brushes, pocket change, cooking equipment, pencils, and markers—in their everyday practice. These objects are often used in the usual ways; sometimes, they are not. Therapists adapt objects or activities so that the person can best use the object or accomplish a task in the easiest fashion, given the limitations of the disability. This adapting process often takes considerable effort and imagination, and usually several adjustments. Therapists are always adjusting things to get them to fit right or to work better. They like to combine objects and ideas in new ways. "Hey, how about this?" or "Shall we try it this way?" or "Maybe this will work!" are phrases overheard in OT practice settings on a daily basis. Therapists have a willingness and ability to engage in open-ended problem-solving activities, and involve themselves and the patients in active strategies in order to find a new way, perhaps the only possible way, for the person to accomplish an everyday task.

This ability to adapt activities and objects and to teach new ways to do ordinary activities seems to be a central part of their professional identity. Patty told a story about a nurse coming to her "in a dither saying this person just can't dress himself. He just can't. You have to come see him and figure something out." Patty went in and spoke to him. She adjusted the mirror, rearranged the objects and clothes, and helped him learn how to put on his shirt with one hand. "Problem solved!" At the end of the story Patty gave a satisfied smile and said, "They always ask us to do things like that and they are amazed that we can figure these things out and they are really quite simple." Kathy commented, "Yeah, they always say, 'Get the OTs to figure that one out.' "

This willingness to use usual objects in a setting where technological sophistication is valued poses some problems with the therapists' image, but not their effectiveness. A willingness to use usual or unusual things in unusual ways is taken for granted by both the therapists and the patients. Not only do occupational therapists use commonplace objects in this uncommon world of the clinic, they also borrow the specialized materials of the clinic in a surprisingly irreverent way. This is a function of their practical natures, not a purposeful disrespect for the materials or their medical purpose. In any case, no one seems startled to see x-ray film used to make stencils, or IV tubing to tie something in place, or tongue depressors for a variety of uses. This use of part of the technical apparatus of the clinic for very common purposes seems acceptable in the OT room. We have commented on this many times in various presentations to occupational therapists and they readily confirm this observation. Many contributed examples of their own. One of our favorites is from an occupational therapist in Pennsylvania who commented that he works in a psychiatric hospital where he and the other occupational therapists find urine sample containers (unused ones) to be very convenient paint jars.

Common Sense as a Legitimate Mode of Reasoning

HOWARD GARDNER'S NOTION OF COMMON SENSE

This willingness to deal in everyday activities and a readiness to adapt objects and actions in new ways seems central to the practice. It also seems that these are characteristics that the therapists value and identify with. What therapists do, or get their patients to do, are not dramatic acts. They do not stand out as significant performances or events, or difficult procedures. Their actions are small steps requiring a lot of, not trial and error, but fine adjustments, and revisions and repetitions. Their thinking is also not dramatic. It is not based on elaborate statistical probabilities or precise measurements of unusual substances; but it is complex. Therapists consider many factors, seemingly simultaneously, while thinking about a complex problem, or a potential solution. Their thinking is reasoned and makes sense. Perhaps the best way to characterize it is to call their approach common sense. In speaking of common sense, Howard Gardner says:

> Common sense ... I define as the ability to deal with problems in an intuitive, rapid and perhaps unexpectedly accurate manner. (1985, p. 287)

He goes on to explain that common sense is neither very common nor a simple phenomenon. In examining the intellectual components of that skill, he continues:

> In order to account for this highly desirable form of competence, it proves necessary to bring to bear a number of other considerations. To begin with, the ability to engage in calculations about the proper ordering and orchestration of multiple lines of activity involves logical-mathematical intelligence. Then, if an individual is to engage in considerable planning about his life (or the lives of others) it is necessary to posit a highly developed personal intelligence, or more simply, a mature sense of self. Finally the movement from the ability to plan a line of action to the actual achievement of actions (from dreams to deeds) transports us away from the realm of cognition, in a strict sense, to the arena of practice, or effective action. Here we impinge on the sphere of will—certainly a critical component in the ways in which we actually lead our lives. (pp. 287–288)

It seems that the day-to-day practice of therapists does involve this sort of complexity of thought and action. However, the problems that are addressed—eating, grooming, and so forth—are rather mundane, in most people's view. Their solutions are achieved through the use of common objects and actions. This makes the OTs and their thinking appear rather ordinary in the glamorous high-tech world of the teaching hospital. The therapists in the Clinical Reasoning Study seemed to "take this as a fact of life." In general they seemed quite secure about the quality of their work and of its importance to their patients. They felt that their judgments were sound and that they could "figure it all out" in a way that was both knowledgeable and clever. Within and among themselves, occupational therapists seem to feel that their practice is viable and valuable and that their common sense makes for good clinical judgments in many ways.

COMMON SENSE IN TRANSPORTING ANN BACK
TO THE COMMUNITY

In Maureen Freda's story of Ann, Maureen demonstrates many of the components of common sense that Gardner discusses. She expresses the "intuitive, rapid and perhaps unexpectedly accurate manner" of dealing with problems, in her immediate insight that caring for her baby would be Ann's central goal. She quickly thinks to borrow the "recus-a-baby," she thinks of adding weights to simulate the weight of the child as it grows, and simulates "squirming" as well. This expresses not only an intuitive understanding of the real situation that Ann will face, but a rather complete understanding as well. No amount of "chart talk" type of goals for Ann—such as strengthening, balance, and co-ordination—would quite capture just what skills Ann would need to walk with a 10-pound squirming infant. Maureen constructed a close-to-real, whole situation that provided practice in a task that could not be effectively learned as a series of several subskills. She created a whole, where a sum-of-parts collection of activities or skills would not be effective. Maureen also demonstrates the ability to "engage in cal-culations about the proper ordering and orchestration of multiple lines of activity" in her ability to manage the overall progress Ann makes in OT treatment. She negotiates favors and permissions from nursing staff and administrators, involves Ann's husband at a particular point when she senses that they are both ready, decides when and how to rein-troduce the actual baby in Ann's treatment, and even finds a neighbor to help care for the baby in the afternoons. This orchestrating and integrating of "services" for Ann, perfectly timed to match Ann's emo-tional and physical gains, demonstrates an ability to "see" the whole problem complex, and to manage the treatment of different aspects of it in a logical and meaningful sequence. Maureen's "mature sense of self" that Gardner thinks is necessary if one is to be helpful to others is not as obvious in the story, until you reread it and notice how per-ceptive Maureen was about Ann's feelings and how carefully she ap-proaches Ann's sense of loss, and her fear and frustration. You also sense her concern for Ann and her husband and the engaging, yet respectful, way she has of talking with and working with them. What is very obvious in this story is Maureen's ability to transform "dreams to deeds" through the very "effective action(s)" that she guides Ann through in the course of her treatment.

Summary

Occupational therapy is a health profession that is constituted to help restore people's ability to engage in the tasks of everyday life.

Therapists recognize the importance of these life tasks and the constitutive role that these tasks play in making meaning of our participation in the everyday life-world. By reteaching many of these tasks OTs help a person reconstruct a meaningful life that has been disrupted by disease or disability. Thus, their role is often one of transporter, helping the person across the difficult terrain called "rehab" and back into the community.

Reteaching everyday tasks in the uncommon world of the clinic is not an easy task, nor is the therapy easily understood. The tasks that OTs take on, and the problems they help solve, require many forms of thinking and many kinds of action. The thinking is often complex, and the actions often precise. Much of OT requires that therapists "adapt" or invent the particular therapy that will best meet the patients' needs and goals, and will contribute to the construction of a new sense of self. To do this sort of inventing requires knowledge and cognitive skills; but often the critical element in solving problems of everyday life is common sense.

Since daily activities are executed by the biological self, prompted by the psychological self, evaluated by the social self, and made meaningful by the phenomenological self, the therapist must attend to several levels of human endeavor simultaneously in order to help the person to make the changes necessary to return to the community. Therapists analyze the functional limitations, determine their probable biological, psychological, or social causes, imagine possibilities for change, and design and execute programs to help the person to bring about the projected change. Therapists reason about several aspects of the condition, drawing on different, and sometimes disparate areas of knowledge in order to create a fairly complete picture of the problem, as well as to project and evaluate possible resolutions. They also employ a broad spectrum of psychomotor, mechanical, and artistic abilities. Part of the "know-how" of the therapist is a willingness or ability to make new objects, or design new procedures, or use common things in uncommon ways. The therapist is often in a situation where "figuring it all out" results in a new and unusual solution to an uncommon problem encountered in executing ordinary tasks. More frequently, "the problem" is a somewhat novel collection of problems. Thus, the focus—and usual result of practice—is the creation of an "adaptive" way of participating in everyday activities for the person who might otherwise be unable to do so. The problem complex is transformed into a set of adaptive objects and routines that permit the person to perform everyday activities and participate in the physical and social world.

■ P A R T ■
III

Clinical Reasoning: Taking the Client from Structural Limitation to New Formulations

■

The Therapist with the Three-Track Mind

■ MAUREEN HAYES FLEMING

Introduction: Multiple Modes of Reasoning

Early in the Clinical Reasoning Study, we began to realize that occupational therapists were using several reasoning strategies. Different modes of thinking were employed for different purposes or in response to particular features of a problem. One reasoning strategy that therapists frequently employed was very similar to the hypothetical reasoning typically discussed in the medical problem-solving literature. We called this "procedural reasoning." Therapists tended to rely upon a hypothetical, or procedural, style of thinking when considering the person's physical ailment. This is probably because therapists' knowledge of clinical conditions is frequently acquired through medical lecture courses—which may or may not be taught by physicians, but are almost always presented within the philosophical framework of the medical model. This type of reasoning was similar, but not exactly like medical problem solving. The focus of OT treatment is different from medical treatment. For physicians, the problem to be solved is the clinical condition. For occupational therapists, the problem is to help the person solve problems of daily functioning incurred as consequences of the clinical condition. In a procedural mode of reasoning therapists search for techniques and procedures that can be brought to bear on the physical problem.

A second type of reasoning was employed when therapists interacted with the patient as a person, a social being. We called this "interactive reasoning." When the therapists were interacting with their patients as people, their interactive style would change. Their interactions were clearly guided by some sort of reasoning. As one therapist said:

> When we interact with patients we are honest and real, but we think about how we are acting and why. It's not just some enthusiastic, but unguided interaction like . . . like say—a hairdresser. You know how they are, they just talk about anything. There's no purpose behind what they are talking to you about, or how they react to what you say, except to make the time pass more pleasantly. When therapists talk to patients there is a reason behind what they say that is more than just conversation. When we interact with patients we think about what we are going to say and why.

We could see that the therapists interacted with their patients in a way that was purposeful and structured by some sort of tacit plans and guidelines. We knew that some parts of occupational therapy education are focused on developing therapists' interactive skills. Lectures and assignments are designed to develop various aspects of interaction, such as interviewing skills or group process techniques. The tradition of "therapeutic use of self" (Fidler and Fidler, 1963, p. 40) probably also influences OT practice. Perhaps the primary place where interactive reasoning is acquired is clinical education. The clinical education of occupational therapists includes objectives and experiences aimed at improving students' interactive skills; and part of the evaluation of the affiliating students' clinical performance considers interactive skills. The notion that interaction is guided by a different type of reasoning than hypothetical reasoning is supported by a growing body of literature in psychology and philosophy. Although we developed the idea that interaction was guided by a particular form of reasoning ourselves, it was not difficult to find similar concepts in the current literature. Many authors have postulated the idea that there are several forms of reasoning. Many of them will be referenced throughout this chapter and Chapter 8.

Both procedural and interactive reasoning were employed to address different aspects of the whole problem. The procedural reasoning strategy was used when the therapist thought about the person's physical or emotional limitations and what procedures were appropriate to improve function. Interactive reasoning was used to help the therapists interact with and understand the person better. Although these reasoning strategies are distinctly different, therapists shifted rapidly from one form of reasoning to another. Reasoning styles changed as the therapist's attention was drawn from the clinical condition to another feature of the problem, and to how the person feels about the problem. Therapists could process or analyze different aspects of the problem, almost simultaneously, using different thinking styles; and they did not "lose track of" their thoughts about aspects of a problem as those components were temporarily shifted to be the background while another aspect was brought into the foreground.

Later we realized that there was a third type of reasoning that therapists employed when they thought of the whole problem within the context of the person's past, present, and future; and within personal, social, and cultural contexts. This was an especially useful form of reasoning, which therapists used when they wanted to, as they say, "individualize" the treatment for the particular person. We called this "conditional reasoning" because it took the whole condition into account.

Procedural Reasoning

Therapists used procedural reasoning when they were thinking about the disease or disability and deciding on which treatment activities (procedures) they might employ to remediate the person's functional performance problems. In this mode, the therapist's dual search was for problem definition and treatment selection. In situations where problem identification and treatment selection were seen as the central task, the therapists' thinking strategies demonstrated many parallels to the patterns identified by other researchers interested in problem solving in general, and clinical problem solving in particular. The typical medical problem-solving sequence—diagnosis, prognosis, prescription—was commonly used. However, the words the therapists used to describe this sequence were "problem identification, goal setting, and treatment planning. Experienced therapists used forms of reasoning similar to the problem-solving strategies identified by many investigators studying the reasoning strategies of physicians. For example, therapists used all three problem-solving methods described by Newel and Simon (1972): "recognition, generate and test, and heuristic search." They also displayed characteristics identified by Elstein, Shulman, and Sprafka (1978), such as "cue identification, hypothesis generation, cue interpretation, and hypothesis evaluation" (p. 277). They interpreted patterns of cues, in much the same manner that Coughlin and Patel (1987) identified among physicians and medical students. A detailed description and analysis of these characteristics of occupational therapists' procedural reasoning appears in the next chapter.

Interactive Reasoning

Interactive reasoning took place during face-to-face encounters between therapist and patient. It was the form of reasoning that therapists employed when they wanted to better understand the person in particular or, as Oliver Sacks says, "this patient" (1988). There are many reasons why a therapist might want to know the person better. The therapist might want to know how the person feels about the treatment at the moment or what the patient is like as a person, either out of sheer interest or in order to more finely tailor the treatment to his or her specific needs or preferences. Further, the therapist may be interested in this person in order to better understand the experience of the disability from the person's own point of view. When colleagues and students in our courses and workshops have analyzed videotapes of therapeutic practice, the complexity of interactive reasoning strategies is always striking. There are a number of fairly distinct purposes for which interactive reasoning is employed. Some of these are listed below.

1. To engage the person in the treatment session. Mattingly (1989) identified six such strategies.
2. To know the person as a person (Cohn, 1989).
3. To understand the disability from the patients' own point of view (Mattingly, 1989).
4. To finely match the treatment goals and strategies to this particular person, with this disability, and this experience of it. Therapists call this "individualizing" (Fleming, 1989).
5. To communicate a sense of acceptance, trust, or hope to the patient (Langthaller, 1990).
6. To use humor to relieve tension (Siegler, 1987).
7. To construct a shared language of actions and meanings (Crepeau, 1991).
8. To determine if the treatment session is going well (Fleming, 1990).
9. To show interest in the persons and their concerns without indicating a distaste for or disapproval of the condition (Bradburn, 1992).

Although the therapists in the Clinical Reasoning Study did not initially recognize interaction and interactive reasoning as central to their practice, they saw developing good interactions with their patients as at least adjunct to practice and as necessary for a variety of "good reasons." The particular therapeutic reasons listed above prompted therapists to use different types of interactive strategies, which were, in turn, guided by different aspects of the interactive form of reasoning. Some of the reasoning styles or strategies identified, and the hypothesized reasons for using them, seem to be similar to new concepts about reasoning that have been proposed by various psychologists and philosophers. These theorists have proposed that there are many useful ways to think, and that hypothetical-deductive reasoning is not necessarily the only, or even the best, reasoning method. Many of these forms of reasoning are proposed by investigators who study how individuals think about themselves and their experience within the cultural context. They concern themselves with how such elusive processes as values, norms, and symbolic meanings are used to guide, gauge, frame, and formulate thought and action. Others examine properties of problems and relate them to problem-solving strategies. Most theorists who explore these forms of thinking propose that particular features of the problem will influence the individual and, in effect, direct him or her to select a particular problem-solving method. Such features may include salient characteristics of a task or problem (Hammond, 1988), the context (Greeno, 1989), individual interests and talents (Gardener, 1985), and degree of interest in individual uniqueness (Silverstein, 1988) or past experience (Dewey, 1915).

The notion that characteristics of the presumed problem will prompt a particular thinking process was borne out in our observations of the therapists in the Clinical Reasoning Study. The therapists shifted from one form of thinking to another. They often "picked up" subtle cues and responded to them rapidly and then returned to another task and thinking mode without, "skipping a beat," as one observer commented.

If such numerous reasoning strategies exist, and if the therapists had different purposes in mind for using interaction, then would it also be likely that the purpose of the interaction would prompt the use of a particular reasoning strategy? It seemed so to us. For example, in trying to understand the person as a person, the therapists' reasoning looked like the mode that Belenky, Clinchy, Goldberger, and Tarule (1986) describe as "connected knowing," which these authors link to empathy. In trying to understand the disability from the patient's point of view, they used a phenomenological approach similar to that advocated by Kestenbaum (1982) and Paget (1988). Their interaction with patients produced an understanding of the person as an individual within a culturally constructed point of view, as they shared what Schutz (1975) calls a "reciprocity of motives."

When individualizing the treatment, therapists appeared to be functioning intuitively rather than analytically. Hammond (1988) has proposed that intuitive reasoning is indeed as effective and complex as analytical reasoning, but that it is employed in response to a different form of problem, one that is not well defined and has a large number of facets. Tasks in which there are a large number of cues, from a number of sources, and which require perceptual rather than instrumental measurement, Hammond argues, induce the person to use intuitive methods of problem solving. He further asserts that in these situations analytical reasoning would be less effective than intuitive reasoning. Therapists often employed intuitive reasoning in response to problems that they suddenly saw as more multifaceted than they had initially assumed.

Mattingly's strategies, discussed in Chapter 8, indicate that therapists have several ways of engaging the patient in treatment. Some of these require very complex interpretations of subtle interactive cues in order to be effective. The 23 interactive strategies that Langthaller (1990) identified in one therapeutic encounter seem to be partially influenced by the work of psychoanalytical theorists such as Carl Rogers (1961), and by occupational therapy theorists such as Fidler and Fidler (1963) and Mosey (1981). This is not surprising, since reading the works of these theorists is part of the therapists' educational preparation. The complexity, subtlety, and facility with which some therapists used numerous interaction forms, however, suggests processes far more complex than could be accounted for by professional education alone.

We also had a strong sense that therapists' reasoning about and interaction with patients was directly related to their values. Their sense of the importance of patients as individuals and the degree to which the practice was guided by a complex set of deeply held humanistic values lead us to draw parallels to work on ethical and moral decision making, such as that expressed by Gilligan (1982), Kegan (1982), and Perry (1979), among others. The task of monitoring the patient's feelings about the treatment and yet managing that treatment (which is often difficult and sometimes painful or distasteful), seems to require a considerable amount of what Howard Gardner (1985) refers to as "interpersonal intelligence." Gardner postulates two interpersonal intelligences. One is "the capacity to access one's own feeling life." The other is the ability to notice and make distinctions among other individuals, in particular among their moods, temperaments, motivations and intentions" (p. 239). Interactive reasoning requires "active judgment" (Buchler, 1955) on several levels simultaneously. This requires that the therapist "read" the patient, that is, assess the patient's "cues" to determine mood, intentions, interests, and so on. Next the therapist conveys this interpretation to the patient and interprets the patients response to that interpretation. This reciprocal process of evaluation, interpretation, and ultimately confirmation is one that Erikson (1968) considers essential to identity formation and to the person's future social interaction capabilities.

It may be that the ability to interact successfully and therapeutically is strongly linked to the therapist's personal and professional identity. Gardner (1985, p. 275) hypothesizes that interpersonal intelligence is predicated on a well-developed sense of self. It seemed to us that good interaction skills were linked to professional self-confidence, combined with a mature personality and a clear sense of self. Novice therapists reported that in their first year of practice they had neither the confidence nor, they believed, the right to interact with patients as individuals. They reported that they "stuck to the procedural" until they were confident in their use of those skills. Indeed, even in the second year of practice, we observed therapists negotiating a sort of halting course back and forth between the procedural and interactive modes of thinking about and treating their patients. In the senior therapists, procedural and interactive forms seemed to flow together, each enhancing the other. Interaction is an important aspect of occupational therapy, and necessary for engaging the patient in therapy. Interactive reasoning, in its many forms and intents, was used quite effectively by most therapists to guide their interactions with their patients.

Integrating Procedural and Interactive Reasoning

ROLE PERCEPTION INFLUENCES REASONING

We have mentioned here, and in earlier chapters, that the therapists seem to have taken on the difficult task of working with the patient both as a physical body and as a person whose sense of self has been disrupted by illness or injury. We have also pointed out that concepts and perceptions of how one treats the physical condition are often different from perceptions about how one treats the *person who has* the physical condition. Experienced OTs seem to have the uncommon ability to treat the physical condition objectively, while simultaneously understanding the person's subjective experience of his or her condition. The novice therapists did not seem to do this as often, or as smoothly, as the experienced therapists.

One fairly obvious difference between new therapists and seasoned ones was that the new therapists seem to vacillate back and forth between attending to the clinical condition and attending to the individual person in a discontinuous manner, whereas experienced therapists smoothly integrated these two levels of attending to the clinical condition and the person. One can readily make some guesses as to why this might be so. First, the experienced therapists knew their craft well. The procedures they used and the reasoning that guided them were easy for the experienced therapists. Knowledge of anatomy, neurology, and so on, and treatment techniques had "sunk" to the tacit level. Therapists could execute procedures or construct adaptive equipment almost, but not quite, without thinking about it. The day-to-day treatment techniques became "second nature" (Hayes, 1978) for experienced therapists. One could say that they had the time and energy "left over" to talk with and interact with patients. However, the variety of styles of interaction that any given therapist could use, and the clearly obvious variety and complexity of the reasons and reasoning behind those interactions, led us to believe that this skill was developed by other factors not related to mere time on the job.

We began to see that there were different styles or types of therapists and that these differences could not be accounted for by the simple distinction of years of experience. A greater difference was noted in relation to therapists' values and the different perceptions therapists had of their role. Some therapists strongly valued their interaction role with patients. They believed it was part of their professional responsibility to understand their patient's perceptions of themselves and their illness experience (Kleinman, 1980). These therapists tended to talk with their patients about what one patient called "deep subjects." These deep subjects concerned patients' feelings about their injuries, their anger and sadness about their losses, their frustration about not being able to do basic simple tasks, their depression, their fears for their future and their drastically altered life and self-image.

The most common pattern of "deep subject" interaction emerged in the following way: The therapist and patient would be working together on a therapeutic exercise or task, the therapist would signal a level of acceptance and comfort with the patient, and this, in turn, would trigger a readiness by the patient to disclose something about how she or he was experiencing the disability or illness. Generally, the patient would, verbally or otherwise, express some feeling, and the therapist would allow the person to continue the discussion, either by simply listening or by participating in the conversation. The tone of the participation was accepting, and, through words or facial expressions, therapists would convey empathy for the patient and the situation. Often the discussion would end with the therapist trying to point out some positive quality or skill that the patient still had. The skillful therapist was able to do this in such a way that the patient's negative feelings were not denied, but given credence even while a positive point of view about the person and the future was offered. These sorts of therapists also made a greater attempt at using and understanding symbolic meanings that the patient offered or that the therapist thought were implicit in the words or actions used in the therapy sessions. They saw their role as helping the person reconstruct a new sense of self and a new life, and they saw interaction as one of the therapeutic skills they possessed.

Other therapists saw their role as much more strictly tied to the procedural concerns. They perceived themselves as having specialized knowledge that could be used to help patients learn the skills and tasks they needed in order to function in the home and community. Their focus was much more on the physical body than on the person. Some therapists thought that their role was fairly strictly guided by what the hospital and insurance companies defined as "reimbursable service," for example, improving range of motion (ROM); increasing sitting or standing tolerance; improving independence in eating or dressing; driver training; perceptual retraining; or helping people to learn safety precautions during ADL tasks such as cooking. These therapists saw interaction as peripheral to treatment, whereas other therapists saw interaction as central to therapy. So it turned out that the integration of the procedural and interactive aspects of therapy and reasoning was not so much a matter of experience or time on the job as it was of values and role perception. Two novice therapists rapidly became proficient at addressing the biomechanical aspects of the problem complex and at interacting with the person, whereas others were slower at acquiring the knack.

COMMON STRATEGIES EMPLOYED REGARDLESS OF PERSONALITY STYLE

There were also differences among the experienced therapists in their seeming ability to address these two concerns simultaneously. At first this looked like a simple difference in personality. For example, Liz is tall, with a short, brown, stylish hair cut, a large collection of artistic earrings, and an outgoing personality that she describes as very "New York." She liked the challenge of patients with conditions that were new to her. Cathy has soft curls, green eyes, and a quiet melodious voice and a calm demeanor. She thought carefully about each infant and child she treated. Christa, a willowy strawberry blond with the formal and reserved manner that is part of her German heritage, was very secure in her professional knowledge and experience. Yet all of these therapists, who on the surface seemed to be very different, had many common qualities that immediately intrigued us. One was that they had a wide range of interactive styles and skills. They could be supportive or almost demanding. They could encourage a person to work harder, or commend or console them if they worked too hard. They could be absolutely silent, yet present, or run a continuous line of verbal background such as talking, humming, making encouraging noises, or even singing. Cathy often softly sang or hummed lullabies to sooth the distressed infants she worked with. Liz, in the informal atmosphere of the spinal cord unit, sometimes sang bits of popular songs with or to patients, as a way of encouraging the person or to form a bond or express some "message." Christa, who worked with people who often had very diminished capacities to understand their condition or what was happening to them, gave quiet, encouraging directions and reports to people as she evaluated their motor capacities or asked them to participate in a therapeutic activity.

What interested us even more was that these therapists, and others, varied their interaction in direct response to the patient. They always "took their cues" from the patient and managed the mood of the session based on their perceptions of the patient's mood, interests, physical status, and so forth. There was an immediate responsiveness to the patient. This sort of interaction was very subtle and very complex. It seemed automatic and uncontrived and was variable. Often the therapist's facial expression and posture "mirrored" that of the patient and reflected an immediate involvement in their concerns. At other times, therapists took a slightly different tone or stance, as if trying to give some of their own energy to the patient or to invest some of their enthusiasm in the project they were doing together. This variation was carefully calibrated so that it was different, but not too different from the patient's. If a patient with a spinal cord injury was depressed, Liz would talk with the person about his or her feelings. She would begin with a look of concern and a quiet, deep tone of voice. Gradually as she skillfully guided the conversation to a brighter (if only slightly) side of the problem or point of view, her tone, and posture elevated too. Invariably she would end the conversation with a look in the eye and a comment that more or less said "Is this settled for now?" or "Is this a good point to stop?" and a smile and a comment like, "So what should we do today?" Nearly all of the therapists matched their tone and actions to those of the patient and were responsive to the person's moods. Often, therapists changed what they were doing in therapy specifically to adjust to the patient's moods or wants. Such fine-tuning of interaction and response to the patient was characteristic of those therapists who took the phenomenological approach, regardless of their personality style, or the type or age of patients treated.

UNDERSTANDING PATIENT AND THERAPIST AS PEOPLE

We have mentioned earlier that therapists need to understand "this person" as a person and not simply a patient whose most interesting quality is his or her disease. It also seems that it is important that the patient understand that the therapist is a person too. A favorite example from one of the videotapes will illustrate this point. We call this vignette "Cindy and the Deviled Eggs." Cindy, an experienced therapist with a reserved yet warm interactive style, was working with Alice, who was dependent upon a ventilator in order to breathe. Alice was becoming increasingly more anxious that if she did the exercises Cindy requested she would not be able to breathe. No amount of Cindy's calm reassurance and concern for Alice would soothe her and enlist her cooperation. Cindy, rather than mirror the patient's mood, "switched gears" entirely and complimented Alice on the deviled eggs she had made in OT the day before. Alice smiled and they had a conversation about Alice's favorite recipes. Here, in a moment, Cindy not only distracted Alice from her fears, she also complimented Alice on her considerable culinary skills. This directly "validated" Alice as a real person and symbolically said, "you are valuable and talented." A few minutes later Alice and Cindy were calmly engaged in the original, somewhat dull, but necessary exercise routine. The seemingly meaningless and frightening exercise was transformed into a therapeutic experience because Cindy saw Alice as a person. Alice returned the recognition by giving Cindy a brief recipe for lasagna.

Sometimes the patients had to see therapists as real people in order to consent to participate with them at all. While watching a videotape of Debbie (the department chief and an experienced hand therapist) and her patient (a neurologist from a nearby hospital), we realized how important it is that the therapist not only have procedural expertise but also be perceived as a real person, at least by some patients. In this tape, the patient has come for his weekly occupational therapy treatment, which is aimed at reducing the effects of scarring, and increasing the range of motion in the affected fingers. The patient, Dr. C., seems to be disappointed with his progress and has recently seen his surgeon, who also seemed, according to the patient, to be disappointed in the progress. Debbie is engaged in preparing for the session and is seated at a table across from the patient and listens to and responds to his concerns with words, "uh-huhs," and facial expressions. Throughout several minutes of this discussion, Debbie is expecting Dr. C. to put his hands in hers so that she can begin treatment. Several times he seems about to give her his hand and then withdraws it, often looking at the hand with a sort of puzzled expression on his face and an intense examination of the scar. More comments about the hand follow. Then the conversation becomes more general and he again attempts to "hand over" his hand to the therapist and again withdraws. There is a constant back-and-forth pattern: As the conversation is less intense he becomes more ready for the treatment; as he comes closer to the treatment he withdraws and returns to the discussion of the hand. Each time he returns to the discussion, it seems that his comments become increasingly more "medicalized," jargon-filled, and concentrated on hands and healing processes in a depersonalized way, seemingly avoiding the fact that this is his hand. Debbie, in the meantime, tries a number of interactive strategies to get him to give her his hand. She listens and confirms or offers alternate opinions. She changes the focus slightly to splints and splint making. Suddenly, Debbie comments, "You know there are other things you can do for exercise besides this [coming to OT]. For example, holding tools like gardening tools and working your hand like this would help. It's going to be a good weekend . . . maybe you could rake leaves, that would be good. Or golf . . . that's good." He comments that he likes golf. She comments that she and her husband like golf, especially in Bermuda. "Me too," he says, and suddenly gives Debbie his hand. She takes the hand and begins the long-awaited preparatory massage. The therapy continues, as does a simultaneous discussion about golf, leaf raking, and furniture refinishing, and the need to clean out one's garage on crisp autumn days.

We saw many examples of patients having to trust the therapist and see the therapist as a "real" person before they were willing to entrust the therapist with the care of their bodies, and especially their feelings. This example was particularly notable because it was so clearly visible in the offering and retracting of the patient's actual hand, and also because the social situation was so different from the usual. Most of the time the therapist is more knowledgeable about the medical aspects of the condition than is the patient. Here the patient was presumably more knowledgeable about his medical condition, and furthermore was higher up in the social structure of hospital personnel, than was the therapist. These two issues made the situation more difficult for the therapist, and apparently the doctor-client as well, but they also made the interaction one in which the need for trust could be clearly observed on the videotape.

The ability to treat the person's problem with professional and expert knowledge, and the ability to interact with the patient as a person, are both important in occupational therapy. The degree to which therapists possess these skills seems to vary with the experience, personal traits, and points of view of individual therapists. The question of procedural expertise can probably be accounted for by education and experience. Studies, such as those conducted by Dreyfus (1972), and Dreyfus and Dreyfus (1986), Benner (1984), and Benner and Tanner (1987), postulate a continuum of learning and skill that practitioners acquire through experience. These studies have begun to enlighten our understanding of how procedural expertise evolves and develops. The question of how interactive skill and interactive reasoning evolve and develop in practitioners is not yet sufficiently addressed in the professional development or clinical-reasoning literature. It is our perception that a great part of this skill is linked to personality and sense of self, factors that are difficult to influence. On the other hand, interactive styles and skills can be improved. Perhaps recognizing the importance of interaction to therapy is a first step in developing the skill.

A Perception of Other Reasoning Styles

Although we began to see quite clearly that interaction was an important part of therapy and were confident that particular reasoning skills and strategies were employed to guide that interaction, we still thought there was "more to it than that." We kept struggling for a way to capture what the "it" was that we knew was there in some therapists' minds. This unidentified "some quality," we were convinced, was the cause of a certain intriguing sense of the therapeutic interaction between therapists and clients. This perceived "something" seemed to be more characteristic of some therapists than others. It was a quality that seemed to differentiate OT from similar fields such as physical therapy or social work. This quality was clearly there; we saw it more and more in treatment sessions, in videotapes, and in the way OTs talked to and about their patients. We thought that we might be able to capture this elusive quality by examining the culture of OT, especially some of its important values. Such values are often not articulated directly but are embodied in habits of action and language (Bourdieu, 1977).

Occupational therapists have a few rather curious phrases that they use frequently. These phrases seemed to be very much part of their culture and seemed to mean a lot to them. One was that therapists talked about keeping the "session on track" or not wanting to "lose" the session. This was related to their concern to "make something happen" in the session. They always wanted to be sure that the session was worthwhile in some significant way. This was not simply a concern that some physical progress or, as they say, "gains" would be made. It was a concern to "make something click," that something should "fall into place," that the session would have some significant meaning for the patient. Therapists in all our studies have commented that many sessions with patients are absolutely draining. They put tremendous emotional and physical energy into "keeping the session on track," constantly watching for cues, making small variations in their own and their clients' actions, evaluating, interpreting, adjusting, revising, re-interpreting, always trying to manage or mold the session so that something happens. Usually something does happen. The patient makes some physical progress or has some insight, even gives up an impossible goal or, perhaps, accomplishes something more than had been expected. When they "lose" a session or nothing "clicks," therapists are disappointed and even more drained. When the session is a "good one" therapists are tired, but pleased.

All of this gave us the idea that therapists might be engaged in some sort of monitoring and evaluation process while they simultaneously conducted treatment. They seemed to be deeply involved in directing the therapy session, while simultaneously making a distant evaluation of it. This realization lead us to postulate an idea that therapists thought along several "tracks" simultaneously. We began to see that therapists were conducting and monitoring the procedural aspects of their treatment of the physical body. They were interacting with patients both to elicit their cooperation and to understand the person's response to the treatment at both physical and interactive levels. In addition, they were not only observing and analyzing their patients' behavior, but their own as well. Therapists were thinking of themselves as director, actor, audience, and critic all at once. No wonder they found some sessions exhausting. "Making something happen" or "keeping the session on track" is a very dynamic, almost moment-to-moment process. It is more than simply knowing the correct procedure and executing it well. There is a quality about the practice in which "individualizing" is not simply making a few adjustments to the usual procedure to suit it to the particular peculiarities of this patient. There seems to be a deep-seated expectation that a therapist should actually create a particular therapeutic experience for this person as an individual. Therapy in some ways is not simply applying a solution to a problem. It is very much a process of creating an experience, a "lived experience" (Dewey, 1929), for the client. The experience is created so that the patient can learn something or have some insight into problems and possible solutions. At a deeper level, the experience is a way of creating and recreating meaning for the patient. Some therapists seemed to evaluate their own performance based on the degree to which a particular session was an experience for the person.

A dietician who participated in one of our workshops spoke of the need to look for "the teachable moment." She said that dieticians are attentive to the patients, and look and wait for the right moment when the patient will be ready to hear, or learn from, what the specialist has to say about eating habits and nutrition. Occupational therapists who what to "keep the session on track" and provide "just the right challenge" (Parham, 1987) seem to have an eye out for the opportunity, as the dietician implied, but they seemed more actively involved in creating a situation where something could "happen." Therapists want the condition to change in some way, some dynamic way in which they can "feel something click." We borrowed the therapists' term "track" to illustrate this new insight. Therapists seemed to be thinking in many tracks simultaneously. There was the procedural track, the interactive track, and then a track that followed, that observed and interpreted, what was "happening" with the patient.

Another phrase therapists use often is "putting it all together." Whatever this "putting together" is, it seemed to be important, and something therapists thought of as uniquely their own role. What is the "it" that therapists "put together," and how do they know when they have accomplished this elusive task? To make a long story short, experienced therapists seem to have very vivid images in their mind of who the person is and what the person can be like, given time and therapy. Therapists' visions of this future person guided their evaluation of the day-to-day, as well as the overall, treatment. Therapists know that the session is "on track" when it seems to be moving a patient toward becoming like that image. "Putting it all together" means having a person develop a set of insights and skills that will allow her or him to live the life the therapist thought was possible. These images guided the therapists through the process of both "creating an experience"

(Dewey, 1929) and monitoring the session to ensure that it was "on track" and that "something happened." The image is a possibility that the therapist "sees." This is not simply calculating a likely outcome, given knowledge of the effects of a particular treatment procedure; it is a sense or understanding of the clinical condition as it has affected this particular person's ability to act and interact, in the particular personal and social worlds, with a particular sense of self. Since this sort of reasoning was concerned with possibilities, we called it "conditional reasoning." We postulated that this reasoning was managed by what we called the "conditional track."

Conditional Reasoning

The concept of conditional reasoning is the most elusive notion in our proposed theory of a "three-track" mind. Yet we are firmly, if intuitively, convinced that there is this other form of reasoning that many therapists use. This reasoning style moves beyond specific concerns about the person and the physical problems and places them in broader social and temporal contexts. We use the term "conditional" in three different ways. One is that therapists think about the whole condition; this includes the person, the illness, the meanings the illness has for the person, the family, and the social and physical contexts in which the person lives. A second is that therapists need to imagine how the condition could change and become a revised condition. The imagined new state is a conditional, that is, a proposed state, which may or may not be achieved. The third sense is that the success or failure of reaching a point in life that approximates that future image is very much contingent upon (or conditional upon) the patient's participation. The patient must participate, not only in the therapeutic activities themselves, but also in the construction of the image of the possible outcome, the revised condition. Conditional reasoning seems to relate to and guide the phenomenological aspects of practice. We observed this sort of reasoning only among the therapists who took (however intuitively) the phenomenological point of view. Therapists who were less interested in the patient, and more interested in the medical condition or the OT treatment procedures, did not seem to use this reasoning style. We found that most of the experienced therapists found this idea very congruent with their practice, whereas novice therapists did not identify this idea with their practice.

Conditional reasoning seems to be a multidimensional process, involving complicated, but not strictly logical, forms of thinking. We postulate that in using conditional reasoning, the therapist reflects upon the success or failure of the clinical encounter from both the procedural and interactive standpoints and attempts to integrate the two. Thinking then moves beyond these concerns to a deeper level of interpretation of the whole problem. The therapist interprets the meaning of the problem in the *context* of a possible future for the person. The therapist imagines what that future could be like. This imagined future is a guide to bringing about a revised condition through therapy. There are at least two thinking processes at work here: imagination and interpretation. This form of reasoning, we propose, is best suited to addressing the whole condition from the phenomenological perspective. Through attention to the ailment, the person, and the personal and cultural meanings the person attaches to the experience, the therapists were able to create the best solutions for the particular patient. "Individualizing," it seems, is complex and requires both the phenomenological perspective and conditional reasoning.

The therapists tried to imagine what the person was like before the injury. Similarly, they tried to estimate or imagine what the possibilities were for the person's future life. By imagining, therapists mentally placed the person in contexts of current, past, and future social worlds. The therapists used imagination in order to best match the treatment selections to the specific interests, capacities, and goals of this person. Thus, therapists were able to make today's treatment relevant to "this" person. The present treatment therefore was not simply a link to future performance. It was placed in the context of a life in process.

Perhaps this form of reasoning is best described by example. Cathy, a pediatric therapist, was the most articulate of the therapists we studied about using this form of reasoning. It was conversations with her that first sparked our interest in this aspect of clinical reasoning. Cathy usually treated very young children who lived in the community and came to an outpatient early intervention program, so that the mother, or another person, was usually present. Cathy invariably included the mother in the session. The mother might be enlisted to hold the baby in an advantageous position, or to help get the child's interest in the session or a toy. Cathy would often talk to the mother while simultaneously working with the child. She often asked questions like, "Does he do this at home?" "Does she usually cry in this sort of situation?" "What does he like to do?" "Does he usually have difficulty calming himself down?" These were not diagnostic history-taking questions in the medical or procedural sense. These were questions that Cathy asked to help her, as she said, "construct an image" of what the child was really like on a day-to-day basis. She said she used that image to structure her treatment and imagine possible goals for the child. As she said, "I see this little child, and his movement patterns and his difficulties, and then I imagine what he will be like in two years, and then when he is 5 and maybe going to school. I think of what I can do to help him develop the skills that he will need to function in school and in the community, and what he will be like, and how his family will be with him." Here Cathy describes a process of imagining and integrating images of past, present, and possible futures for this child, given the variables of the child himself, the developmental delays and disabilities he displays now, his family situation, the social and educational opportunities available to him, what he might be able to do in the future, and how she might enable that future condition to come about.

Clearly, it takes professional experience to be able to project the possible developmental pattern and potential rate of success in attaining it. It also requires a mind that is imaginative, curious, and interested in future possibilities. This is a way of thinking that moves beyond an analysis of present abilities and interactions to envision how those interactions might help to construct a better life for this child.

Having constructed these images, which of course changed slightly over time and throughout the course of treatment, the therapists used images as a way of interpreting the significance of treatment for the patient. Therapists would mentally compare the patient's abilities today, and the relative success of today's session, against the image of where they wanted the person to be in the future. Therapists would "see" the patient today and estimate how close he or she was to "where I thought he should be" at this point in the course of treatment. They would mentally check to see how far the person had come toward attaining the future they had in mind. The evaluation of today's treatment was made in the context of past and future possibilities, and the particular state of things today would serve as a sort of mental mile marker, indicating progress toward a distant, and perhaps only dimly perceived, future.

One reason that we called this conditional reasoning was because a change in the present situation was "conditional upon" the therapist and the patient participating in effective therapy. This condition was dependent upon, not only the therapist's ability to engage the patient in treatment in the sense discussed in the interactive section of this chapter, but in addition, the ability to build a shared image of the person's future self. This image building was often accomplished through stories, or narrative, as described by Mattingly (1991). However, in many aspects of therapeutic interaction the images the therapists helped to build were often based in action and through visual images. They often included having the mother share a mental-visual image of the child in the future. The therapists constructed images on a long-term basis, such as wondering what an infant who is now being treated will be like in school, several years later. They used images on a short-term basis as well, as a way of extending the therapy and the images back into the home setting. Cathy says to Jean, Nicholas's foster mother, "Would he do this at home?" "Could he just sit quietly and look at something and have this nice position?" "Could the kids maybe hold him like I am doing while they watch TV?" Here, she creates a visual image, based on action in the present, of the child in a near-future situation. She does this in order to enhance the therapy, but also to build an image of the child as a participant in the family, rather than just a problematic baby.

One technique that therapists often used was to tell patients that they were getting better and to produce a sort of evidence of this by saying such things as, "Remember when you couldn't do this? Now you can." Sometimes therapists would also use this technique for themselves. They commented that when they were discouraged with a person's progress they often had to remind themselves "how far they had come." This technique helped both the patient and the therapist focus on the importance of their joint participation in this enterprise. It helped them through difficult, frustrating, and boring times and allowed them to place the moment in a more positive, though abstract and distant, context. But, most of all it seemed to remind them both that the condition was changing. Such changes were often quantitative, such as increased range of motion, and would be noted in the person's chart. But qualitative changes and their meanings were often more important to the therapists and patients. These changes were not reported in the chart. These important changes were progress toward that shared future image that the therapists and patient jointly constructed and worked toward. Such meaningful progress was best measured through memory, their collective memory. So the therapists were not simply saying, "This is progress. Remember how bad things were before." They were saying, "If you have come this far, maybe we will get to where you imagined you would, even though you are discouraged today."

Summary

Occupational therapists have an investment in "treating the whole person." They manage to treat many aspects of the person—sometimes simultaneously, and sometimes a piece at a time—addressing the physical limitations, the person as an individual, and the person in the contexts of past and future self-image and social, cultural world. To attend to all these aspects of the person and "put it all together," that is, to make a sufficiently complete package of the therapeutic processes that the person is able to engage in meaningful tasks, the occupational therapist uses several types of reasoning. We called those general types procedural, interactive, and conditional reasoning. Within these types there seem to be several styles or variations of reasoning strategies. Each of these three types of reasoning will be addressed in the following three chapters.

■

Procedural Reasoning
Addressing Functional Limitations
■ MAUREEN HAYES FLEMING

Introduction: Selecting Procedures to Suit the Problem

Procedural reasoning is the term we gave to the type of reasoning that therapists used when they tried to identify their patients' functional problems and to select the procedures that might be employed to help people reduce the effects of those problems. Procedural reasoning is similar to the hypothetical or propositional reasoning advocated in the medical problem-solving literature. This similarity is not surprising because parts of the problems that occupational therapists address are similar to the type of problems addressed by physicians—problems of the physical body.

Since procedural reasoning is very similar to some of the reasoning strategies reported in the medical problem-solving literature, this chapter will present several concepts from that literature. Examples of how occupational therapists employed various aspects of this type of reasoning will be presented later in the chapter so that the reader can begin to understand how features of problem solving are employed in occupational therapy practice.

A word of advice regarding terminology is probably necessary before we proceed. The term "problem solving" is used in the medical problem-solving literature somewhat differently than OTs tend to use the term. In medicine the biggest and most relevant problem to solve is "What is the diagnosis?" or "What is causing the person to have problems?" So problem solving in medicine is to a great extent *problem identification*. This problem identification process is what Rogers and

137

Holm (1991) refer to as "diagnostic reasoning." They encourage OTs to develop more skill in that area. We contend that OTs use several types of reasoning in clinical practice. Certainly all professionals need to continually improve their skills, and OTs are well advised to improve their problem identification skills. In this chapter I explain aspects of what physicians call problem solving, or diagnosis, and later illustrate how OTs use similar strategies to identify the physical aspects of their patients' problems. Since the OT's task is to work on functional performance and to find meaningful solutions to problems that may involve such complexities as a sense of self-worth, problem solving in OT often involves the invention of unique solutions for particular patients. This requires aspects of reasoning that are discussed in other chapters in this book. For the sake of convenience, in this chapter I will use problem solving as an umbrella term that includes two broad phases: problem identification and problem resolution. Problem identification will comprise the vast majority of the content of this chapter.

Aspects of Medical Problem Solving— a Brief Overview

The medical problem-solving literature and the literature regarding clinical judgment by psychologists began in the 1950s, with the hope of improving practitioners' clinical judgment (Goldberg, 1970). A particular concern was improving prediction. Psychologists were interested in improving their rate of accurate prediction, especially in regard to serious matters such as the potential for suicide. They hoped to predict whether or not a person was likely to commit suicide, given particular personality characteristics, history, or behaviors, and thus to be better able to prevent such acts.

With the notion of prediction came the discussion typically referred to as "clinical versus statistical prediction" (Meehl, 1954). This was a debate about whether physicians' clinical judgments were superior, or inferior, to diagnoses made using statistical probabilities generated from records of numerous cases. Of course, both types of analysis are important.

Today, three somewhat different types of research are conducted on clinical reasoning in medicine. One is concerned with identifying the *cognitive processes* that physicians employ when making clinical judgments. This type of research is essentially psychological research and is generally referred to as medical problem solving. The work of Elstein, Shulman, and Sprafka (1978) is central to this area of research.

The other two types of research on clinical reasoning among physicians rely heavily on the use of computers. They are medical decision making (decision analysis) and artificial intelligence. Medical decision-making research is an extension and elaboration of the original actuarial or "statistical" research developed by Meehl (1954) and others, and develops databases relative to the statistical probabilities of a disease being present, or treatment being effective, given various other factors.

Artificial intelligence research, or "modeling" of expert decision making, is elaborate, expensive research aimed at developing sophisticated computerized programs for ideal decision making. This seems to us to have very little bearing on occupational therapy and so will not be further discussed in this book. The *medical problem-solving literature* will be the primary focus of this discussion.

THE PURPOSE OF MEDICAL PROBLEM SOLVING

Reasoning in medicine has long been characterized as a three-part process involving diagnosis, prognosis, and treatment. The physician's most essential task is diagnosis. Diagnosis is often a search for invisible causes of diseases and discomforts; it is an attempt to identify a hidden source of a problem. Since one cannot see the the disease directly, one searches for "manifestations" of the disease. These manifestations have typically been cast in two broad categories: signs and symptoms. Early research in medical problem solving was based on an assumption that diagnosis is more or less an elaborate matching task. Researchers attempted to track physicians' thinking processes as they took medical histories, sought signs, identified symptoms, and matched these to particular diseases or organ dysfunctions. The better diagnosticians were thought to be those who were familiar with a greater array of medical conditions and who could readily match lists of signs and symptoms to those conditions. Identification of signs and symptoms was, and still is, "thought of as a critical task in medical problem solving" (Kessera, 1990). Diagnosis is the foremost task of the expert physician.

Today there are many devices, procedures, and laboratory tests that enable physicians to literally "see" what could not previously be seen. There are laboratory tests that can identify all sorts of minute aspects of the person's biochemical condition. It may seem that such advances would make the diagnostic process easier, because the physician is no longer dependent only on memory and sensory cues to make a diagnosis. But this additional information places even more weight on the physician's ability to process and manipulate that information. Therefore, research in diagnostic reasoning has shifted away from the assumption that clinical judgment is a matching skill and views this more as a process of analysis. Both signs and symptoms are called "cues" in the medical problem-solving literature. Cues may be arranged in differing patterns and subjected to various interpretations. Analysis and interpretation have become an even more important task, now that more conditions are known and more measurements of physical elements are possible.

A second, critical problem-solving task is prognosis, or prediction of the likely course of the disease. Two important features of the early and current work in studying prognosis or prediction are the recognition of the importance of hypothetical reasoning and the usefulness of generating and evaluating statistical probabilities. In much of the medical decision-making research, probabilities are calculated, recorded, and modified to guide physicians' thinking about probability that a person with a given set of symptoms, demographic characteristics, or history has a particular disease or condition. Probabilities are also calculated for risks and survival rates given various treatments at particular stages of the disease, or considering other aspects of the person's overall physical condition, such as nutritional status or the presence of other medical or environmental factors. Demographic characteristics such as gender, age, and ethnic origin.are also relevant factors.

Treatment is the ultimate goal of medical intervention and, in clinical medicine, is the third traditional step in the reasoning process. Treatment selection is guided by the physician's own cognitive processes and is usually enhanced by statistical information regarding the effectiveness of a particular intervention, in light of the various characteristics of the patient and the disease. The possibilities for treatment selection, too, have increased over the years, as new treatments are developed and tested. Again, analysis has become more important than simple recall in all aspects of medical problem solving.

Problem Identification and Problem Solving

PROBLEM SOLVING AND GOALS

Newell and Simon (1972) view problem solving as a goal-oriented activity. "A person is confronted with a problem when he wants something and does not know immediately what series of actions he can perform to get it" (p. 72). They comment that the "desired object" can be tangible or abstract, and the actions can be physical, perceptual, or mental. They are primarily interested in problem solving that involves mental rather than physical solutions and remark, "the critical activities, at least in human problem solving of any complexity, are symbol manipulating activities" (p. 72). They attempt to break the process down into smaller elements.

> Instead of defining directly what it means most generally for a human to have a problem . . . let us try the following strategy. To have a problem implies (at least) that certain information is given to the problem solver; information about what is desired, under what conditions, by means of

what tools and operations, starting with what initial formulation, and with access to what resources. The problem solver has an interpretation of this information—exactly that interpretation which lets us label some of it as a goal, another part as side conditions, and so on. (p. 73)

It may be useful for us to dissect this representation of the aspects of problem solving in order to gain a fuller understanding of it. There are several elements to the problem situation and its potential solution. They seem to be

1. The person's initial *perception* of a problem. The person recognizes that something is needed or wanted. This may be information, an object, and so on.
2. The *goal*. This is a clearer representation of what it is that the person needs or wants.
3. *Information*. The person has some information that can be brought to bear on the problem, or seeks additional information.
4. *Resources*. The person has internal resources such as information or concepts stored in memory. There also may be external resources from which additional information, objects, or assistance may be gathered.
5. *Means*. The person has intellectual, motor, and perceptual skills and intellectual operations that are used to gather additional information, objects and so on.
6. *Actions*. The person has the skill and ability to take particular actions toward reaching the goal.

Problem solving may take place entirely within the mind of the problem solver, or may require transportation of information and objects from external sources. Problem solving can be entirely abstract or may include some observable action.

TASK ENVIRONMENT AND PROBLEM SPACE

Newell and Simon also proposed the concepts of "task environment" and "problem space" as elements of problem solving. The term "task *environment* . . . refers to an environment coupled with a goal, problem, or task. It is the task that defines a point of view about an environment" (p. 55). By environment, they mean the real (concrete) environment. The situation as it is, "the environment itself" (p. 56). The task takes place in a particular environment.

"Problem space" refers to the individual's "internal representation of the task environment" (p. 59). This is a process of interpreting the problem and mentally structuring an understanding of it. Newell and Simon hypothesized that problem solvers store and retrieve information based on how they characterized or categorized that information in the first place. They felt that a person imagines a problem and/or its resolution to exist in a conceptual space, the problem space. They comment about "problem space" in the following paragraph.

> We need to describe the space in which problem solving activities take place. We will call it the *problem space.* . . .This is not a space that can yet be pointed to and described as an objective fact for a human subject. An attempt at describing it amounts, again, to constructing a representation of the task environment—the subject's representation in this case. The subject in an experiment is presented with a set of instructions and a sequence of stimuli. He must encode these problem components— defining goals, rules, and other aspects of the situation—in some kind of space that represents the initial situation presented to him, the desired goal situation, various intermediate states, imagined or experienced, as well as any concepts he uses to describe these situations to himself. (p. 59)

The distinction between the task environment and the person's representation of it is a useful one for understanding the sometimes complex interaction between the *problem representation* and the *problem-solving* skills of the individual who attempts to interpret the situation in the external world given the information available.

PROBLEM SPACE IN MEDICAL PROBLEM-SOLVING LITERATURE

The notion of "problem space" has been incorporated into the medical problem-solving literature in a way that seems to include both Newell and Simon's concept of a mental space, or category in which the person assumes the problem exists, as well as the concept of physical space. Feinstein (1973a,b, 1974) suggested that the physician should imagine the body to be divided into particular systems and subsystems, each occupying a particular space, for example, chest cavity, abdomen, cranium, and so forth. Feinstein recommended that physicians organize their analysis of medical problems so that they first identify the general area or system to be considered, and then direct their thoughts to ever more specific subsystems in a descending hierarchy, a process leading to increased specificity of the locus of the problem.

Elstein and colleagues (1978) use the notion of locating the problem space in both senses: the *cognitive space* in which individuals have organized their stock of knowledge, and the *body space* or *organ system* or *physiological process* in which the specific medical problem may be located. They propose that early cue gathering and hypothesis generation are an attempt to locate the appropriate problem space, both physically and conceptually.

Types of Problem Solving

RECOGNIZING THE ANSWER VERSUS SEEKING A SOLUTION

Newell and Simon (1972) were interested in creating models of human problem solving that would be applicable to physicians and other experts. After considerable research they proposed that there are three main methods of problem solving: the recognition method, the generate-and-test method, and the heuristic search method. They proposed that individuals either immediately recognize a problem and the answer, or else they have to think about it. Recognition, they say, is "one universal method of solving problems—by recognizing the answer" (p. 94).

> Recognition processes are important for solving problems, but not because they can be used for solving hard problems. . . . They are important because problem solving often proceeds by reduction: a hard problem is solved by replacing it with ostensibly easier problems. (p. 95)

When one has to think about problems and search for solutions, Newell and Simon suggest that two strategies are useful. One is the generate-and-test method, the other is heuristic search. These will be discussed later in the chapter. The concept of recognition has been elaborated by other researchers to include not only simple recognition, as in "recognizing the answer," but also to recognizing aspects of the problem. This is generally referred to as pattern recognition.

PATTERN RECOGNITION

Recognition, sometimes called pattern recognition (Coughlin & Patel, 1987), is a problem-solving strategy commonly used by many types of practitioners (Schön, 1983). It is especially useful in the *problem identification* phase of problem solving. Research in pattern recognition as an element of problem solving goes back at least to World War II, when the Department of the Navy did extensive research on what was then called "signal detection" (Swets, Tanner, & Birdsall, 1961). People's abilities to perceive patterns and to develop them into images of a possible whole are also the focus of other research, especially Gestalt psychology. For the sake of this discussion we will limit ourselves to studies of pattern recognition in medical and health-related professions, even though there are many useful insights into pattern recognition in other bodies of literature.

There is evidence that physicians' expertise in pattern recognition improves diagnostic accuracy (Papa, Shores, & Mayer, 1990; Norman, Rosenthal, Brooks, Allen, & Muzzin, 1989). Pattern recognition is similar to Newell and Simon's concept of recognition; however, the term is often used to refer to the specialized form of recognition that experts have developed through years of experience. Experts immediately recognize a problem without having to analyze single aspects of the problem configuration; they "recognize" this pattern as representing an instance of a familiar problem or category of problem. Much of the academic portion of the education of health professionals is aimed at describing these patterns, usually called "clinical conditions." Much of clinical education helps the student to recognize these patterns in real patients (Cohn, 1989). Pattern recognition is thought to be the ability to observe a phenomenon quickly and perceive a configuration of features as a representation of a particular entity.

In reading the literature, one has the impression that either there are two different interpretations of how the process works, or there are two types of pattern recognition. One interpretation is that people perceive patterns as a whole. The other is that patterns are perceived as sums of parts. Those who take the latter point of view seem to propose that people observe a phenomenon and select particular features of it that are perceived to be relevant. These features are referred to in the literature as "cues." The features are interpreted as being both important to identifying the phenomenon, and related to each other in some way. Since in medicine, as in other types of problem solving, the task is to see the observable behavior or physical characteristic and infer a relationship to an invisible process, the relationship between cues in a perceived pattern is considered important. Medical students are taught about diseases and diagnoses through lectures, slides, and observations that focus on describing the particular features (cues) and patterns that are "manifestations" of particular diseases or processes. Several researchers theorize that this process serves to develop "templates" (Hammond, 1988) or "holons" (Koestler, 1967) in the student's mind, which are stored in memory and then called upon later to match to a particular perceived pattern in a patient. Coughlin and Patel (1987) have proposed that if this diagnostic information is presented in the same pattern and sequence as was learned, and to which the student or physician has become accustomed, diagnostic accuracy is improved. If the same information is presented in a different pattern, however, identifying it is much more difficult. In this chapter we will assume that pattern recognition is the ability to

1. Observe a phenomenon.
2. Identify significant characteristics (cues).
3. Perceive a relationship among the cues (a configuration).
4. Compare the present configuration to a previously learned category or type (template).

A sequence such as that below is often offered as a diagrammatic illustration of the events in pattern recognition.

$$\text{OBSERVE} \rightarrow \begin{matrix} \text{IDENTIFY} \\ \text{CUES} \end{matrix} \rightarrow \begin{matrix} \text{PERCEIVE} \\ \text{CONFIGURATION} \end{matrix} \rightarrow \text{COMPARE TO TYPE}$$

This simple sequence does not adequately reflect the actual number of events in pattern recognition, nor does such recognition actually proceed in a strict linear sequence. Many cues can be part of more than one pattern. A person usually does not follow this sequence literally, but imagines several possible configurations of the cues, then mentally arranges and rearranges them into several possible known patterns, and compares and contrasts these with a variety of learned types of templates. The pattern recognition form of reasoning is a more complex process than can be illustrated by a linear progression such as that shown above. Good pattern recognition seems to include a shifting of attention among sets of cues and then a mental reconfiguring of them in several potential patterns until a "best fit" between the possible patterns presented and the learned templates is perceived. It seems to require not simple recognition of wholes, but a willingness to remain attentive to subtleties and to entertain a variety of possibilities as to how given parts or cues may contribute to a variety of patterns.

THE GENERATE-AND-TEST METHOD

Newell and Simon state that the generate-and-test method is a "set-predicate formulation" (1972, p. 92). To "predicate" means "to affirm as a quality or an attribute or a property of a person or thing, or affirm or base (something on or upon given facts, argument, conditions, etc.)" (Webster, p. 1121). So, a set-predicate formulation is simply a matter of affirming that some object, characteristic, and so on, is a legitimate member of a particular set. Newell and Simon comment that this type of problem involves

> being given a set and the goal of producing or determining a member of a subset of that set—this latter identified most generally by a test that can be performed on the elements of the set. (pp. 95–96)

Thus it seems that the generate-and-test method involves fewer steps. One way to characterize these may be to

1. **Identify** (or perceive) a problem.
2. **Locate** a set (space) in which the problem potentially lies.
3. **Generate** potential **subset(s)** of items that may be legitimate members of the set.
4. **Identify inclusion criteria** for legitimate membership in the set.

5. **Test** the attributes of the problem to determine if they meet the inclusion criteria.
6. **Select** members of the proposed subset that conform to the inclusion criteria.
7. **Predicate** (affirm) that these attributes are indeed members of the subset.

Newell and Simon give an example of a simple generate-and-test problem-solving event:

> An extra chair is needed from the living room to seat an additional guest at dinner. Here the set is small (say four chairs) and accessible; furthermore the test is rapid (reject large stuffed chairs, reject tacky chairs, any others will do). (p. 97)

Although this is offered as an example, it might be useful to be more precise about how it illustrates this type of problem solving. Using the steps above, we can analyze the example as seen in Table 7–1.

TABLE 7 · 1 Analysis of Generate-and-Test Problem-Solving Event

Step	Example
1. Identify problem.	I need one more dining chair.
2. Generate set.	All potential dining chairs.
3. Identify subset.	The chairs in the house which could serve as dining chairs.
4. Inclusion criteria.	A dining chair must be moveable, of sufficient height, have a relatively straight back, and be attractive.
5. The test.	Evaluate (look at) each living-room chair to see if it meets the selection criteria.
6. Select members of subset.	Any chairs that seem to meet these criteria. (Suppose there are two such chairs in the living room.)
7. Predicate.	Decide that these two chairs are legitimate members of the subset. Grab one of the two chairs.

The generate-and-test method usually requires that the person generate or identify several sets in which solutions may be found, and that each set and each potential solution be tested. Thus, most problems are solved, not by going through the above sequence once, but several times. Clearly it is important to identify the appropriate set in which the problem lies. It is also important to know and carefully apply the inclusion criteria. Medical diagnosis, for example is a set-predicate (or generate-and-test) process whereby the physician attempts to identify the set in which the patient's problem lies. Given the symptoms and history, the physician identifies the set of which this particular condition may be a subset. So she or he inquires, "Is this a disease? A degenerative process? A reaction to some substance?" and so forth.

HEURISTIC SEARCH

Heuristic search is a similar strategy, except that more cues are sought before hypotheses are generated. The term "heuristic" means to invent or discover. It also means to use rules of thumb to find solutions or answers (Webster, p. 659). Often, when people use the term heuristic, there is an implication that there is a search for a path, such as using rules of thumb like "moss grows on the north side of trees," or the "sun sets in the west," to find a new path through the woods. In heuristic search, the search is for the best path to the solution. Newell and Simon speak of heuristic search "as a path from the initial element in the problem space to the desired element" (1972, p. 98). In heuristic search, new hypotheses are generated, not simply recalled from past experience. Often the problem is perceived as a novel problem, and not as one that easily stimulates the memory of a standard hypothesis. Frequently, several interrelated chains of hypotheses are strung together in the person's mind to try to account for a new or unusual condition or set of problems. Sometimes there is a greater focus on the search for solution than on identification of the cause. Heuristic search is usually employed to solve problems with which the person is unfamiliar. It is also useful in seeking novel solutions to a familiar problem, or in reanalyzing a problem in a new way. Heuristic search, when successful, usually results in the person discovering something new. This may be something new altogether, but is usually something new to this person. For example, a person may be familiar with a condition but feels the characterization or explanation of it is insufficient. The person then analyzes the problem using the heuristic search method to develop a better model of the problem, to achieve insight into it, or to find a better solution. Since occupational therapy is often a process of inventing a particular solution for the individual patient, OTs often use the heuristic search method in the problem resolution phase of problem solving.

A FOUR-STAGE MODEL OF MEDICAL INQUIRY

Procedural reasoning usually begins with problem identification. Much of the research that has been conducted regarding problem solving in medicine has focused primarily on the diagnostic, or problem identification, phase of problem solving. Elstein, Shulman, and Sprafka (1978) identified what they referred to as a "four-stage general model of medical inquiry" (p. 277). This focuses primarily on the diagnostic phase of problem solving by medical students and physicians. The four stages are "cue acquisition, hypothesis generation, cue interpretation, and hypothesis evaluation" (p. 277).

A sequence of useful steps to analyzing problems is discussed throughout their book, *Medical Problem Solving: An Analysis of Clinical Reasoning*, and is summarized below.

1. *Cue Acquisition*

Elstein, Shulman, and Sprafka refer to cue acquisition as

> the process of collecting data in clinical problem solving. Medical problems differ from many others traditionally used by psychologists to study problem solving, in that all the information needed to solve the medical problem is typically unavailable at the start. Consequently, medical problems are not usually solved by restructuring or drawing implications from available information, as are so many puzzles in the Gestalt tradition. Not only must one go beyond the information given by employing logical inference, but one must also go gather data at certain specific points. Effective cue acquisition proceeds according to a plan that permits and facilitates selective data acquisition. (1978, p. 277)

First, the careful practitioner identifies cues. These may be bits of the patient's history, or a present report of feelings, physical indicators (such as a rash), or reports from laboratory tests. Cues are gathered and at that time the physician does not evaluate them or hypothesize about them. They are collected as separate elements, as if on a list. They may begin to "fall into patterns" in the practitioner's mind, because of prior knowledge of clinical conditions, but there is often a conscious choice to suspend interpretation of the cues until all relevant cues are gathered.

Good Cue Identification Skills

There are several important aspects to good cue identification skills that the Elstein group and others have discussed. Some of these are

- A practitioner should gather several cues without wasting time searching for every possible cue. This is a matter of gathering enough cues, but it is difficult to know how many are enough.
- A practitioner should also be able to determine which cues are relevant, irrelevant, central, or peripheral. This is not easy to do, and the skill is apparently acquired through experience. The ability to judge the relevance or centrality of a cue is what Benner (1984) refers to as having a "sense of salience."
- A third judgment the practitioner must make is the relative importance of a cue. This is sometimes referred to as giv-

ing "weight" to a cue. The weight of a cue has to do with its importance in signaling a particular clinical condition. The practitioner asks how important is this cue in making the diagnosis. Some cues are relatively "light-weight" cues. For example, nausea and vomiting are common cues. They are a strong cue that the person is sick, but they are common to a great number of problems and are therefore relatively weak cues when it comes to determining a particular diagnosis.

- Cue gathering is not a passive activity. The cues are gathered with the aim of detecting and later evaluating them. They are made within the context of a vast knowledge base ready to be accessed. They are gathered within the clinician's perspective. Taking an open-minded perspective on the problem often increases the person's ability to perceive or gather numerous cues.

- Cue recognition is greatly influenced by prior knowledge. Many cues are so subtle that they are not perceived by the untrained eye. Conversely, innumerable cues become obvious signals to the experienced practitioner. Some of these cues can be described or communicated in technical verbal terms, but many are part of the clinician's stock of prior knowledge.

2. Hypothesis Generation

The practitioner next creates possible hypotheses about potential relationships among the cues and/or the relationship of cues to possible diseases or physiological disturbances. At this hypothesis generation stage, the most successful problem solvers generate several hypotheses. Hypotheses will pose a relationship between the observed cue and some underlying process. The Elstein group posit that "hypotheses are retrieved from memory with a goal in mind" (1978, p. 45).

Several sorts of hypothetical relationships are possible. Examples include

- An hypothesis posing a *causal relationship,* such as a cue caused by the condition itself. For example, the cue "fever" or "elevated white blood count" is a sign of infection. Therefore, the cue "fever" is caused by the condition "infection."

- An hypothesis postulating *an association,* such as a cue that is a result of a disrupted physiologic process that is secondary to the actual cause. For example, spots appear on the skin of children who have chicken pox. The cue "spots" is a result of disruptions to the child's system and were caused by this particular type of infection.

- A hypothesis posing a *situational relationship*. For example, an elevated blood pressure is a result of the person's anxiety over his physical condition, not the condition itself.
- The *null hypothesis*, that is, the cue is not related to the disease.

The hypotheses should be "held in abeyance" and not evaluated immediately. Good diagnosticians can hold multiple possible hypotheses in their minds at the same time. Each is temporarily held "suspended" in the mind while the practitioner carefully evaluates each one systematically. This is done through processes Elstein, Shulman, and Sprafka refer to as "cue interpretation and hypothesis evaluation."

3. Cue Interpretation

The practitioner selects one of the previously generated hypotheses in order to reevaluate the cues, asking "Will these cues make sense if this hypothesis is legitimate?" Then, the next hypothesis is selected and the cues reevaluated. This process takes place (rapidly), until some cues or patterns of cues seem to be much more important than others. These cues are examined individually, as potential elements in the hypothesized patterns.

4. Hypothesis Evaluation

Next, the clinician rearranges the question and asks which of these sets of cues best supports the remaining viable hypotheses. An hypothesis is judged to be important if it seems to be supported by (1) the presence of cues thought to be central and/or necessary for determining a diagnosis of the hypothesized disease or (2) nonabsence of critical symptoms or cues. In addition, the hypothesis is evaluated for its own plausibility and potential veracity.

STRUCTURAL FEATURES OF INITIAL PROBLEM FORMULATIONS

Chapter 7 of Elstein, Shulman, and Spafraka is based on the doctoral dissertation of Linda Allal, who identified four features of the structural organization of what she called "initial problem formulations" (1978, p. 176). She states, "We may propose that a set of problem formulations defines the dimensions of the functional problem space in which a physician's search for a diagnosis is conducted" (p. 176). These features seem to be very useful in understanding problem solving at a detailed level and to be particularly relevant to the kinds of problem solving that occupational therapists engage in; consequently, we have included most of Allal's description of these structural features (Fig. 7–1). Of these four features, only "competing formulations" was present in all instances studied. "Functional relationships" (pp. 176–177) was employed the least often of the four features. This is not surprising as it is a more conceptually complex task.

One characteristic of reasoning common to all the physicians and medical students by Elstein et al. was "generation and evaluation of competing hypotheses" (1978, p. 148). Physicians always looked for more than one potential cause of the problem presented. They devoted a considerable portion of their reasoning efforts to seeking additional cues and rearranging hypotheses in their minds, in order to either support or negate more than one possible cause of the presenting ailment. This is probably because medical education is structured specifically to encourage competing hypothesis generation. Such competing hypotheses are useful for keeping the thinker focused on the task of interpreting cues and evaluating hypotheses and avoiding any tendency to settle too soon on a favorite hypothesis.

Procedural Reasoning in Occupational Therapy

GOALS, PROBLEM SPACE, AND TASK ENVIRONMENT IN OCCUPATIONAL THERAPY

Problem identification and resolution in occupational therapy is goal-directed. The overall goal, as we have stated before, is to help the person function as well as possible in everyday tasks, given the consequences of the disease or disability. Particular goals for individual patients are important directors of problem solving by occupational therapists and their patients.

Occupational therapists are willing to examine a wide variety of potential problem spaces to identify potential sources of a problem or its solution. In fact, they see part of their professional task as one of addressing "all areas of concern." They typically analyze a problem by considering factors in many problem spaces, such as cognitive, emotional, cultural, neurological, and situational aspects of the person.

The task environment of occupational therapists is a bit nebulous. The therapist addresses the patient's problems and develops solutions in the task environment of the hospital, but these solutions are expected to be carried out later in the home environment. This is sometimes not

Structural Features. An examination of the physician data indicated that the result of the physician's information-processing activity during the early part of the workup is not a undimensional list of problem formulations. Rather, it is a structured set of formulations that may be described in terms of four features: hierarchal organization, competing formulations, multiple subspaces, and functional relationships.

A. *Hierarchal organization.* A set of problem formulations may include formulations organized into a general-to-specific hierarchy that pertains to a single diagnostic category (an organ system or a disease mechanism, for instance). A physician may generate a problem formulation such as gastrointestinal (GI) disorder and, as subcategories under this formulation, one or several more specific formulations such as inflammatory bowel disease or intestinal malignancy, or both.

B. *Competing formulations.* A set of problem formulations may include some that provide alternative explanations for some group of symptoms. For example, a physician may generate inflammatory bowel disease and intestinal malignancy as competing problem formulations.

C. *Multiple subspaces.* A set of problem formulations may include subsets of formulations that pertain to different types of diagnostic categories (such as different organ systems or different disease mechanisms). Each of these categories may be considered to designate a subspace within the functional problem space in which the physician is operating. For example, a physician may generate a set of formulations that consist of four subspaces: GI disorder, diabetes mellitus, anemia, or cardiovascular problem.

D. *Functional relationships.* A set of initial problem formulations may include functional relationships that the physician hypothesized to exist between certain problem formulations. For example, a physician may consider anemia to be secondary to GI disorder.

FIGURE 7 ▪ 1. Linda Allal's four features of the structural organization of problem formulations. (From Elstein et al., Medical Problem Solving, copyright 1978, Harvard University Press. Reprinted with permission.)

effective because the solutions the therapist devised in the hospital may not necessarily work at home. A classic example for many practitioners is a typical scenario of the person with an upper extremity amputation. Often, professionals spend time constructing a prosthesis for a person and go through lengthy training sessions with the person.

The person then returns home and finds the prosthesis cumbersome and uncomfortable. The person abandons the prosthesis, learns to perform many activities with one hand and the stump, and dons the prosthesis only for a formal occasion, such as a wedding. The therapist in these situations might have better spent the treatment time helping the person to do one-handed activities in the first place.

The task environment in which occupational therapists work is often only a "stand-in" for the task environment in which the actual problems of daily living need to be solved. This is a problem that therapists often point out when they are complaining about the "shortened length of stay" necessitated by some reimbursement systems. They feel that, not only do they not have enough time to teach patients what they need to teach them, but that also there is not enough time for the repetition necessary to ensure that there is "transfer" of the skills learned to the home environment.

PATTERN RECOGNITION

Like all experienced practitioners, senior occupational therapists often recognize familiar patterns instantly. They do not have to subject the pattern to any particular analytical skill or process of inquiry. For example, a pediatric therapist instantly recognizes a child's posture and movement patterns as those produced by cerebral palsy. The therapist needs only a quick glance at the child to recognize the characteristic movement pattern. Usually, this sort of pattern is recognized as a whole and not as a combination of individual cues.

In other instances, patterns may be recognized, but some analysis or interpretation is required. This involves consideration of the cues in relation to a known pattern or type of physiognomy, or behavior, or both. For example, a therapist may observe a person behaving in an unusual or socially inappropriate manner. The therapist would not necessarily be able to tell immediately whether the behavior was a result of a psychotic process, confusion, or apraxia. A therapist gave an example of this from her experience.

> I was doing an ADL evaluation with a lady who had been newly admitted. She was slow, but doing OK. Then she took her hair brush and raised it off the bedside table and put it in her mouth. I didn't know what to think of this. Then I saw the look of righteous indignation on her face. She was more surprised at this behavior than I was. Then I realized this must be apraxia. She had motor planning problems. She expected to brush her hair but the motor plan that was actually triggered was for tooth brushing.

Pattern recognition is important for all clinicians because it makes practice more efficient. If a professional can quickly recognize a problem or condition, then he or she can move into deeper levels of analysis more quickly, and move on to the problem resolution or treatment phase.

As useful as pattern recognition is, it is also important to know that this is not simply an automatic process. The ability to recognize many patterns of cues and behaviors quickly becomes part of the proficient therapist's fund of tacit knowledge (Polanyi, 1966). Practitioners need to both trust and question their pattern recognition skills. Therapists need to be attentive to many features of their patients' problems and to continue to learn to recognize new, more subtle, and more complex cues and patterns throughout their lifetime of practice. Below are two examples of pattern recognition. In the first example, the therapist, Marie, is simply communicating some of the behavior patterns of a child with cerebral palsy, with whom she worked in a public school setting. These patterns are so familiar to her (and, she expects, to the occupational therapists who would read her story) that they are simply "taken for granted" in her narration of the story:

> I usually arrive at Jackie's classroom as he is finishing math. I greet him where he is seated in his electric wheelchair with his aide nearby. Once he spots me, he often goes into a total extensor pattern. He usually does this when he is interrupted or excited, and he begins to maneuver his chair erratically, upsetting the group around him. Sometimes he giggles and screeches (overflow), and by now the entire room has been disturbed and the teacher looks perplexed. As the school year passed, Jackie's movements became slightly less erratic and he was able to leave the classroom with less fanfare. Jackie knew that once he was in the corridor he was responsible for good, safe driving. Typically, he did not demonstrate the head and upper extremity control needed for lengthy trips in the chair. Extensor and reflexive patterns often interfered. A crowded hallway continued to be a disaster for most of the year. Increased muscle tone, reflexes, et cetera, often made wheelchair operation very difficult. After direction, and sometimes redirection, Jackie slowly made his way through the hall. I was often witness to some of his best driving performances because he knew it was what I was watching for. In the hallway, we often encountered a variety of circumstances, such as kids stopping to pat Jackie on the head or touch his wheelchair or ask me a question about him.

This example is simply an introduction to a clinical story that Marie wrote. As a means of introducing the reader to the child, Marie notes eight patterns that are typical of children with cerebral palsy: extensor pattern, overflow, erratic movements, limited head control, limited use of upper extremity, reflex patterns, increased muscle tone, and distractibility. These are mentioned not as a description of the clinical condition, but to paint for the readers (other occupational therapists) a picture of the child and the events in the day that the child and the therapist shared. They provide us with an illustration of pattern recognition. They also illustrate how much pattern recognition is a part of therapists' everyday working knowledge or tacit knowledge. This is an example of the sort of pattern that can be taught fairly easily. Classroom descriptions in a clinical conditions course, and observations or videotapes, would probably serve to introduce the student to the pattern. Other patterns are more subtle and require lengthy descriptions or more direct experience.

CASE EXAMPLE

The next example is taken from the story of an experienced therapist, Carol, working in a psychiatric hospital. She titled the story "My Worst Stuck Moment in Practice." This is an example of the sort of pattern recognition that comes only from experience and requires much more analysis. This is a story about a new patient included into a group that Carol generally leads along with another therapist who spends much more time with the patients on the wards. The other therapist was not there on that particular day and has not been able, as is their custom, to "fill Carol in" about new patients or events on the unit. Here, Carol comments about what happened part way through the group session.

My Worst Stuck Moment in Practice

by Carol _____

At this point, I noticed that Laura (a new patient) looked different. She had a blank, staring or fixed expression on her face. My first thought was that she was having a petit mal seizure. That thought was quickly abandoned when she began to grimace and have facial tics. I was not sure what was going on, but I didn't think it was a seizure. It went from bad to worse when she suddenly yelled out—the sound ripped through my chest. To say I was startled would be an understatement! Of course, I was concerned, but I was also feeling frightened and not sure what was going on. My heart was pounding, while outwardly I tried to appear calm and in control. I looked around at the others, and they appeared anxious. Laura tried to say something but was having immense trouble getting it out. I thought of a speech problem such as stuttering when someone can start a word but can't finish it. She said "I'm so fff. . .fff. . .fru. . .fru. . .fru. . .FRUSTRATED!" She rapidly repeated this, running her words together, "frustratedfrustratedfrustrated-FRUSTRATED," emphasizing each word with rapid side-to-side shakes of her head. After a fashion, she was able to slowly, painfully express herself (her goal) and explain to us that she has Tourette's syndrome and that when she "stuffs it" or holds her feelings in, the only way she can get rid of them is to "go with the flow," so to speak. She continued to try to "express it," while I was thinking that it doesn't seem to be helping at all. She appeared more agitated; she was getting louder; and any minute I expected someone from Security would be knocking at the door to investigate what's going on in the gym. I asked her if it might be helpful to return to the unit for medication.

"No," she said, "the doctor is trying to treat this behaviorally because she thinks it's OCD." I desperately tried to remember the class where they talked about Tourette's. All I can come up with are vague memories of a "Quincy" episode. I tried to return the focus to the activity.

Case Discussion

Here we see Carol, an experienced therapist, become a temporary "novice" (Benner, 1984) because she is faced with a situation that is new to her. Her commentary is very interesting because she simultaneously talks about her emotional reaction to the situation, as well as giving us some insight into her cognitive search for the classroom description of the typical pattern of this clinical condition. Interestingly, she searched another source, a television program she had once seen. Judging that to be an unreliable source, she wisely returned to coping with the situation in the here and now and learning about Tourette's syndrome later. Carol can hardly be faulted for not recognizing this very rare syndrome. The example is included here to emphasize the usefulness of pattern recognition and the importance of experience in developing pattern recognition skills.

NONEXCLUSIVE CUES AND PATTERNS

Therapists are taught to recognize many patterns. In clinical practice these patterns become more vivid to therapists because they see actual patients exhibiting the patterns. Therapists learn to recognize fine nuances of these behavioral patterns as their experience increases. This refined pattern recognition is especially useful in cases where a particular configuration of cues may be present in more than one diagnosis or clinical condition. In these instances, particular cues are not in the exclusive domain of a given condition. They may also not be exclusive to a particular problem space.

CASE EXAMPLE

Below is an example of a therapist's reasoning about a patient who exhibited cues that could be present in more than one clinical condition. The therapist's ability to assess the *quality* of the patient's movement patterns and his affect lead her to a deeper insight into the clinical problem.

Conflicting Cues

by Sonja Bradburn

An elderly, widowed, Caucasian man was admitted with the diagnosis of major depression. His concerned children brought him to the psychiatric unit because they were afraid that he might commit suicide because he had become so listless, and wished to die. In the past he had taken great pride in caring for his home and cooking meals for his girlfriend. For no apparent reason, he had become more depressed and sedentary, with a loss of interest for all previous activities. Now most of his days were spent in a recliner chair. Their acute awareness of his current useless state completely overwhelmed both him and his children.

I first met this patient in the hallway. He stood alone in the unit crossroad, between the dining area and the nurse's station. He was well dressed and groomed with the exception of noticeable dandruff. Lunch was over, so all of the other patients had left the area. Meal times are short because patients usually retreat to the safety of their rooms before treatment groups begin again.

I introduced myself by name and extended my hand to him. He hesitated for a few seconds while looking into my eyes, then firmly shook my hand and pleaded for help to return home. His anxious voice did not match the flat, almost masklike affect. This odd combination of anxiety and a blank facial expression reminded me of a previous home health patient of mine. We walked to the interview room together. His slow, stop-and-start, shuffling gait clearly did not seem like psychomotor retardation from an affective disorder. Some side effects of antipsychotic medication can mimic Parkinson-like symptoms in some patients, but this was the first psychiatric hospitalization for this man. He had never taken antipsychotics. Even before we reached the interview room, I suspected that this man might have more than just major depression.

When I asked about his self-care and home management he said, "I feel tired all the time. Lately I don't seem to have the motivation to do anything at all. It seems that I'm taking the corners more slowly. . . . Maybe I'm getting too old."

He seemed to be a good historian, clearly describing symptoms of depression with a passive wish to die. He was very depressed about his increased difficulty to be productive, and therefore had lost motivation to work. Losses in some form often precipitate prolonged grief reactions and a major depressive episode. In this case, it appeared that his loss was the ease of movement.

Immediately after the interview, I recommended a referral for neurology, which later proved to confirm my suspicion that he had Parkinson's disease.

Case Discussion

In this story Sonja recognizes cues and patterns that make her question the diagnosis of major depression. One of the cues is "slow gait" or "psychomotor retardation." This behavior or cue might be produced by depression, but it might be caused by some other disturbance. So slow gait is not an exclusive cue. It may be present in any number of conditions. She also sees patterns, such as the "anxious voice," that seem to be in conflict with the assumption that this is depression. Here, she questions whether the configuration of cues—slow gait, sadness, and anxious voice—represent a pattern that is common in major depression. While psychomotor problems such as slow gait can accompany depression, Sonja notes the the *quality* of his gait is not like the quality of the gait patterns of other depressed patients whom she has known. She sees this and other patterns of behavior that remind her of patterns that she has seen in patients with Parkinson's disease. She then returns to the notion of depression and reasons that possibly his depression is related to his diminished energy and motor capacity, which in turn were caused by the Parkinson's disease. Sonja did not just accept the diagnosis of "major depression" and close off her observational skills and clinical reasoning. She observed cues and questioned their meaning and their relationship to one another. She noticed their patterns and matched these patterns to what she had seen previously with patients with this and other diagnoses. She maintained an open mind and a sense of inquiry. She then thought that the depression that she and other staff members had observed was not the primary ailment, but it was secondary to the Parkinson's disease.

This story illustrates at least *three* important aspects of cue interpretation and pattern recognition.

1. The need to search multiple subspaces. The cue, "slow gait," would have been interpreted as just a slow gait, or a gait that was slow because of a number of other reasons. Such reasons might have been
   - He was cautious, fearful, or both, and purposefully moved at a slow pace. This too would be the emotional subspace, but a different category of emotional problem.
   - He was tired, and therefore had little energy and was simply "dragging his feet." This would be a somewhat different subspace— fatigue.
   - He was depressed and this gait was due to "psychomotor retardation." This would be an example of searching the emotional subspace.
   - He had a neurologic problem that interfered with his motor production. This would be searching the subspace "neurological" with further specification of motor production, versus, for example, sensory difficulty.

Sonja interpreted this cue as neurologically based because the patient's slow gait resembled the particular shuffling gait of people with Parkinson's disease. Her past experience provided her with this qualitative, or nuanced, practical knowledge. She represents an excellent example of procedural reasoning because she searches many subspaces for templates or patterns that may match this particular person's gait pattern.

2. A sensitivity to competing cues. Sonja observed a "flat affect" in this man. Flat affect is a common cue or symptom of depression. However, she also noted "an anxious tone in his voice, a pleading for help to return home," and "eye contact," all of which are cues that are not particularly consistent with depression. Sonja noted the conflict when she commented, "His anxious voice did not match with the flat, almost masklike affect." She comments that this is an "*odd* combination." Here, by being sensitive to competing cues Sonja avoids four common errors in problem identification:
   - Settling too soon on an interpretation (or hypothesis).
   - Exclusion of relevant cues.
   - Failure to recognize the presence of cues that would negate or challenge the initial hypothesis.
   - Reinterpretation of cues to fit the early hypothesis.

3. Use of a qualitative interpretation of a cue. Sonja noticed two cues which, though present in both depression and Parkinson's disease, are *qualitatively* different in each. They were "flat affect" and "psychomotor retardation." By observing and interpreting these behavioral

patterns carefully and matching the nuances of these patterns to previously observed patterns, she "interprets" the cues as ones that support the Parkinson's hypothesis more strongly than the major depression hypothesis.

THE FOUR-STAGE MODEL OF PROBLEM SOLVING AND OCCUPATIONAL THERAPY

Occupational therapists also use the four-phase strategy proposed by Elstein, Shulman, and Sprafka (1978). This process moves beyond simple pattern recognition or matching, to a more analytical level, through the inclusion of hypothesis testing and evaluation. Here, the practitioner gathers cues (cue identification), forms them into potential patterns, and then advances two or more hypotheses about what the problem might be (hypothesis generation). The therapist then returns to an analysis of the cues in light of the hypotheses generated and rechecks the potential usefulness of the cues (cue interpretation). Finally, the hypotheses are reviewed and the most likely one selected (hypothesis evaluation).

For example, a therapist might ask a child to color a picture and observe that the child does not take the offered crayon and simply looks down, possibly at the paper. Given these two cues, "doesn't take the crayon" and "looks down," the therapist might generate the following hypotheses or questions:

> Is the child shy, afraid, embarrassed? (emotional space)
> Does she understand the task? Know how to color? (cognitive subspace)
> Is she deaf? (neurological space)

Since none of these questions or tentative hypotheses can be tested without further inquiry, the therapist takes additional action in order to elicit more cues and to interpret the initial ones. The therapist might try asking the child to take the crayon again, or might offer a different activity, or change position in relation to the child. Each of these variations in the therapist's behavior would be chosen to elicit some behavior on the part of the child, in order to support or reject one or more of the above hypotheses, or, in some cases, to construct new ones. When the therapist feels enough cues have been gathered to support a particular hypothesis, that hypothesis is held as a working hypothesis. Then the cues are again interpreted in light of that hypothesis (cue interpretation). In this hypothetical case, the therapist might have assumed that there was some emotional reason for the child's behavior. The therapist might try the request again, only this time using a more supportive tone of voice and perhaps changing posture slightly. If the child then proceeded to color, the therapist could assume that she had interpreted the cues correctly.

This, then, is a way of interpreting the emotional cues. If the child did not respond, however, the therapist would have to try another way of testing other hypotheses regarding those cues. The therapist might demonstrate what the child was expected to do—color a particular shape on the page, perhaps. If the child responded and colored a similar shape, the therapist would know that the child had not responded at first because she did not understand the task. The therapist still would not know whether this lack of understanding was a cognitive, language, or hearing problem. This would be a good time to move on to eliciting some more cues and advancing more precise hypotheses in the various cognitive subspaces. The therapists would try asking the child to do other tasks in order to determine whether she could hear, recognize simple English words, or understand commands, in order to interpret the new cues and evaluate the remaining hypotheses and any new ones.

STRUCTURAL FEATURES OF PROBLEM SOLVING IN OCCUPATIONAL THERAPY

Occupational therapists demonstrated all four structural features of problem solving as proposed by Allal (in Elstein et al., 1978). Later in this chapter we carefully analyze a problem-solving sequence by one therapist, in which all four of these features were displayed. First, we discuss some of these features individually. Generating competing formulations was a strategy commonly used by the occupational therapists. Experienced therapists in the Clinical Reasoning Study and others typically generated two to four possible hypotheses regarding the cause and nature of aspects of a person's problem. They generated several hypotheses about potential treatment activities as well. There was a tendency among the newer therapists to seek the "right answer" rather than to generate hypotheses, but they soon learned that thinking about the problem was more important than knowing what it was.

Case Example

Here is an example of competing hypothesis generation.

Jon

by Jane Clifford O'Brien

I work in a diagnostic outpatient clinic. Jon, a 26-month-old boy diagnosed as having cerebral palsy [CP], was referred to occupational therapy for evaluation of his poor motor development. The purpose of his evaluation at the clinic was to qualify him for services.

Jon came to the evaluation with his paternal great-grandmother (Doris) and grandmother (Bert) who care for him. Jon's mother had left him, so his grandmothers had taken over his care. His father lived with them. They were from rural South Carolina. They told me Jon rolled, sat up, walked, and started talking normally and then, at 15 months, he got sick and went to the hospital. The doctors said he had a stroke. He was hospitalized for a few weeks and then sent back home, where his grandmothers took up his care. In the early part of the interview Bert said that Jon seemed to be "getting worse." I wasn't sure whether she meant Jon himself was "getting worse," or whether it was becoming more difficult to care for him as he became larger. When I asked them what they thought was the problem, Doris said, "Everything was going well until he started teething." The first time I saw Jon, I did not question this comment, but continued to evaluate Jon's motor skills.

I completed his evaluation and, although he experienced tonal abnormalities, I did not feel he looked like a child who had only problems associated with stroke or cerebral palsy. Doris and Bert were concerned that Jon did not eat a lot and could not sit up independently. They did not know what to do with him and were having trouble handling such a large child. I provided Doris and Bert with techniques to improve Jon's feeding abilities and motor skills and made a follow-up appointment to measure Jon for a stroller.

I spoke with the physician who had evaluated Jon and reviewed his medical record. I told the physician I felt this child looked like something else was going on; his tone pattern was "different" than what is typical of stroke and CP.

The next visit, Bert and Doris said Jon was not eating as well as he did last time. They said he was more irritable. Doris said she was beginning to have back pain from lifting Jon. We ordered a Snug Seat for Jon. During our conversation, Bert said again that she was sad about Jon's condition because he was doing well until he started teething. I asked her to elaborate on this and documented exactly what she said in my notes. Doris came to the session towards the end, and I asked her the same questions. Doris agreed with Bert and said that Jon was walking when he left the hospital after having the stroke, and when he started teething he stopped walking, talking, started drooling more, and so on.

I reported this to the physician, but it was dismissed as information from poor historians.

The next visit we provided them with a Snug Seat. Jon was having a difficult time holding his head up. The techniques used in the first session to improve his feeding would not work and Jon was not able to do things he did at the first session. I spoke with the physicians at the clinic and we decided that since Jon was going to his primary care physician tomorrow, we could talk with him. I expressed concern that Jon was getting worse.

Jon was hospitalized for failure to thrive the next day. His diagnosis in the chart continued to be cerebral palsy. I visited with Bert and Doris, who stayed with him. I documented in the chart the history Bert had given me of his decline in functioning. One day Bert cried to me that she just wanted to know what was going on and showed me a picture of Jon at 20 months, walking. I suggested that she show the picture to the physician to show him that Jon had declined in functioning. After she showed them the picture they started evaluating Jon for progressive disorders.

Later that week, Jon was diagnosed with adrenoleukodystrophy. This is a very rare condition. Jon got worse rapidly and died shortly thereafter. Bert and Doris thanked me for staying with them through the process. It made me realize the importance of listening carefully to the caretakers.

Case Discussion

Here Jane, the therapist, illustrates the concept of competing hypothesis generation, or competing formulations. This is a tricky situation and one not necessarily likely to induce competing hypothesis generation, because Jon already had a diagnosis—two in fact. But Jane was experienced enough to know that the cues she was interpreting about his tone and the reports by the grandmothers were not cues and patterns that in her experience, were typical of a child with either of these diagnoses. This made her feel that "something else" was happening. She did not have a clear hypothesis about what that something else might be, but she did have a tentative hypothesis which gained strength over time. On follow-up visits Jon seemed to her to have "lost ground" rather than proceeding, however slowly, through the developmental steps and improved motor control that Jane expected of a child with either cerebral palsy or stroke. The "big" cue came when the grandmothers pointed out that even after the stroke he could walk, but now clearly could not. Then Jane knew that there must be some sort of significant problem. Not only was Jon not progressing, but he had lost a developmental skill, walking, that he had once had. Further, his lack of ability to walk, which Jane had assumed to be a result of the stroke, clearly was not a problem produced by that stroke. Jane succeeded, on the third try, in getting the physicians to listen to her hypothesis that something else (probably progressive) was happening to this child. This is an example of competing formulations in that she had at least two hypotheses that were in conflict with one another: (1) Jon's inability to walk is a more or less stable and permanent condition and his motor behavior and development are as expected for a child with an earlier CVA [cerebrovascular accident] and CP [cerebral palsy]; (2) Jon's inability to walk and perform other motor tasks is worsening, and his muscle tone and motor performance are not like that which is typical of children with CVA or CP. The hypotheses were not about whether or not he had a stroke or cerebral palsy. Jane did not doubt these diagnoses, nor was she making hypotheses about diagnosis. Her hypotheses were about the child's motor performance, and developmental progress. She hypothesized that these behaviors were not consistent with her expectations and that possibly something else was affecting the child's functioning and development. Thus she indicated her concerns and observations to the physician for further examination and diagnosis.

There is another interesting point regarding hypotheses in this story. The grandmothers noted that the child seemed to get worse ever since he started teething. It may be that the teething was a noticeable event and thus a sort of marker for the women to remember times when he was both teething and "getting worse." They associated these two events that seemed to coincide. They may not have been posing a hypothetical relationship, but the professionals may have assumed that they were making such a causal hypothesis. The professionals may have immediately dismissed the information because it came couched in what they thought was an erroneous hypotheses, that teething could somehow cause the deterioration in motor and developmental skills. When Jane heard the presumed connection between these events the first time she dismissed the information. When she heard this as a historical fact of a developmental event, "We have a picture of him standing and walking after the stroke," then the nature of the information essentially changed. It was easier to pay attention to this cue, presented in this fashion.

In essence, all these hypotheses took place in one subspace, that of developmentally appropriate motor performance. Even from a medical decision-making point of view, they were in the same subspace, the central nervous system. However, when the critical question, for the grandmothers and the OT, was asked —"Is he getting worse"?—then the cause for concern became clear. The same could be said from the medical point of view. When the question of whether this was a stable condition or a deteriorating one was asked, then the corollary question of whether this was a progressive disorder could be raised.

Competing formulations may take place in a single problem space, as we saw above when the neurologic space was the problem space but the subspace shifted from brain damage to progressive deterioration. Formulations may be postulated in a number of different problem spaces. It is fairly typical for occupational therapists to generate hypotheses in a number of problem spaces and subspaces. This is probably because OTs concern themselves with human functioning, which often involves many aspects of the person, both biological and social. Sometimes, therapists set up competing hypotheses in different spaces, wondering, for example, if a person's behavior was influenced by a central nervous system condition or an emotional one, as in the example Sonja wrote about the man with Parkinson's disease. Such queries are often used to help the therapist select the proper type of activity or avoid something that would be inappropriate, given the condition. More often, therapists seem to generate hypotheses in many subspaces in order to postulate a relationship among events or functions in a number of subspaces. Sometimes these relationships are postulated as *functional relationships*; sometimes they are organized, or reorganized in an *hierarchic relationship*.

The following example was read to a group of experienced therapists. Together they came up with competing formulations in multiple subspaces, organized as a hierarchy, and postulated some functional relationships. Here is an excerpt from an early observation that we presented to a group of therapists. "A pediatric therapist working with a boy who was performing an activity improperly had to decide how much she should correct the child. Here was the interchange (Mattingly, 1989):

Therapist: You know how to make a square, right?
Child: Circle! Square!
Therapist: Uh oh, we're losing our square.
(The child seems to be veering from square to circle)
Child: Is that better?

We asked the therapists to tell us some of their thoughts (hypotheses) about what might be the problem here and what the therapist might be thinking about the child as the event was unfolding. Here are most of their responses, which were given as simple phrases and written on the blackboard.

1. Did the child understand the task?
2. Was it a perceptual/motor problem?
3. Did he have poor self-esteem?
4. Did she think he had a motor problem?
5. Did she think this was a conceptual problem?
6. What was the response of the child?
7. Was she trying not to interfere with his sense of accomplishment?
8. What would be the cost of correcting him?
9. Were there time constraints?
10. What is his baseline performance?
11. Was she building rapport?
12. Was she trying to generate a collaboration process?
13. What did she think about his ability to take risks?
14. What is OK here? (meaning what sort of performance is acceptable)
15. Is the kid testing the therapist?
16. If so, does she know he is testing her?
17. Is she trying to assess his ability to self-correct?
18. Is she trying to develop trust with child?
19. Maybe she doesn't want to lose the session?
20. Where is this in the session?
21. What is his history?
22. What is his context—what's going on at home?
23. Is she assessing his skill in fine motor tasks?
24. Is she trying to build a skill?
25. Is she trying to evaluate a particular skill such as drawing particular shapes?
26. Does she see a difference in cueing and correcting?
27. Diagnosis, age—is she wondering about these?
28. What is the setting or environment (i.e., clinical setting)?
29. What is her energy level?

These therapists generated several competing formulations. The formulations were generated in three problem spaces: perceptual/motor function, cognitive processing, and emotional influences. There is also an implicit hierarchy in these formulations. They may be illustrated as seen in Tables 7–2 and 7–3.

TABLE 7 · 2   Competing Formulations in Three Subspaces with a Hierarchy

Motor	Cognitive	Emotional
Can he produce circle/ square?	Did he understand the task?	Is he trying?
Does he have fine motor problems?	At what level?	Is he testing?
How old is he?	Does he know circle/square?	Self-esteem? Cost of correcting?

The implicit hierarchy of hypotheses may be described as such. Therapists generated several possible functional relationships:

1. The child was old enough to understand and execute the task; therefore something was interfering with the production of the square.
2. There may be a neurological problem.
3. There may be a central nervous system problem that interferes with his perception of the shape.
4. There may be a motor production problem interfering with his ability to execute the shape.

One hypothesis was that the child did know what a square was, but knew he could not draw it very well and that this reduced his self-esteem so that he lost his enthusiasm for trying to draw. Thus, the functional relationship was drawn between poor self-esteem and inability to produce the square. A converse hypothesis that included a functional relationship was that he did not know what a square was, but he wanted to please the therapist and therefore gave it a try but did not succeed. Here the functional relationship was drawn between lack of understanding and lack of ability to produce the square. A third hypothesis was that he knew what a square was, wanted to make a sincere effort, but that his motor planning problems prevented him from being able to do so. Here, the functional relationship is drawn between motor planning (neurological) problems and the lop-sided square.

TABLE 7 · 3   Considering Multiple Aspects of the Situation

Therapist	Context	Child
Does not want to lose session.	Setting	Trust
Elicits cooperation. Cue or correct?	Time in session	Rapport

An Analysis of the Hypothetical Reasoning of one Therapist

The following example is given to illustrate how one therapist employed all of the reasoning strategies and features discussed in this chapter. They are:

> Goal-oriented problem solving
> Task environment
> Problem space
> Recognition
> Pattern recognition
> Generate-and-test
> Heuristic Search
> Four-stage model of problem solving
> > Cue identification
> > Hypothesis generation
> > Cue interpretation
> > Hypothesis evaluation
> Structural features of problem formulations
> > Hierarchical organization
> > Competing formulations
> > Multiple subspaces
> > Functional relationships

THE SITUATION

The patient, Tony, is a 26-year-old male truck driver who drove his motorcycle into a brick wall and sustained a closed head injury. He was residing on the neurological floor of a large medical center. He had been there approximately 3 weeks. Originally he was confined to a wheelchair, but at the point of this session was able to walk some, though his gait was not normal. He had made some gains over his initial memory loss, but memory and judgment problems remained.

The therapist, Christa, is an experienced occupational therapist who has had several years of work with patients with serious neurological conditions. She has earned bachelor's and master's degrees and has taken certification courses in neurodevelopmental techniques. She has seen this patient briefly on a few occasions. Tony was generally treated in OT by Christa's student.

The research process for this particular incident included (1) a pretreatment interview by the author (Cheryl Mattingly) with the therapist, (2) a session where the therapist evaluated the patient for about 40 minutes, and (3) a posttreatment interview with the therapist for about 15 minutes. All of these were videotaped. A few weeks later the therapist and the author viewed the videotape. At that time the therapist commented on what she was doing, and why, during a segment of the evaluation session. This commentary was recorded on audio tape. The audio was dubbed over the videotape. The comments from the interviews, the session, and the commentary were also transcribed onto a computer disk and printed on paper.

During the pretreatment interview, Christa stated that she was concerned about several aspects of Tony's functioning. His muscle tone, balance problems, and judgment problems were her major concerns. The analysis of her reasoning process will focus on these three concerns. These issues were concerns within the broader context of what training and guidance Tony would need in order to be safe, functioning alone within the community. A central concern was whether or not the judgment and balance problems were temporary, and therefore not a great problem, or whether they would be long-term or permanent. If permanent, they would influence whether or not he could work (and if so at what), and whether he could drive or use public transportation, and be able to read transportation maps or routes if necessary. Would he use caution during his daily activities, job, interests, and so forth, or would he need supervision? Christa's principle focus in conducting the evaluation was to determine the likelihood of his being able to perform his daily life tasks, possibly including work, with little or no supervision (although we will see that she explores many other problem spaces in order to address this overall goal). The *problem space* was concerned with safe daily performance of work and daily living tasks. The *task environment* was his future living and working situation.

The session included about 10 minutes of Christa talking with Tony before they did any of the more active evaluation procedures. Christa asked him how he was feeling, what progress he was making, and so on. While this was a pleasant and seemingly casual conversation, it was clear that Christa was making numerous observations, and probably interpretations. Tony seemed to accept and expect her professional judgment and inquiry. Next, Christa asked Tony to take off his shoes and stand. Then Christa led Tony through a series of moves on the mat, mostly in supine position, presumably to test his reflexes, balance reactions, and muscle tone. After about 20 minutes of this, Christa asked Tony to sit on the mat. Later she did some balance tests on a balance board. Tony had difficulty with these, and fell forward in the test in which Christa asked him to close his eyes. Christa anticipated this and caught him quickly and easily. The final test was to ask him to catch a tennis ball, and to bounce a Ping-Pong ball with a paddle. A brief conversation followed, and Tony was escorted back to his room by the OT student.

The posttreatment interview followed immediately in a room nearby. Christa began with, "Well Tony is unpredictable," and gave a wry smile and a sigh. It is clear that Christa learned a lot and considered this a challenging and interesting session. She talked about several issues, her hypotheses, and her interpretations and expectations for Tony. The following analysis will interpret what she said, not in the absolute sequence in which her ideas advanced, but as an illustration of the concepts presented earlier.

TRANSCRIPT FROM A SECTION OF THE POSTTREATMENT INTERVIEW

Maureen: When you left you said it's so hard to say anything about a patient before you see him, and now it's after the session, and it's such a surprise. Just tell us what you think.

Christa: Well, Tony is unpredictable. Tony is different every day. So you don't really know what to do. At least you can plan your treatment roughly, but you always have to change things.

When I first started out, Tony was actually much better than I expected. His muscle tone was close to normal. But that's one reason why I checked out the myoclonus in his ankles, just to be sure that I'm not seeing the wrong thing; and I checked it out, and he really did have myoclonus in both ankles. Therefore, the tone hadn't disappeared. It was there, but it was not visible just looking at him. So I knew at some point he was going to have trouble with it.

Then I was working on the quality of his movements, initially doing some in-between range movements because Tony, as I told you earlier, does not have any awareness of his right side being different from his left side. Well, his right side is quite different. But it has improved quite a bit, and is beginning to catch up with the left. So I still want to look for in-between range controls, and he's beginning to get that. He's not as spontaneous on the right, but I can pretty much predict as to what he will do, and that worked out just nice. But when I then introduced more axial rotation, I still felt that there was some retraction obligation on the left scapular region. But that also has gotten better.

As you bring Tony up against gravity, I know from his pathology he's losing it. Tony moves a lot. He moves a lot spontaneously, and as he moves, it's hard to control his movements. And you don't see this too often with patients; usually you have to really drag them across the mat. And yet Tony wants stimulus and he moves in a big wide range, which is sort of typical for somebody who has high tone.

And not only that, but I discovered something about Tony I never knew when I treated him today. Number one, Tony is ataxic. I've never seen ataxia in Tony before. That would explain his sudden wide-range movements at times. Although he has spasticity in his legs, it is a mixed picture. He has a low tone in his trunk which I always felt was present, but I couldn't really prove it because he wasn't well enough to drag him across the mat the way we did today. So today I'm convinced, yes, he has low tone in his trunk, yes, he does have truncal ataxia. And he has some high tone in his legs. He has low tone in his arms. So, that gives me a very different picture than I thought before we started training him.

Maureen: Tell us about what this means in terms of what his injury was or what his potential is.

Christa: Okay, it fits the picture of Tony I had originally. When I first saw him he had a very low-tone trunk, low-tone arms. But because he was also medicated, that made me think that maybe his tone is normally high, but with the medication it is reduced, and therefore his lack of trunk control is probably medication induced. But I couldn't prove that. In the meantime, they have taken him off most of his medication; I think they were going to take him off Haldol completely this week. But it tells me that he does have more than just cortical involvement, which we pretty much thought at first. And that really points much more to the cerebellum as well. And also he has got some brain stem involvement, which was very clear today. Number one is because at the end of treatment, I saw nystagmus, spontaneous nystagmus, which I had not seen in Tony before. Which makes me think that all that vestibular bombardment triggered that nystagmus, which I've never seen before, but I didn't have to test before because there wasn't evidence of it. There was nothing documented, and also his injury was not supposed to be brain stem cerebellum. And he complained about some nonspecific eye problems that nobody really knew what to do with. But without testing him I could see that he had nystagmus, that spontaneous lateral gaze. Therefore that would sort of go along with his ataxia. That would pinpoint his deficits more to lower center, brain stem, cerebellar connections. That would explain why he does the wide-range movements. That would explain his truncal ataxia in kneel standing and in standing. That was quite striking today, I thought.

Maureen: Is motor control mediated from higher centers?

Christa: At first when we worked with Tony, because we didn't really challenge him as much, we did gross motor stuff on the mat, but we really did not get him fatigued. Fatigue increases your symptoms right away to begin with, but also you see more symptoms as the patient does higher level activities because they lose control. And it was very clear today; Tony lost control several times and also he moved more than the average patient would move, because his lack of control made him want to move to regain control. That was sort of unexpected. I know that Tony moves spontaneously a great deal, but he moved much wider ranges right from the start; and I think now that we're getting rid of his spasticity, or decreasing it significantly, you see more of the underlying weakness. You see more of the ataxia and more of the low tone. So, in other words, you're bringing it from above normal to below normal very fast and he hasn't gotten that middle range yet.

So, I think our treatment after this session has to change. And that would mean doing more facilitation to his trunk. We have done some inhibition, which worked fine for his legs, which gave us just enough decrease of muscle tone in the lower extremities, but it has affected his trunk also. His trunk, which was close to normal, is now below normal and gives us new problems such as ataxia and instability of the hip. So that is significant. It also—since Tony does not have good body awareness—that new vestibular awareness on my part makes me think, "Oh, if Tony responds to vestibular stimulation by getting a nystagmus, he must have something wrong in the brain stem area." It confirms again the ataxia and the nystagmus, so he becomes a slightly different patient for future treatments.

Maureen: How about the balance? He's working a lot on that. You saw a real dramatic problem there.

Christa: Tony, at first, did quite well, extremely well, with controlling his right trunk in side-lying and partial-supine, something he had not been able to do before. So I saw very spontaneous, maintained trunk extension against gravity, with good quality, some abduction of the leg which is all high-level stuff. But when it came to higher level, more antigravity positions, he had to broaden his base. He has a harder time maintaining co-contraction of the hip. Again, that was new. He says, "My right leg feels stronger," when in fact he is saying, "I have more spasticity in my right leg. It feels stronger to me because it's different. It's supporting me more." When in fact, when you have taken the spasticity away (so some of the movement), it was quite clear that he has much more weakness underneath it.

So, up against gravity I was trying to get him to balance his right hip and lower extremity against gravity, which was very difficult to do. I didn't even attempt, or attempted but I gave up on it, trying to balance his left hip on his right hip. That was difficult only because I felt at that point, if his tone is really as low as I think it is, he won't have the stability to hold himself up. His whole body weight would have been on his right knee, and he must have had good hip and knee control in order to be able to take that weight and to take that movement that I was planning on introducing. So I felt that was not going to be a smart move because Tony was not controlling his movements as well as I expected it. So I had to really scale my expectations down.

Maureen: When you asked him to close his eyes, were you looking for vestibular stuff as well as the motor control, or . . .

Christa: Yes, I was, I had never had him do anything like this, and because of his ataxia. Sometimes you find patients that really do better with their eyes closed, unless you have significant sensory involvement. Now Tony has no known sensory deficits that I'm aware of. But with his eyes closed, number one, it was a new experience, he didn't know what to expect. I'm sure he hasn't tested himself out either. It was certainly unexpected to me. I expected him to

	have some trouble, but I didn't expect this sudden movement, and again that explains the ataxia. Ataxic people are very sudden, unpredictable. And that ties in again.
Maureen:	. . . with the loss of higher control.
Christa:	Yeah, he just cannot judge the range of movements that he is going to do. So the timing of his co-contraction is off.

ANALYSIS OF PART OF THE INTERVIEW

Problem-solving steps and features as described by Elstein, Shulman, and Sprafka (1978) were employed by Christa as outlined below.

Cue Identification

She elicits and observes 23 cues:

1. Muscle tone close to normal
2. Myoclonus in the ankles
3. Quality of movement
4. Right side "catching up"
5. Axial rotation and retraction obligation
6. Balance against gravity—"losing it"
7. Moves in a big, wide range
8. Ataxia
9. Decreased spasticity in legs
10. Low tone in trunk
11. Truncal ataxia
12. Some high tone in legs
13. Low tone in arms
14. Nystagmus
15. Eye problems
16. Wide-range movements
17. Lost motor control
18. Co-contraction
19. Instability at the hip
20. Spontaneous, maintained trunk extension against gravity
21. Broad base
22. Hard time maintaining co-contraction at hip
23. Cannot balance right hip and L.E. against gravity

Hypothesis Generation

Christa generated several hypotheses as she went along. Here are two examples taken from the tape which illustrate Elstein's four-phase model.

Hypothesis 1

Cue: Muscle tone.
Hypothesis: Muscle tone close to normal.
Cue interpretation: Check for myoclonus.
Hypothesis evaluation: Myoclonus was there, therefore the tone (high tone) had not disappeared. Therefore she rejected the hypothesis that his tone was close to normal.

Hypothesis 2

Cue: Low tone in trunk.
Hypothesis: Ataxia.
Cue interpretation: Low tone in trunk versus high tone in leg and wide-range movements are indeed both present.
Hypothesis evaluation: Yes. Ataxia is present—the mixed tone and ataxia would account for the wide-range movements.

Overall Christa generated four competing hypotheses in the neurological problem space, in different problem subspaces. They were all related to trying to determine the nature of Tony's balance problems. The problem subspaces examined were

1. Muscle weakness in trunk and hips
2. Fatigue
3. Medication
4. Brain stem "involvement"

Cue Interpretation

Listing cues by possible problem subspace we see the pattern shown in Table 7–4.

Larger Hypotheses

Christa's four competing hypotheses regarding the reasons for poor balance can be framed as follows:

1. *If* he has weakness in trunk and hip muscles,
   then he cannot currently execute the motions needed to walk properly.

Therefore his walking looks unsteady, because the weak muscles are not providing enough support.

If so the problem is temporary and can be remediated through strengthening and practice.

2. *If* he is fatigued and he has some minor problem in strength and/or balance,

   then fatigue may also depress his spatial awareness, interest in the task, effort, and attention.

   Therefore an underlying minor problem may be exacerbated by the fatigue.

   If so it is indeterminate whether or not the balance problem will be a long-term problem.

3. *If* he has received some medication,

   then it might have affected his balance, coordination, and/or spatial awareness, attention, and so on.

   Therefore this balance problem may be only a result of the medication.

   If so, this may be a transient problem.

4. *If* there is some damage to or dysfunction of the brain stem,

   then this could influence his sensorimotor processing.

   Therefore he may have diminished balance reactions.

   If so this is probably a permanent problem which may affect his safety and influence his ability to work.

Cue Interpretation

Cues were interpreted as to whether they did or did not support a hypothesis (see Table 7–4).

Four cues might contribute to any hypothesis:

1. Quality of movement
2. Loss of balance against gravity
3. Low tone
4. Increase in symptoms

They are nonexclusive cues; therefore they are weak cues.

Three cues support the weakness hypothesis:

1. Tone close to normal
2. Right side catching up
3. Decreased spasticity

If they support the weakness hypothesis, then they also tend to indicate that he is improving. Further—they tend to negate the medication and fatigue hypotheses.

TABLE 7 • 4   Cues Considered in Four Problem Spaces

| | Problem Space | | | |
Cues	Muscle Weakness	Brain Stem	Medication	Fatigue
1. Muscle tone close to normal	*			
2. Myoclonus in the ankles		*		
3. Quality of movement	*	*	*	*
4. Right side "catching up"	*			
5. Axial rotation		*		
6. Balance against gravity—"losing it"	*	*	*	*
7. Moves in a wide range		*		
8. Ataxia		*		
9. Decreased spasticity in legs	*			
10. Low tone in trunk	*	*	*	*
11. Truncal ataxia				
12. Some high tone in legs				
13. Low tone in arms				
14. Nystagmus		*		
15. Eye problems		*		
16. Wide-range movements				
17. Lost motor control		*		
18. Co-contraction		*		
19. Instability at the hip		*		
20. Spontaneous, maintained trunk extension against gravity				
21. Broad base		*		
22. Poor balance		*		
23. Increased symptoms	*	*	*	*

*Indicates this cue may contribute to a hypothesis in this problem space.

Eleven cues support the brain stem problem (neurological problem) hypothesis:

1. Myoclonus in the ankles
2. Quality of movement
3. Axial rotation
4. Balance against gravity—"losing it"
5. Wide-range movements
6. Ataxia
7. Low tone in trunk
8. Nystagmus
9. Eye problems
10. Loss of motor control
11. Broad base
12. Co-contracture is difficult

13. Instability at hip
14. Poor balance

Hypothesis Evaluation

Christa applies the cues to each of the possible hypotheses. The four cues that could apply to any hypothesis are useless, as they do not separate one hypothesis from another. Three cues support the weakness hypothesis. So that hypothesis is still viable. Those same three cues negate the fatigue and medication hypotheses, and those two hypotheses are dropped. Eleven cues support the brain stem hypothesis, which becomes the leading hypothesis.

Structural Features

Christa actually concerned herself with several other issues regarding Tony and his future including his emotional state, family structure and situation, his prior work, and life habits and skills. She generated many more hypotheses in more problem spaces and subspaces. However, in the section of the transcript analyzed here, Christa generated four competing formulations. They were in several subspaces of the overall problem space of the neurological system. The nature of the influences that the different hypothesized causes would have on Tony's balance problem, however, are different and are examined from the point of view of different subspaces within that system. Determining these differences is important because they will influence how Christa thinks about Tony's problem, and the functional abilities and disabilities that would result. The medication and fatigue subspaces are explored to determine whether Tony's balance problem is a merely temporary or transient problem, and of no great concern. If the balance problem is temporary, then Tony's future functional capacity will not be compromised. However, if the brain stem subspace hypothesis is correct, then the problem is not simply a balance problem. It is a problem of loss of *balance reactions*. Thus Tony will continue to have poor balance and be unsafe in many situations. He will not be able to return to his former occupation as a truck driver, nor work as a house painter, as he had speculated in an early part of the session. Therefore, OT is required to help him develop skills that will enable him to make judgments about what sorts of activities he can participate in, and to develop compensatory methods to deal with his lack of balance reactions.

The functional relationship that Christa draws is that the wide-range movements, the ataxia, the poor balance, the nystagmus, and the myoclonus are all related to an injury to the brain stem. Such an injury is likely to affect the speed and quality of one's balance reactions.

Summary

Using only one treatment session and interview we have illustrated several features of clinical reasoning that occupational therapists employ when considering the patient's clinical condition and the performance limitations which may result. Many of these features are similar to those identified by Newell and Simon (1972) and by Elstein, Shulman, and Sprafka (1978). All occupational therapists may not employ all of these features in every situation, but we did observe repeated instances of therapists using a variety of these strategies and approaches to problem solving.

■

Interactive Reasoning
Collaborating with the Person
- ■ **CHERYL MATTINGLY**
- ■ **MAUREEN HAYES FLEMING**

Introduction: Doing with—
Active Collaboration

THE NEED FOR COLLABORATION
WITH THE PATIENT

Expert therapists become extremely skilled at reasoning about how to interact with their clients. This skill is particularly essential in occupational therapy because effective therapy demands a high level of commitment by clients. The need for and belief in a very collaborative practice was voiced by therapists in the Clinical Reasoning Study. When we asked them what made occupational therapy different from other health professions (say, physical therapy or nursing) they would say two things. One, occupational therapists cared about function. Two, occupational therapists "do with" their clients. Therapists would say, "Nurses do for patients. We help patients do for themselves." "Good nurses" are ones with the patience to let the patients do what they can. We were surprised that the *process* by which therapy was conducted seemed to be as essential to the professional identity of occupational therapy as the kind of problem therapists addressed or the procedures employed. In the hospital setting where patients are not in the middle of ordinary lives, "doing with" patients often means that therapists have patients conduct their own self-care as much as possible. Therapists sit or stand near the patients and coach, encourage, and help.

They often do not seem to be actually doing something themselves but are "doing with" the client to help them in the transition from dependent patient to (as they say) "independent living." Doing with patients also means having patients practice exercises in the hospital during the times when they are not being seen by the therapist. Clients are asked to take an active role in their treatment. This contrasts with the comparatively passive role they generally assume as patients of other practitioners in the hospital.

This concern with a patient's experience of disability derives in part from deep beliefs which belong to occupational therapy's professional culture. The meaning that the patient makes of an illness enters directly into the therapeutic process, because this process is built on a practice of "doing with" the patient. This requires therapists to devise treatment goals that are meaningful enough to patients that they are willing to work hard as partners in the therapeutic process. The therapists thus find themselves constantly confronted with the interpretive task of translating between their way of seeing and the patients'. If the goals that the therapists pursue are too far afield from the patients' perceptions of their functional needs, therapy is likely to be stalled.

Therapists also continually refer to their interpretations of patient meanings, to modify treatment directions or to attempt to persuade patients to see their disability in a different light. They often see possibilities where patients see none, and commonly attempt to help patients fight despair and passive resignation in the face of their disabilities.

Robert Murphy, commenting on his own resistance to therapy and his enormous depression as he faced a deteriorating body, notes that "[rehabilitation] therapists must breach imposing psychological barriers to reach their patients and enlist their cooperation in the long tedious process of reconstructing their bodies" (1987, p. 54).

Effective therapy requires that patients be committed to a long path, where gains are so slow they are difficult to perceive, or are counteracted by a faster rate of deterioration. This means that therapists must address the problem of motivation. They must tap into commitments and values deep enough within patients to commit them to such a process. No matter what the technical expertise or theoretical orientation of the therapist, effective collaboration requires treating the disability as more than a biomechanical matter that can be separated from the experience of the patient.

Even when therapists would like to ignore the patient as a "whole person" the cooperative nature of the practice compels them to acknowledge the patient's meaning world at some level, simply to induce the patient to take the therapy seriously. This clinical reasoning in practice means reasoning, not only about what is wrong and how to fix it, but also about how to engage the patient in that fixing process.

This, in turn, involves understanding enough about the meaning of the disability from the patient's perspective to develop a shared account of what "fixing" the problem could amount to in terms of their lives. Even therapists who prefer to avoid delving into a patient's life and try to restrict their practice to more narrowly construed physiological problems find themselves taking on the "whole person," as the quest for collaboration makes this unavoidable. If therapists cannot succeed in getting the patient to collaborate with them, they may discontinue treatment. So, for instance, one therapist tells the staff in a planning discharge meeting, "If Leo doesn't make some treatment goals, I'm going to discontinue therapy."

More Than Just Being Nice

Creating a collaborative relationship goes far beyond being "nice" to the patient. It involves a subtle interpretation of what a person wants from therapy. Therapists must interpret motives and meanings from the cues based on what patients do and say. Often this reading of what matters is not easy to ascertain. Clients may have mixed feelings about therapy, their bodies, or health professionals in general. They may not know how they feel. They may not want or be able to talk to the therapist. Therapists often see people at critical, rapidly changing, and frightening times of their lives. There are times which confuse and anger the best of us. Skilled therapists often become adept at helping patients clarify the meaning of their disability and their aspirations for the future.

CASE EXAMPLE

The following case illustrates how collaboration is a necessary starting point for effective therapy, and it also shows that being collaborative is more than being nice.

Mr. Tattoo

by Dawn Dale

Working for a large home health agency can generate many "stories," but one generally learns several basic concepts in this practice arena. First and foremost, you are on the patients' turf, not the converse. Your creativity and treatment media become stretched to the maximum. However, the pervading feeling most patients exhibit is relief in knowing you are there to nurture a positive change, although the methods to your madness are not always clear.

It struck me as strange to be summoned by an office director to open a particular OT case. The field staff usually do this, and do it well. However, I was assured it was absolutely necessary for me to open this case.

Behind the closed door of her inner sanctum, this director began to relay the following tidbits: "We have a particularly tough case right now."

"Go on," I said.

"We have an OT referral on a patient who has already kicked out two nurses, two physical therapists, and one home health assistant. Over the weekend, this man saw Dr. A. in the ER [emergency room] and was diagnosed with pneumonia. He is a C-7 quad who became this way due to driving under the influence and blames everyone but himself. He signed himself out of the ER against medical advice. Three weeks ago, he signed himself out of the rehab center as well."

"What is it that I can offer this man?"

She responded, "Dr. A. prescribed IM [intramuscular] antibiotic injections, and he is allowing Betty (our RN) to administer them. Mr. T. has expressed concern to her that his legs are drawing into flexion and that he is not getting therapy. She thought an OT referral might be appropriate. I agreed, because you all seem to be able to manage even the worst problem patients."

My initial thoughts were along the line of, "Why me?" I agreed to take on Mr. T., and with more than slight reluctance I called his home to set up an evaluation time.

As I drove out to Mr. T.'s home, I kept running thoughts and ideas of how I could successfully approach this man and get my foot in the door. I felt the usual nurturing approach would not work. I was expecting some large, ogre-type individual with a loud mouth and broad shoulders.

When I arrived at this address, I was somewhat surprised to see Mr. T. lived in a house trailer. There was no ramp and no car. I knocked on the door, and Mrs. T., a very slow-moving and slow-speaking woman, opened the door. Introductions were pleasant, but it was easy to see that the "light was on and no one was home."

She led me to the door where the patient was resting quietly in a hospital bed. He was a slight man, wet with sweat from the 85-degree temperature indoors and the fever he was carrying. Short of breath and short of stature, this scrawny little man seemed very unimposing.

Before I realized, I spoke exactly what I was thinking, "So you're the one who's been causing all of this trouble?"

"What do you mean?" he responded.

"I understand you have kicked out five of our personnel already. I'm here to do a job, which is what I intend to do. Let's get an understanding up front. I'll help you any way I can, as long as you make progress and show some carryover here at home. The first time you are short with me or my staff or fail to cooperate with the program, I'll pull out. You won't have to worry about kicking me out or demanding that we leave. Do we understand each other?"

While I was waiting for his response, I couldn't help but notice the stump on his left arm, which was what was left of a below-elbow amputation. I was later to learn this injury occurred 14 years ago and that he had long since thrown away that "good-for-nothing" prosthesis. The tattoo on his right shoulder caught my eye. It read "Born To Fuck" in bold Roman script.

He tugged at his beard with his right hand as if in deep, reflective thought, constantly eyeing and sizing me up. Short of a leather jacket, I was sure God had delivered me to a Hell's Angel.

Finally Mr. T. said, "It's not the therapists I'm fed up with. It's those d—— doctors. They don't know nothin'. Everybody from your outfit has been nice. I'm just frustrated."

I realized I had successfully cracked his shell. The assistant sees him now and reports he is dressing UEs [upper extremities] independently and has begun LE [lower extremity] dressing with a dressing stick. The scrawny little devil has turned out to be one of our brightest stars and nicest angels. Despite the fact that this approach worked, I still wonder if there was a better approach I could have used.

COLLABORATION WITH OTHERS

Collaboration also goes beyond treating the designated "patient." Therapists routinely consider how to work with other essential members of a client's world—a wife, a teacher, a daughter, for their cooperation is essential to the success of therapy. Nowhere is this more evident than in home health. The following case illustrates how a home health therapist worked not with a single patient but with his wife as well. This cooperation particularly matters when therapists care about improving not just function given the bimechanical deficits.

CASE EXAMPLE

Mr. S.

by Karen F. Barney

This story retells a practice experience that I had during the spring of 1989, while I served as a faculty member at Eastern Kentucky University, with some follow-up contact (postassessment) during October 1989. The experience was part of the geriatric research project of which I was a member, under the direction of Ruth E. Levine and Laura Gitlin of Thomas Jefferson University. This pilot project seeks to determine whether "low tech" cure of chronically disabled older adults is feasible in the community, so as to prevent institutionalization.

As one who met all of the appropriate criteria for candidates, Mr. S. had been referred by the collaborating home health agency and randomly selected to be a part of the student group in the project. The course of events leading up to my seeing him included his having experienced an extensive CVA affecting his left side. He had a residual lack of motor function and sensation, and his expressive components of speech were affected. He had been treated first in an acute care setting, then in a rehabilitation hospital, and then in home health. My involvement followed his last series of treatments by home health occupational therapists several months later.

I had been told by the nursing director at the home health agency that this man lived with his wife of 50 plus years, and that both of them were fairly disabled. She felt that they could both benefit from OT intervention as proposed in the research project.

In the course of our first conversation, Mrs. S. interjected many comments about what they had experienced, what their current situation was, and what their aspirations were. It became clear to me that a critical aspect of any intervention that was planned needed to be collaborative effort on the part of all of us (Mr. and Mrs. S. and me). That collaboration, I believe, is the essence of quality care in most home health intervention programs, in order to ensure appropriateness and effectiveness.

Mrs. S. articulated most of what was discussed in response to my questions. The couple had lived in this community all of their lives. Mr. S. had worked for 35 years for the same employer who is still in contact with them, they had raised several adopted children, and they were currently living below the poverty level. It was very difficult to ascertain whether Mr. S. could not or did not want to respond to my questions—he verbalized very little, and his overall affect was flat.

Mrs. S. seemed very confused about my role—she had been accustomed to having occupational therapists perform biomechanic functions with her husband (what she described appeared to be ROM, use of the airsplint, splinting, etc.). As a consequence, over the series of several sessions that I spent with Mr. and Mrs. S., I had to repeatedly clarify that I was there to see if there were any activities which her husband might need or want to do to enable him to function better and to assist both of them in maintaining their independence.

The elements of living that appeared to be very important to both of them centered around their being involved with their family, and independent in the community. Mrs. S. showed pictures of their family throughout the series of interventions, and recounted the contacts that they had with their children and grandchildren. On one occasion when I came to their home, the bed where Mr. S. slept was in a back bedroom with his wife's bed, the living room was cleared of extra furniture, and the entire home appeared to be free of clutter. Mrs. S. exclaimed with pride that they had had a family reunion and many of their children and grandchildren had visited them the weekend before. Mr. S., though customarily nonverbal, appeared to be in better humor than usual—his wife stated that he had thoroughly enjoyed his grandchildren.

The aspects of living which Mr. S. seemed to greatly value, in addition to those shared with his wife, were the idea that he would like to try to shave himself and to garden again—he had spent his work life assisting an affluent family with a complete range of household duties, and had taken great pride in maintaining their lawn and garden.

Since the electric razor which he had used in the past needed to be "found," (source—Mrs. S.) I decided to work with him on the planning of a garden—I could immediately visualize him outside in the back of the house with a garden plot—if we were able to overcome the accessibility limitations of his getting outside in his wheelchair. I then thought that in light of the multiple limitations that I was observing—both his and her mobility and accessibility problems—that it would be more practical to have a raised garden developed on their porch. In a subsequent session, it was clear that Mrs. S. did not like the idea of converting some of the porch space, so that we all agreed that a galvanized tub on a stand could serve as his "garden." I was delighted to see that they discussed this idea with their son who was visiting from another state, and who immediately purchased a tub and potting soil for that purpose prior to my next visit. Mrs. S. and I discussed obtaining seeds for the garden; she exclaimed that she had a special course from which she could arrange for free seeds. We agreed that this would be a logical source for them. My interventions ended before they were able to obtain the seeds; however, I felt that it was very important to have Mrs. S. invested in the project in order to ensure Mr. S.'s participation. He definitely needed her support in every respect for him to be able to participate.

In the meantime, the electric razor was found, and I discovered that it needed a new head—the reason Mr. S. had not been using it was that it "pulled on his beard" (source—Mrs. S.). Therefore, I located a supplier for the head and purchased it on their behalf. When the new head was positioned and a mirror set up before Mr. S., he very willingly used his unaffected right hand to shave at the kitchen table. For the first and only time in all my sessions with him this far, I saw him smile.

Strategies to Encourage Collaboration

If therapy is going to work, patients must form an alliance with the therapist and agree to play their part in the therapeutic effort. How does the therapist go about proposing this contract? There is strong evidence that the therapist's interest in building rapport with patients is linked to this need to gain the patient's cooperation. The importance of this cooperation is evident in the number and variety of strategies that therapists in our study had developed to engage the patient more personally in the therapeutic process. The strategies most pervasively used in the group of therapists that we studied are enumerated below. We found that therapists working with quite different patient populations had devised or borrowed a similar repertoire of such strategies.

CREATING CHOICES

One common strategy involved structuring a situation in which the patient had to make a choice about what to do, generally among a limited range of options. The therapist would often say something such as, "What do you want to do tomorrow—put on your shoes and socks, more work on transfers, or brush your teeth?" Sometimes therapists wanted patients to continue working on an activity, but also wanted to allow them some choice in the matter, as one pediatrics therapist did with her 4-year-old patient who had just finished coloring a drawing: "Now what one should we do?" The general strategy of presenting options within a range allows the patient to make some decisions but also gives the therapist room to structure the overall treatment plan. Some of the more experienced therapists who participated in our study would allow their patients to do things outside the list of choices they presented. For instance, in response to the pediatric therapist's question above, the child responded, "I want to show my drawing to my Mom," and the therapist agreed.

The need to give clients choices arises because therapists often ask them to face difficult situations in therapy. Clients are not always able to deal with disability or its meaning for their lives. Giving a choice may mean letting a client do nothing, or not chastising a client for "noncompliance," as sometimes clients are not ready to embark on treatment programs, however beneficial. And sometimes, of course, therapists are not given this choice. It is enforced by the client's "disappearance."

CASE EXAMPLE

The following case, while titled "Diane's Realization," could be just as aptly titled "Ellen's Realization" for the therapist (Ellen Berger) describes her own discovery about why a parent chooses not to carry out a feeding program with her child. This is a humbling case with a happy ending, and reveals how the therapist cannot control cooperation but must rely upon the client's active choice to take it up. It also vividly shows how therapists can easily miss the deep and difficult phenomenological issues surrounding disability.

Diane's Realization

by Ellen Berger

I was working in an early intervention program (birth to 3-year-old).

I received a telephone call from a woman I knew from the local community. She was a pediatric nurse at the local hospital. Her husband was an engineer at the General Electric plant. They had two children: Brian, 3½ years old, with severe cerebral palsy-quadriplegia, possible mental retardation, and seizure disorder; and Anthony, an 18-month-old, who seemed to be developing in a typical fashion.

Diane, the mother, wished assistance with feeding Brian. She reported concern with adequate caloric intake and medications being insufficiently consumed due to Brian's oral motor problems. It was summer. Brian had PT—no OT—and they requested my services as a "personal favor."

I went to their home to observe Diane's interactions with both her children while discussing their daily routines and the identified problem. I observed that Diane was not only exceptionally adept at "therapeutic handling and positioning" with her son, but also she clearly had a pleasant, warm and loving relationship with both her boys.

After some "playtime," we went to the kitchen to review Brian's diet, and for me to observe Diane's present feeding technique. Having had a reasonable amount of training in oral motor dysfunction I believed that I could see the problem areas and where Diane would benefit from therapeutic technique changes.

So, I suggested and demonstrated some oral feeding techniques which yielded immediate results. (Imagine!) Diane demonstrated what she had observed and all seemed fine. We agreed to check back with each other in a few weeks unless there were problems.

About 4 weeks later, I called Diane. She seemed a bit distant or distracted but reported that all was going well. She agreed to another home visit in a few weeks.

At the scheduled visit, Diane was warm and friendly but it was clear that my recommendations had not been followed through on. I made some of the same and a few new suggestions and told Diane to call me any time. School was about to start for Brian and he'd have OT available there.

I did not hear from Diane again, aside from a hello in the grocery store, until about 6 months later. She called and when I picked up the phone and said hello, she said "Ellen, Anthony picked his nose today." I said, "Diane? How are you?" She repeated "Anthony picked his nose today." I thought to myself, "Hmm, perhaps she's not as well put together as everyone thinks— or maybe she's snapped."

Finally, Diane said "Ellen don't you get it? I love Anthony, I've never doubted that. He's perfect, he's beautiful, his body works, his hands work, he speaks, but today he picked his nose and it disgusted me. It really disgusted me—made my stomach turn, but I still love him." She went on to say, "And Brian, I love him too, I can help him move, and learn and play and interact and I don't care that his body doesn't work right or that he doesn't speak. But Ellen, I must confess, when he eats it disgusts me. And when I did those feeding therapy things it was even worse. But now I know that it's possible to be disgusted, even repulsed by something someone you love does—and still love them. I'm ready to work on feeding now—when can you come out and visit us again?"

INDIVIDUALIZING TREATMENT

A second strategy went beyond giving patients choices among a generic set of treatment modalities and involved therapists in creating individualized treatment activities. Ingenuity is required to devise treatment activities that fit the patient's individual interests and also achieve the overall physiological or skill-building goals that have been set. The goals themselves may not vary much among patients with the same disability, but the way the therapist structures treatment activities to achieve those goals must be adapted to the particular patient. For example, one therapist had worked with an artist whose injured hand was worsening as reflex sympathetic dystrophy (RSD) seemed to be setting in. The therapist was very worried about this, because reflex sympathetic dystrophy is a serious condition, difficult to remediate and very painful for the patient. The artist was highly motivated, since the use of her hands was essential to her work, which she cared about. One of the treatments the therapist devised was having the woman make dough sculptures. Stirring the dough was an especially good strengthening exercise and may have worked against the RSD, and the patient was also doing something that had special significance for her.

Another example involves a hand therapist whose young male outpatient had not been improving and did not seem motivated to do the exercises that had been assigned to home. In one of the treatment sessions we observed, the therapist began thinking aloud about activities he could be doing in his daily life that would exercise his hand and yet be more interesting to him. Her first suggestion was activities that could help around the house, "folding things or vacuuming." When the young man did not respond to these suggestions (not surprisingly), she then had the idea that he could do a project in which he would make something for the children in pediatrics. Her office was right next to the pediatric occupational therapy room and she had mentioned to me before the session that he liked children.

Her suggestion of a project did not have the intrinsic fit that sculpting in dough had for the artist, but it illustrates a common move, from routine to nonroutine treatment activities, in the thinking of therapists when a patient has refused to cooperate with earlier proposals. In this session, the therapist considers abandoning her standard program of exercises; suggests housework, which the patient resists by his silence; recognizes that resistance; and finally suggests doing a project for the children. She may have stopped short of arriving at a project closely fitting the patient's sense of identity and pride in occupational skills, but she did break out of the standard treatment framework she had been unsuccessfully trying to impose on him for several months.

STRUCTURING SUCCESS

A third common strategy for promoting alliances with patients involved structuring successful treatment sessions. All the therapists in this study were concerned with devising activities that the patient could successfully perform. They saw this as important for maintaining motivation. Each could discuss at length the need to structure activities so that they could push the patient as far as she could reasonably be expected to go without pushing her so far that she failed. In occupational therapy terminology, this is the "just right challenge" (Csikszentmihalyi, 1975).

Success depends not only on judging the patient's physical ability but also on how far he might be willing to push himself. Such clinical judgment becomes extremely fine-grained and necessitates sensitivity to subtle cues from the patient. For instance, a pediatric therapist working with a child who was performing an activity improperly had to decide how much she should correct the child. This was the interchange:

> **Therapist:** You know how to make a square, right?
> **Patient:** Circle! Square!

> **Therapist:** Uh oh, we're losing our square. (Patient seems to be veering from square to circle.)
>
> **Patient:** Is that better?
>
> **Therapist:** Much better. (Mattingly, 1988)

The therapist decided to correct the first time, and not to correct, but validate, the second. She was asked after the session how she learned to judge when to correct and when not to. She said:

> It's something you learn by trial and error, by reflecting on the sessions that went badly afterwards and trying to isolate what went wrong and correcting for that the next time. In correcting a child, you have to set your acceptable limits, have an idea of the child's limits, what you'll accept for now, what you think they can do. As you get to know them, you learn what they can tolerate, how much they can stand to be corrected, and how much you have to let go for now. It varies with the kid. With some, there's always a contingency plan, "OK, five more, then we'll do something else."

Therapists described such reasoning in peripheral terms, as a critical but intuitive and a theoretical aspect of practice. The considerations involved in making this kind of small, ordinary decision are quite elaborate, based on the therapist's understanding of the patient's inner world of motivations, commitments, and tolerances. In this example, the therapist had to refer tacitly or explicitly to a number of theories about the child in answering such questions as "What are her limits for this task, based on past experience with her and other children like her?" "What can the child do in the context of this task?" "How much can the child stand to be corrected?" "How much do I have to let her go for now?"

This theoretical structure is refined when the therapist's decision does not give her the results she had expected—if trouble arises. This therapist is clear that much of her learning comes from past problems. However, what she characterizes as a "trial and error" method appears, upon closer examination, to be more systematic. What she tries is driven by theories about the patient and what the patient can handle; she is not merely randomly experimenting, she is employing her "theories-in-use" (Argyris and Schön, 1981), applying her "tacit" (Polyani, 1966) professional knowledge.

Patients were regularly told by therapists that they were performing successfully and they were often asked to validate that success. Validating success is another strategy, sometimes an explicit one, for trying to strengthen the patient's commitment to therapy. An example that we looked at in an earlier chapter serves as a good illustration of this strategy.

> **Therapist:** At first you couldn't sit up at all. Now you've learned to sit up by yourself.

Patient:	Yes, yes.
	(Pause)
Therapist:	Is that as hard as it was?
Patient:	(response unclear)
Therapist:	Not too bad. Because you really couldn't do it for the longest time.
	(Pause)
Patient:	I wish God could do a miracle on me. I can't use my arm as I should.
Therapist:	Well, you are doing much better. You can give yourself a lot of credit. You and others have been working hard.

The therapist was asked after the session about these validation points. She felt that his agreement (as in the first two interchanges) was an important confirmation from him that things were improving and that such a confirmation mattered because it showed some active involvement on his part. She recounted her description of the session. "I was saying to him, 'Last week you had more difficulties. Now it is easier. You must be feeling easier.' Before, everything was lousy in his view. I want confirmation from him that things are improving." The concern for confirmation and the tacit theory that the patient's pessimistic view will prevent him from improving is probably what drives her to directly contradict the one personal statement he made during the treatment session quoted above, in which he portrayed his disability as not having changed sufficiently.

CASE EXAMPLE

Interestingly, different strategies sometimes run into conflict with one another. Strategies are not necessarily harmonious or additive. Clinical reasoning gains subtlety when therapists must choose between different values they hold about involving clients in therapy. An excerpt from the following case story illustrates a therapist's need to sacrifice giving the patient choices in order to structure successful treatment sessions.

A.J.

by Anonymous

"The patient was a talker. By this I mean he loved to keep an ongoing dialogue with anyone in close proximity. At times, he needed to be redirected to his task. Besides range of motion activities for his right upper extremity, I also worked with A.J. on identified cognitive deficits. Areas of concern were his difficulty with planning and organizing. I gave him a series of tasks to complete that had a fixed end point. You could see the progression in his ability to plan, organize, and execute these tasks.

"He began treatment on the twenty-third of May. At that time I knew his priority was to move his right dominant upper extremity. This was his primary concern in all our discussions. The next treatment sessions consisted of neuromuscular facilitation of wrist extensors with a vibrator. A.J. enjoyed this activity as it was relatively easy to solicit wrist extension. Once he began to see that I could get his wrist to move, I had him hooked into treatment. We used the skateboard to increase his right shoulder motion. In addition, we used the overhead pulleys to eliminate gravity and to increase shoulder abduction and adduction. Although he fatigued easily he was an active participant in his 45-minute treatment sessions.

On the twenty-ninth of May (after a full week of occupational therapy and physical therapy treatment), I increased his treatment in occupational therapy to two times per day. His first treatment session was strictly bathing and dressing. At first he was very nervous about this and passive. He wanted everything done for him. However, after five bathing and dressing sessions the patient had gained significant confidence. Using a grab bar, tub transfer bench, and adjustable shower hose, he had progressed to where he was able to bathe with minimum assistance, versus maximum assistance when we had begun. In addition, he had made the same gains with his dressing and undressing abilities. Initially, he had been adamant about not shaving himself; however, with the proper setup, he was shaving himself independently. I had learned that A.J. did best when you told him what was expected rather than giving him choices.

GIFT EXCHANGE: "DOING FOR" PATIENTS AND "DOING FOR" THERAPISTS

A fourth strategy which therapists used to build alliances with patients led them to treat disability in an even more personal way. This was "doing for" patients, going outside their formal role to help the patient with a task and in this way create a strong social bond. A hand therapist called up the insurance company to find out why one of her patients was not getting his work compensation benefits; a pediatric therapist knitted a sweater for a patient's mother; a psychiatric therapist noted that the patient she was evaluating had an arm in a cast and promised to get her some adaptive equipment (a personal move here since she is going outside her formal responsibilities, hence "doing a favor").

In each of these examples the therapist goes out of the line of duty, stepping out of a narrowly defined professional role to send the message to the patient that he or she is willing to care in a more personal way for that patient. This obligates the patient to, in turn "care" for the therapist by cooperating with therapy. Setting up a personal bond through "gift exchange" is a powerful means for influencing another. Sociologists have done extensive work on the exchange of intangibles. Anthropologists, notably Mauss in his seminal work, *The Gift: Forms and Functions of Exchange in Archaic Societies* (1967), did some early pioneering exploration in this area. Mauss argued that, particularly in societies lacking elaborated formal systems of legal contract, gift exchange was used as a substitute. The giver indebted the receiver, and this gave the giver a kind of social power over the recipient of the gift. The occupational therapist confronts the same problem as members of small societies. Therapists need to be able to obligate patients to do something for them and often use gift-giving as the means for doing so. Mutual gift-giving can create strong bonds—those we associate with families, for instance. Witness the central place of gift exchange in family life—birthdays, Christmas, Hanukkah, and the like.

CASE EXAMPLE

The following case recounts small (but important) gifts the therapist gives to a patient (such as wearing a skirt the patient likes). It especially reveals the importance to the patient of offering a gift to mark the end of their work together.

The Gift

by Heather Moulton

Peggy was admitted to a nursing home from a rehabilitation hospital in May of 1984 at the age of 80. She had suffered a middle cerebral artery infarct with left hemiparesis in February of the same year, 3 weeks after having had surgery at a prominent Boston teaching hospital for mitral myxonea. She was referred to OT and PT for evaluation and further treatment with hopes of returning home.

Occupational therapy goals addressed her mild short-term memory loss, sensory and perceptual deficits, ADL capacity, transfer ability, left shoulder subluxation, developing contractures at the left wrist and digits, left upper extremity pain, and seating. Over the course of three-and-a-half months of therapy at three times a week, it became evident that Peggy would not be returning home.

Peggy was an extremely tall, slender, elegant, and dignified Boston Brahmin who had attended private schools. Peggy was fond of gardening and was also an avid rider. She had owned horses for many years. She had lots of friends who visited the nursing home regularly, and her husband visited daily. Her brother was also very involved and supportive.

One very interesting problem, which did improve, was her memory. Peggy was alert and cognitively intact, with the exception of a mild short-term memory loss. She perseverated on the date "12 February 1984." When asked the date she would consistently say "the twelfth of February 1984." She could correctly state the dates of past surgeries and events in her life, but OT stuck on this one date. Her CVA occurred on 24 February 1984. This date happened to be not long after her cardiac surgery, when she was still hospitalized. Her husband stated that the date held no significance. We spent quite a bit of time talking about all the events which led up to her stroke and events that happened since. Through these conversations, it was revealed that her father and husband's father were prominent physicians. She was proud that an entire building of a prestigious academic teaching hospital was named after her father-in-law.

Peggy was also connected to this hospital in another way, as a very active volunteer in a club named after another building, in which I had worked. We could share a lot of stories about the club (with which I was familiar) and the hospital.

In a further effort to resolve the perseveration on this one date, we would read issues of her favorite magazine, *Town and Country*, from January 1984 to the current issues, to give her a temporal grounding. Flipping through the pages created further conversations about clothes and horses. Peggy loved beautiful clothes and would quite often compliment me on what I wore. Since I also rode horses, we would discuss all the area stables and what was happening at the Hunt Club.

After Peggy was discharged from direct services, I consulted on her with the restorative nursing assistant who provided ROM, splint care, and ambulation twice daily. I would visit Peggy to check in on her. One winter day I wore a black, mid-length, wool crepe skirt, with over 200 crystal pleats in it. Peggy thought it was beautiful. It reminded her of a skirt she used to dance in. She commented on how it flowed, so I showed her how fun it was to twirl in. After that, she would periodically ask, "Heather, next visit would you do me the kindness of wearing that beautiful black skirt and twirl for me?" It was certainly not an inconvenience to do so, so I would make the effort to wear it whenever she asked. I would pop in every week or two, just to chat for 5 to 10 minutes. Throughout the next year, I would also take time to give her husband refresher courses in transferring her into and out of their car. She often went out to tea parties and her husband was not particularly adept at transfers, so he needed reminding about technique.

In October of 1985, hunt season was in full swing. Peggy asked the restorative nursing assistant when I was coming in next. Eleanor told her my schedule and left a note for me to stop by to see Peggy. I did so and found her husband visiting. I offered to come back, but she said no, "I have something I want to give you." Peggy then ceremoniously asked Charles to hand me her riding crop. He did so. She said, "I want you to have this for your riding." I was floored. This worn leather crop had the most magnificent hand-carved ivory and sterling silver handle on it. It had an inscription that read: "To Margaret _____ / _____ Club/1950". My immediate response was, "Thank you so much Peggy, but I cannot accept this." Her eyes filled up with tears as she said in her dignified Boston Brahmin accent, "But Heather, you must take this. You have done so much for me." I immediately knew that I must accept it. It clearly meant a lot for her to give it to me and it would have hurt and insulted her to reject it. I gave her a big hug and said, "Peggy, thank you so much; it's magnificent and I will treasure it." It had been given to her by the club at the hospital where she had volunteered and where I had worked. Charles also expressed her [Peggy's] desire for me to have it, therefore I should accept it.

Case Discussion

The above story involves both tangible and intangible gifts. Many therapists have mentioned intangible or symbolic gifts they have exchanged with patients. In a thesis completed by Beth Courtney in 1992, she indicated that all the therapists whom she interviewed regarding how therapists handle termination of a therapeutic relationship gave their patients symbolic gifts. One therapist baked cookies, another gave her telephone number. One therapist had a patient who was discharged abruptly. She commented "It happened so fast. We didn't have much time I just gave him a big hug and wished him well." One therapist made a comment that we have often heard, "I just gave him a few words of wisdom and wished him luck." Many therapists have mentioned these "words of wisdom," or "just one important thing to remember," as a sort of gift they like to give each patient as a symbol of something to remember us by. These "little" gifts seem to function just as tangible gifts do in society, as a way of signalling a relationship.

EXCHANGING PERSONAL STORIES

A similar strategy for creating personal bonds through exchange was evident in the exchange of stories of personal experience with patients. This was probably the most common strategy for building rapport, and most therapists were self-conscious and explicit with researchers about their use of personal stories in creating relationships with their patients.

Here is a typical example which illustrates the informal and unobtrusive use of this kind of exchange. A pediatric therapist is working with a child who will not stop crying. The mother is looking uncomfortable. They have talked earlier about the fact that the child is teething. The therapist, though concentrating on dealing with the child, glances up at the mother and says, "It's funny how teething affects kids different. To some kids, it's nothing. Now Jamie, my friend's kid, he's young to be getting teeth. And both parents are working. So it's just chronic exhaustion." The therapist does not stop to tell an elaborate story for she is also treating the child. But in this off-hand "story in a nutshell"—an extremely common form of storytelling by therapists—the therapist lets the mother know indirectly that she understands why the baby would cry, and she also simultaneously uses a personal experience about a friend.

Most of the therapists in the Clinical Reasoning Study, especially the more experienced ones, relied heavily on telling personal stories and jokes in their clinical sessions. In using personal experiences, in sharing a personal self as a way to create bonding, the therapists were constantly reasoning about how much of the self to reveal, how to make themselves, rather than the patient, the momentary center of attention, without losing the basic therapeutic structure in which the therapist gives and the patient receives treatment.

JOINT PROBLEM SOLVING

A fifth commonly used strategy for developing cooperative relations was asking patients to problem-solve along with the therapist. For instance, one therapist working in the spinal cord unit described joining the unit with no previous experience in spinal cord injuries. She was unfamiliar with much of the adaptive equipment used; consequently, many of the patients knew more than she did about equipment, though one of her tasks was to teach the use of this equipment to patients who were unfamiliar with it. At first she was embarrassed about asking other patients to help, and about receiving advice from the patients she was supposed to be teaching. But she began to discover how much patients liked having a role to play by teaching her. When working with a new or unfamiliar piece of equipment, I often observed her calling for other patients to give their advice about how to use it. This became a strategy not only for creating a personal bond between herself and the patient but also for creating a social group out of isolated individuals. Many of her patients were adolescent boys, often with some mechanical expertise, and solving such problems allowed them to take a strong, active role, if only for a little while.

Interactive Behaviors

Since the Clinical Reasoning Study, several of our students have done research and written theses related to aspects of clinical reasoning. Some of their findings related to therapist–patient interaction will be discussed here.

Maria Langthaler, an occupational therapist from Austria who completed a master's degree at Tufts University in 1989, wrote a thesis that was the result of a carefully detailed analysis of three 5-minute segments of a videotape of a treatment session that had been made as a part of the AOTA/AOTF Clinical Reasoning Study. She first developed three broad areas of therapist behavior to analyze. They were physical orientation, voice elements, and activity. These were further refined to permit closer analyses. For example, physical orientation was subdivided into six categories:

1. Proxemics
2. Body orientation
3. Gestures
4. Head movements
5. Eye movements
6. Facial expressions

Maria developed a coding system whereby she was able to note each instance of the therapist's behavior in each of these categories and to indicate in detail just what the action was. For example, she first describes the action—"the therapist tells the patient that she wants to move backgammon pieces with her right hand, even though that is the less functional hand, in order to try to improve strength and mobility in that hand. During the game the therapist moves her head and eyes several times." Maria indicates each eye movement next to the point in the transcript that corresponds to the event. During the game the patient slightly loses his balance in the wheelchair. The therapist sees this immediately, prevents him from falling, and helps reposition him. They resume the game but the therapist now constantly, but subtly, glances at the patient. Maria notes each instance and notes such details as "looks quickly at him and then back to the game" (Langthaler 1990, p. 108).

Having recorded hundreds of subtle and obvious behaviors of the therapist, Langthaller then developed a list of 33 attributes that were used to interpret what the meaning of these behaviors might be. Each attribute could possible apply to several behaviors. Some attributes were "reinforce, reassuring, confronting, share meanings" (p. 99). Eye movements and facial expressions or tone of voice may all be used to convey any of those meanings. In an interchange between therapist and patient that took approximately 2 minutes, Maria recorded 33 therapist behaviors; she interpreted that the therapist was conveying scores of meanings constituting hundreds of instances of communication. Karen LaCour, an experienced Danish occupational therapist, viewed the tape several times to determine if her interpretation of what the therapist was trying to achieve through her behaviors was congruent with Maria's. Eventually the therapist's own interpretation was sought. All three interpretations were very congruent. What this research (and others that will be mentioned later) seems to us to indicate is that therapists are very careful about how they interact with patients and further, that they have a vast repertoire of subtle behavior that they employ, for a whole host of reasons, in order to carefully manage the treatment session. This management of one's own behavior and the patient's behavior is so much a part of the practice that it is easily observed and interpreted by other experienced members of the same profession. In experienced therapists this is much more than "management." It is an orchestration of the session in which the behaviors of the therapists influence and reflect the behaviors and moods of the patient.

Sonja Bradburn (1992) conducted a study in which she videotaped interview-evaluation sessions between two therapists and their clients in a psychiatric hospital. These were analyzed and interpreted. Sonja showed the tapes, first to the original therapists and then to colleagues, to verify her interpretations. Here too, there was a great deal of agreement regarding what the therapist might be trying to accomplish when she behaved in a particular way. Sonja identified six general categories of reasons for interacting in particular ways. She referred to these reasons as "strategies." They are "empathy toward the patient" (p. 27), "active listening" (p. 31), "values clarification," "affirmation of the patient" (p. 41), "non-reactive to expressed poor judgment" (p. 44), and "goal setting" (p. 45). Under each category Sonja identified several behaviors that the therapist used to achieve or express her interactive purpose. For example, some of the behaviors she lists under "Strategy I: Empathy toward the patient" are facial expression, silence, direct verbal acknowledgement, and agreement with the patient. Each of these behaviors may, in turn, be used for several reasons. Both therapists, Sarah and Alice, "used facial expressions to convey feelings of identified suffering or pain with the patient" (p. 29). At other times, therapists used facial expressions to express esteem or encouragement for the client. This research, too, seems to suggest that therapists carefully orchestrate their interactions with patients for a variety of reasons.

Summary

These studies and others confirm for us our belief that this careful monitoring and interpretation of one's own and one's clients' behavior must be guided by a particular kind of knowledge and a particular kind of reasoning, which is complex, sophisticated, and essential to therapeutic practice. We chose to call this "interactive reasoning." We propose that it is guided by a type of process that Howard Gardner refers to as "interpersonal knowledge" (1985, p. 239) through which knowledge of one's own feelings can be used to understand and even change the feelings of another. Interaction not only encourages participation in therapy, it is, in many instances, a therapeutic process. Occupational therapists use a great number of types of interaction. The selection and conduct of particular interactive strategies and styles is supported by interactive reasoning.

■

Conditional Reasoning
Creating Meaningful Experiences
■ **MAUREEN HAYES FLEMING**

Introduction

In Chapter 6 we proposed that there is a particular kind of inquiry that therapists use when they attempt to understand the "whole person" in the context of the life-world, given the influence the disability may have on the person's future. We called that inquiry "conditional reasoning." Here we will discuss this in further detail. This type of reasoning we feel is not a strictly cognitive process, nor is it always conscious. This is a form of reasoning that is based in social, cultural processes of understanding one's world, oneself, and others. It is a kind of reasoning that makes meaning in the context of culture, a kind of reasoning that requires imagination and an excellent ability to understand; a kind of inquiry that therapists employ when they wish to understand the patient from a phenomenological point of view. In the next chapter, another form of phenomenological understanding—narrative reasoning—will be discussed. Therapists try to understand what is meaningful to the patients, and to their perception of themselves and others in the physical and social contexts in which they experience their lives. In order to do this therapists need to have an ability to imagine the clients, both as they were before the illness, and as they could be in the future. They also need to be able to enlist the patients in imagining a possible future for themselves. This takes all the therapist's interactive reasoning skills and more. It requires an ability to understand and "see" people as they see themselves, and the ability and energy to project a picture for a person's future, one vivid enough that the person will be willing to participate in the image making. The image needs to be so forceful that the person is able to marshall the energy and courage to participate in the treatment activities that will help make that future image a reality. This requires not only great imagistic thinking on the part of the therapist, but also an ability to construct those images along with the patient. The result is a revitalization of intentionality and an engagement in meaningful experiences. Intentionality is rekindled and directed toward the creation of the person's new life. Meaningful experiences are used in the clinic to stand in for meaning-making experiences in the life-world, the everyday world. These meaningful experiences often have words attached to them; sometimes they do not. Generally, these meaningful experiences are actions or sets of actions that the patient and therapist experience together. In the next chapter, Cheryl Mattingly will discuss her theory of narrative reasoning in which therapists and patients construct a future image in words. In this Chapter I will discuss a kind of therapeutic practice in which meaningful experiences are constructed through actions, actions that often carry significant symbolic meaning. This practice is guided by a form of thinking that therapists allude to when they say that they "treat the whole person," and that we are calling conditional reasoning.

Action and Meaning

Many of the therapists who successfully employed a phenomenological approach to practice were interested in their patients' abilities to make new meanings for themselves. This might be as complex as reconstructing a sense of self, or as relatively simple as finding meaning in an ordinary event. This action taking and meaning-making seemed to be most fruitful when the therapist was using conditional reasoning to help the patient imagine and act out experiences—experiences that might teach tasks that could become one of the many small components which contribute to leading a more meaningful life. We think that conditional reasoning revolves around the ways that therapists think about which of the actions that the patient takes have potential for meaning-making. In this chapter we will look at three aspects of meaning-making relative to action. The first is the concept of intentionality, which is a life force through which the individual focuses his or her energy for being in the world. Intentionality is essential to action. Next is the concept of habit. Phenomenologists believe that habits form an important connection between ourselves and our world. It is through our habit structure that we make meaning. Finally we will discuss symbolic meaning, especially those symbolic meanings that can be apprehended through action in a social context. Occupational therapists use action to elevate and maintain their clients' intentional state.

They develop habits, both motor and mental, that may be meaningful as they are being developed, or may enable the person to make meaning of her or his life in the future. Occupational therapists also provide activities that hold symbolic potential, which may or may not be taken up by the client.

CASE EXAMPLE

The following story illustrates the uses of action to develop intentionality; making meaning through the development of habits of action; and the symbolic meaning of the actions taken, the skills attained, and an object made in occupational therapy. It also illustrates some of the therapist's conditional reasoning processes. The therapist thought about the person's past and future and offered activities that simultaneously helped him develop skill in concrete tasks: knot tying and negotiating spatial directions. These same activities held tremendous symbolic potential as well.

Ben

by Anonymous

One of the most unique treatment experiences I have had as an occupational therapist was being able to work with an individual who challenged my abilities in the areas of physical disabilities and psychosocial manifestations at the same time.

His name is Ben. He was admitted to the acute care psychiatric ward following a suicide attempt (jumping out of a car which was travelling at 60 mph). Ben's story went like this: He had a very successful career in the military. He served a total of 23 years. Upon retirement, he initially found his free time to be wonderful, but his idleness soon became a source of frustration for him. It was very difficult for him to structure his time and develop new and challenging activities. He eventually went to school for another career and began working. After settling in to his new career field for almost a year, Ben suffered an aneurysm. As he perceived it, his life was beginning at the bottom.

He was in a coma for two months, underwent the array of testing, surgery, rehab, surgery, then suffered another aneurysm. After 5 months of hospitalization, he was discharged to live with his second wife in a large city in Europe. This was a difficult situation because he had been previously separated (but not divorced) from his wife.

While in Europe, Ben said he came to the realization of his deficits. He explained that he frequently would just sit and cry because he couldn't tie up the garbage bag, wrap up an extension cord without getting all caught up in it, or even go and get a newspaper two blocks away without getting lost. His time was spent arguing with his wife, watching movies that she had to get for him, crying, and doing nothing.

On the day of his suicide attempt, Ben said he was being taken by his wife to a medical appointment, they were arguing, and he impulsively attempted to jump out of the car. Because the car was going too fast and his physical abilities were limited, the door was immediately pushed back on him, keeping him in the car. (His immediate reflection on the situation was "I can't even commit suicide by myself."

Ben was transferred to our hospital on the acute psychiatric ward. This was not Ben's first episode of depression, however. He had another hospitalization just before his retirement for depression, and two previous suicide attempts. This, accompanied with his physical and cognitive impairment, made Ben a high risk for future attempts.

Ben's physical and cognitive impairments included left-side motor weakness, visual impairment, perceptual impairment, and memory impairment. Not knowing how long Ben would be hospitalized, I had begun to focus on his depression. I knew I needed an understanding of his physical and cognitive impairments. It was 2½ years since his aneurysm and he probably wasn't going to get much return. He needed to adapt himself and start living again.

Ben had a number of interests, but his lack of motivation and lack of confidence in his abilities overwhelmed his ambition to attempt activities. I kept remembering his story about crying when he couldn't tie the garbage bag. Such a simple task he couldn't do . . . why couldn't he do it? The best way I knew to find out was to reenact the situation in a nonthreatening manner. I asked Ben if he had ever tried macrame. He commented that it looked too hard and knew he wouldn't be able to do it. I gently persuaded him so that I could observe his task performance. We had previously sat down a couple of times to talk and I thought he trusted me. I taught him the simplest knot in the book. He attempted the half square knot over, and over, and over.

I used a bright cord and put dark backing down for better perceptual discrimination. I tried written directions. I tried verbal clues. After three frustrating sessions, Ben completed a key chain. He even put a bead in it. One simple key chain. It wasn't exactly perfect, and it took so long that I began to think that it was too much for Ben to tolerate. For him, however, that key chain opened new and exciting possibilities. He held that key chain in his hand, smiled and asked if he could do more.

Throughout the course of the hospitalization, Ben made few physical gains. He completed an already started plant hanger, using the same knot with fewer mistakes and easier performance. He and I worked on his sense of direction and lack of confidence stemming from his visual and memory difficulties. I provided him with a map of the hospital and we spent an evening together identifying cues he could use to get around by himself. I tested him throughout the hospital and he did very well. He began working on a model, participated in some life-skill classes on problem solving, and began a work therapy job in another building before his discharge from the hospital. Ben made very good progress and was able to build his confidence during his hospitalization.

Before he was transferred to another hospital, Ben and I talked about his future. He knew his life wasn't going to be easy. He simply said that he at least felt like trying now. He held out the key chain and verified to me that whenever he felt like quitting, he would hold the key chain, think of me, and remember the day he completed it. It's been about 4 months now since he left. I wonder how often he's used that key chain.

CASE DISCUSSION

This story briefly illustrates the three major concepts that will be discussed in this chapter. First, therapists have an intuitive sense of the importance of a state of being that phenomenologists refer to as "intentionality," and its inextricable link to action. This therapist was able to help elevate Ben's intentional state by helping him to participate in a desired action— knot tying. Second, habits that embody personal and cultural meaning are essential to the building and rebuilding of the self. This therapist helped Ben rebuild his sense of self through building skills, habits, of knot tying and direction finding. Third, symbolic meaning is relevant to both action taking and meaning-making. Occupational therapists offer activities that may be interpreted at several levels of meaning. This therapist suggests that Ben found symbolic meaning in the key chain. Perhaps it held some keys to his future.

Activity, Choice, and Intentionality

MULTIPLE REASONS AND CHOICES OF ACTIVITY

One of the first things that Cheryl noticed in viewing the videotapes in the Clinical Reasoning Study was that "Therapists never seem to be doing something for just one reason." My first response to this was a laugh of recognition. Yes, that is typical of occupational therapists. They always try to choose activities that will lead to meeting a lot of goals at the same time. This is not simply a matter of "killing two birds with one stone." It is more complex than that. Therapists expect to be doing something for more than one reason most of the time. It is part of their professional culture to choose an activity that will serve several purposes simultaneously.

A therapist may use one task or "doing" activity for multiple reasons. Some reasons may be quite superficial and relatively obvious, while other reasons for selecting this same activity may be quite complex. These multiple reasons may even be based upon different types of thinking, bodies of knowledge, and rationales. For example, Liz, a therapist, decided to teach Paul, a man with a high-level spinal cord lesion, how to type on a computer with a mouth stick. Her reasons for doing this included the following:

1. Her knowledge of his neuromuscular status led to a decision to do an activity in order to strengthen the muscle supporting his head.
2. Her understanding of the attention mechanisms and their relation to neuromuscular tone led to selecting a very attractive or compelling activity.
3. Realizing that this is a man in his late twenties prompted her to select an activity which may eventually lead to employment, or is at least a worklike activity.
4. Understanding Paul's very great loss of control over his

body led to the selection of an activity which would give him control over something important.

5. Understanding his tremendous loss of social status and social contact prompted Liz to select a high-status activity for him.

6. Paul was a very social person with a great sense of humor and a lot of friends. Liz selected the use of the computer as a communication device. He could write to his friends. In fact he continued to write to Liz and other therapists and nurses on his home computer long after he left the hospital.

7. Talking with Paul and asking him what he would like to do was also essential.

8. Typing on the computer had the potential for becoming a meaningful experience.

This, a single activity, was used for many different reasons. The therapist might have had this same list of reasons and selected a different activity if she had felt it would meet the criteria that she had set up, based on the goals she and Paul wanted to attain. Conversely, she might use this very same activity for a different set of reasons with another patient.

There are many tasks that therapists use as therapeutic activities. Many of them are used by all or most therapists, and some of them seem to be considered the specific domain of occupational therapy. Those tasks generally fall into the broad categories of activities of daily living (ADL) and the learning or relearning of tasks and behaviors related to a social role. However, the specific task and method of going about learning something, "attaining a goal," is more often selected in relation to the stated or perceived needs of the individual than to the medical condition per se. In other words, there are few fixed one-to-one relationships between the medical condition and the activity chosen. Activities are not "prescribed" based on rules; rather they are selected based on sets of principles that guide the therapist to select activities that meet particular criteria. The criteria for activity choice are linked to the therapist's knowledge of the limitations that the clinical condition will place on the person's activity level, and on an understanding of the patient as a particular individual with particular interests and motives.

MOTIVES FOR THE USE OF ACTIVITY

Schutz (1975) made an interesting distinction between two different types of motive. He called these the "because" motive and the "in-order-to" motive. He comments:

It is frequently stated that actions . . . are motivated behavior. Yet the term "motive" is equivocal and covers two different sets of concepts which have to be distinguished. We say the motive of the murderer was to obtain the money of the victim. Here "motive" means the state of affairs, the end, which the action has been undertaken to bring about. We shall call this kind of motive the "in-order-to motive." From the point of view of the actor this class of motives refers to his future. . . . Motivated by the way of in-order-to, therefore, is the "voluntative fiat," the decision: "Let's go!" which transforms the inner fancying into a performance or an action gearing into the outer world. (1975, pp. 126–127)

The other form of motive that Schutz proposes is the "because" motive. The "because" motive is one that is propelled from the person's past experiences.

The murderer has been motivated to commit his acts because he grew up in an environment of such and such a kind. . . . Thus, from the point of view of the actor, the because motive refers to his past experiences. These experiences have determined him to act as he did. What is motivated in an action in the way of "because" is the project of the action itself. (p. 127)

Distinguishing these two motives seems to be especially relevant to some features of occupational therapy practice. Most of hospital practice is based on the diagnosis-prescription model. It is generally assumed that the person is ill "because" some factor is present (or absent or malfunctioning). Determining the cause of the illness—identifying the "because" aspect of the illness—is the primary motivator for the physician. Once the cause has been determined, a treatment is selected "because" it has been shown to be effective against the offending causative agent. Thus, most of the motivation—the conscious direction of most practitioners—is in the "because" mode.

Occupational therapists use the "in-order-to" motive far more than the "because" motive. The "in-order-to" motive is definitely the primary motivator for occupational therapists. The OT and patient are almost always focused on the future. Therapists are often heard making comments like "You need to keep this hand flexible so it will be ready to use when you regain some strength," or "Practice this so you can learn to hold a fork," or "Will you do this activity this way at home or will it be different?" Activities at any level are always conducted "in-order-to" lead to a higher or smoother level of function. Some possibility of greater skill attainment is held as a future goal, and the present activity is engaged "in-order-to" make that possibility come true.

Sometimes the occupational therapists use the "because" mode, but this is usually for the purpose of determining more closely what the cause of a particular observed behavior might be. To be more specific the OT might notice some difficulty a person has in handwriting or basic balance, or frustration tolerance. The OT might wonder if the poor handwriting (for example) is because of increased spasticity, decreased strength, perceptual disturbance, anxiety, or loss of sensation. The therapist might also wonder, "If so, is the situation transitory or progressive?" The "because" motive is used to analyze or explain present behavior based on past or present possible causes.

Occupational therapists actually combine motives and are typically in what we called a transitional motive state. They frequently are well aware of the "because" aspects of the person's current situation and often use the "because" motive to advantage. Instead of focusing on the inhibitory aspects of the prior condition, occupational therapists often try to find out what the person's interests were in the past and use those prior interests and motivations to design OT activities that have some relevance for the person. An example was a videotaped session between Ed, a patient, and Kathy, his therapist. Ed had been in the hospital for a while. He had a therapist who found him difficult to work with and "unmotivated to do therapy." Kathy was "filling in" for this therapist who was on vacation. Ed did not want to cooperate with Kathy, who wanted him to do some shoulder strengthening and mobilization exercises. She tried checkers, a sanding board, and turning pages in a book with a page turner. Ed attempted these only slightly and complained of pain and stiffness. He asked her to scratch his ear, complained about the hospital food, and read the name of the manufacturer off the margin of the checkerboard. Clearly Ed was not interested in participating in therapy. Then Kathy said, "Wait a minute. I'll be right back." She returned with a car magazine. She sat next to him, showed him how to use the page turner and began talking with Ed about the cars in the pictures. A lively discussion took place as Ed gradually turned pages with slow awkward motions, turning clumps of pages at a time. Watching the tape we became quite enraptured with Kathy's conversation and her extensive knowledge of cars. Kathy, it seems, is the only sister in a large family with a passion for cars. Suddenly we noticed Ed again. He was turning pages with speed and precision, backwards and forwards and—guess what—with excellent shoulder range and mobility. Ed was in the spinal cord unit "because" he had been in an automobile accident. Ed learned to use the page turner "because" he was interested in cars. Kathy had him look at the car magazine, "because" of his prior interest and "in-order-to" motivate him to learn to use the page turner. This was also a motivator to continue ranging and strengthening the shoulder, which is necessary "in-order-to" learn and accomplish other tasks. Ed wanted to learn how to drive a car with hand controls, but it was not clear whether or not he would develop enough function. He did not connect the exercises with that goal and was not "motivated." Kathy created motivation with the car magazine "in-order-to" get Ed to exercise his shoulder.

MAKING CHOICES

In addition to the fact that therapists are always doing something for more than one reason, there is the tradition that therapists frequently ask patients to make their own choices of treatment. "So what do you want to do today?"—or a variant of that question—is a common opening to an OT treatment session. Such a question is a bit astounding in the medical setting, where typically the patient is the passive recipient of the pronouncements and prescriptions of the medical and nursing staff. But few patients and no therapists seem surprised at this approach. Usually the therapist follows this question with a list of possible activities: "Do you want to go to the gift shop and get that card you wanted for your nurse? Or do you want to practice your wheelchair mobility? Or how about going to see Mary down the hall?" The interesting thing about these choices is that they often appear to be quite different activities, but when considered more carefully, are all quite similar. The therapist has set some goals, usually in response to prior discussions with the patient. These goals seem to be transformed into sets of criteria. In the example above some criteria might be

- To practice wheelchair mobility.
- To get out of the bed and room and into a more social situation.
- To begin relating to other people as a "doer" rather than receiver.
- To start working on a sense of independence and self-confidence.

Typically, the patient selects an activity or suggests one. There are some cases when patients say things like "Aren't you supposed to know what I should do? or "I don't know. Do you really think I should?" Therapists usually encourage the patient, saying "Oh sure!" or "You won't know until you try." All these strategies seem to clearly illustrate that therapists believe that patients should make choices and should try things that they have not tried before, at least since their injury. This is so ingrained that therapists appear to ask people to make choices who are seemingly unable to do so.

THE CENTRAL IMPORTANCE OF MAKING CHOICES

A videotape of Cathy and Daryus is a good example. Cathy, the therapist, is working with Daryus, and 18-month-old boy with multiple limitations. She is apparently trying to encourage visual attention, reaching, and trunk balance. Cathy and Daryus's mother are sitting on the floor. Daryus is in his mother's lap, facing Cathy. Cathy has placed a small benchlike table between Daryus and herself. On it are two toys. One is a plastic cube that spins. Each surface has a different picture, response button, mirror, or some other attraction. The other is an oblong box, divided into about eight compartments. When someone presses the lid to any of the compartments a plastic character jumps up. Daryus makes a movement toward the cube. He almost reaches it. The move is not what one would call direct or controlled. It is clear that he has difficulty stabilizing the shoulder or projecting the hand into space. It is not clear that he really was aiming for the cube or wanted to play with it. Cathy responds, "Oh, you like this one. Good we will have this one." Her voice is enthusiastic and somewhat singsong. She crouches to be sure that she maintains eye contact with the child. Simultaneously she removes the other toy, places it out of sight, and centers the "selected" toy in front of him on the bench.

One might wonder,"Why go through all that?" The toys, though different in appearance, could certainly achieve the same ends. Why should a small child make a choice, especially if it is not clear that he really did choose that toy in the first place? For whatever reason, the importance of the patient's making a choice is a strongly held value on the part of most occupational therapists.

INTENTIONALITY—A STRONG BUT IMPLICIT VALUE

I think most occupational therapists would probably say that it is important to make choices because that is how we are individuals or express our individuality. Occupational therapists have a very humanistic philosophy, which centers around respect for the individual. So it is not unusual for them to value choice making as an expression of individuality.

Having observed the choice-making event between Cathy and Daryus, we reviewed other tapes and found that most of the therapists had people make choices. The two hand therapists did not ask for choices. They prescribed the activity. The result was that one patient participated only marginally. The other did so only after elaborate and skillful manipulations on the part of the therapist to get him to participate in the treatment.

So what is this choice making? Is it a strategy? Is it the manifestation of a philosophic belief? Or is it a method employed after an analysis of the situation? It is probably at least all three. It is clearly a very common strategy. It is virtually characteristic of OT practice and is distinctly different from most other hospital practice, including physical therapy. One explanation for this may come from another of Cheryl's observations, something she called "attributed intentionality." She interpreted the interaction between Cathy and Daryus as one where the therapist was not sure if the child was making a purposeful choice of the toy but where Cathy's belief in the importance of choice making led her to attribute intention to this behavior on the part of the child. Cathy said, "Oh, you want this one. Good!" as if to model or praise choice making.

It seems that therapists have an implicit belief in the central importance of what phenomenologists refer to as intentionality. Intentionality is at the very core of all our beings. It is an inner force that directs us outward into participation in the life-world. Schutz defines intentionality as

> The most basic characteristic of consciousness: it is always the consciousness of something; it is directed toward something, and in turn is "determined by the intentional object whereof it is a consciousness." The intentional object, then, is the object intended and meant by the individual, and singled out by him for a perceptional and cognitive attention. An intentional act is any act in and through which a person experiences an object, whether physical or ideal. Through it, the object is cognitively constituted. (Schutz, 1975, pp. 318–319)

Occupational therapists understand and value intentionality at a tacit level. They so strongly believe in it that they are willing to provide a temporary or tentative intentionality until the person can reorganize himself or herself and remobilize his or her intentional being-in-the-world. Therapists, because they have studied more psychology than philosophy, tend to refer to this as "motivating" the patient, but I think it is a lot more than that. I think it is a way of *enabling* intentionality.

ILLNESS AND INTENTIONALITY

One's intentional direction of oneself toward being-in-the-world is what Merleau-Ponty refers to as the "intentional arc." "It is the intentional arc which brings about the unity of the senses, of intelligence, of sensibility and motility. And it is what 'goes limp' in illness" (1962, p. 136). Kestenbaum elaborates:

> If the intentional arc goes limp in illness this means that the integration or interpenetration of habits has been destroyed.... The habits of the human body weave round in the human environment and when these habits lose at least a minimal level of integration, the self loses the capacity of carrying on the interaction or dialectic of self and world and [doing so] in a manner which contributes to the growth and expansion of the present habits. When the tension of the intentional arc is disrupted, the body's manner of being in situations is transformed, and sometimes any manner of being is rendered impossible. (1977, p. 27)

Intentionality is essential to life, it is the life force of the individual self. If intentionality is "broken," as Merleau-Ponty says, in illness, then it makes sense that occupational therapists do what they seem to be doing. That is, when patients are very ill, or very young, therapists do not expect much intentionality, they free themselves from their usual requirement of having the patient make the choices, and make the therapeutic choices and decisions themselves. It is not uncommon for occupational therapists to "range the hands" of comatose patients. They assume that patients would not want to develop contractures and have useless hands "to wake up to." Frequently therapists say that they talk to their patients "just in case" they can hear or understand that someone is caring for them.

An example of a patient who is fully conscious but with minimal intentionality comes from Patty, a therapist in the Clinical Reasoning Study. She was working with a patient, Rob, who, as she says, was "just laying around waiting for a cure" and not participating in therapy. This bothered Patty because she knew this was not good for his physical health, and this attitude just did not "sit right" with her.

> So, one day I just decided that he had to start working or he was not going to get "rehabed" and he would get worse with contractions and things. So, I gave him a little pep talk and told him I wanted him to get moving. It took me a few tries to get him interested in doing anything, but then I remembered that he was sort of artistic. I asked him if he wanted to look at the plans for the apartments that were available in the adapted housing complex he was scheduled to move to in New Hampshire. This was a place he did not want to go to, mind you, but I gave it a try anyhow. He said and did a lot of distracting and negative things, but I just kept working the conversation and the activities back to the plans, and he finally got quite interested in them. He had some good ideas for changes too! Things were really different after that day. He sort of took off.

Rob started participating vigorously in therapy after that. He turned out to be a big "success story." The last we heard of him he was still living in New Hampshire in the specialized housing and had created a business for himself using his computer, phones, and considerable intellectual and social skills to match people with specialized needs to adaptive housing. He is a novel kind of real estate broker.

Patty helped Rob to revive some intentionality by making him focus on the concrete task of planning the room arrangement of his future apartment. Rob's intentional arc could now be directed toward a possible future. Rob's intentional arc could now be directed toward a possible future. Therapists like Patty, Cathy, and Liz seem to be willing to supply a sort of intentionality for their patients until the patients are able to revive or develop some of their own. Therapists often talk about needing to wait until patients are "ready" for a stage of therapy, but also the need to gently push and prod people along. Part of this could be interpreted through motivational psychology; but we found the therapists' actions and perceptions, though not necessarily their words, were very similar to the concept of intentionality.

As therapy progresses, therapists seem to take patients through a series of activities in which the role of the therapist as director of the treatment fades, as the patient is better able to direct her or his own treatment. Intentionality seems to be a common thread throughout practice. It is also a dominant way in which treatment activities are sequenced. The "in-order-to" motive is a strong force here. The therapists ask patients to make choices and engage in successively more difficult tasks in order to have people "take on more responsibility" for their own treatment, self-care, and eventual return to the community.

Therapists are able to get patients to focus on activities long enough—a few seconds—that they "want" to do something that they had not done before or thought of as interesting, a focus that sparks intentionality. Intentionality is essential to action, and if the occupational therapists want patients to act, they need to elicit intentionality. Phenomenologists also believe that choice making is an intentional act that permits motor action and makes action *an act*, a significant experience. Therapists seem to be able to elicit intentionality from people with very reduced intentional status. Here is an example taken from a videotape of senior OT students at the University of New England. The students were working with very developmentally delayed adults using "sensory-integration" (Ayres, 1972) techniques. This involves using large balls and bolsters to play on in particular ways that require balance skills. One client, let us call her Joan, was considered to be a "difficult" person. She often did nothing, but when something angered her she would yell, hit, and even bite. She seldom verbalized. She had poor muscle tone and ligamentous laxity, and the classic waddling gait which results. The students asked Joan to sit on "the mushroom"—a large rounded cushion. With some help Joan managed to get on the mushroom. The next task was to rock the cushion back and forth. Joan was supposed to stay on for the ride, but her balance mechanisms were not up to the task—or maybe her attention flagged. Joan slumped to the floor awkwardly but managed to land in an upright sitting position. For a moment there was complete silence. The same thoughts ran through everyone's head—what would Joan do now? Would she fly into one of her famous rages? What would we do if she did? Suddenly a student said, in an enthusiastic and praising tone, "Oh Joan, you jumped. That's great!" Two students rushed to help Joan up. In a rather imperious manner Joan returned to the starting spot and sat on the mushroom and bobbed up and down, signaling the students to continue to rock the ball. Joan tipped herself off, made some happy sounds, and returned once again to the starting spot. These patient students rocked Joan again and again. Joan actually got better at this and began saying "Jump, jump, jump!" each time she marched around the ball to the starting point.

The students and the staff were delighted. They actually found something Joan liked! The therapists who understand sensory integration techniques have elaborate theories about this behavior and its causes in the central nervous system, and they well might apply to this example. I think, however, that this is also an example of therapists eliciting an intentional state, using activity to bring this person into relation with the life-world, to have an intentional focus on something. The students were exhausted at the end of this session (Joan weighed about 150 pounds and must have taken 20 jumps off the mushroom), but they were delighted with the results. They saw something in Joan that no one had seen before—a spark of intentionality.

Therapists sometimes share their own intentionality with their clients. They "do with" patients, as Cheryl has observed. Some of this "doing with" takes an interesting form. It is not the typical reciprocal interaction, where one person says or does something and the other responds. In these situations both the therapist and the patient are internally focused on the same thing or object of interest. They may be both trying to figure out a better way to do something—adjust a splint, for example—or they may be judging just the right color of paint for a craft project. There are numerous situations in which the therapist and patient both focus on the same object, with the same intensity in the same way, often with the same expression on their faces. The intentional state of each person is heightened to the same degree and focused on the same object. This forms a therapeutic bond between client and therapist. It is my speculation that this is also a technique that therapists employ to heighten and maintain the person's intentional state. It is certainly a consciously employed technique to maintain the person's *attention*, but I think it is also a tacit technique used to elevate and focus the person's intentional state. Therapists talk about the importance of keeping the person "focused on a task," to "stay with it," and not to "lose the session." These are colloquialisms that they use that express an implicit understanding of the importance of intentional states.

SOME PROBLEMS WITH OCCUPATIONAL THERAPY'S VIEW OF ACTION AND INTENTIONALITY

The concept that a simple activity is performed for more than one reason seems to be so much a part of the therapists' thinking that they tend to feel that it is "obvious." "Of course you don't play checkers with a patient just for the sake of playing checkers!" You might play checkers in order to have an activity that is an interesting and intrinsically motivating means to practice and improve finger flexion and extension. You might be evaluating or improving perceptual motor function or eye–hand coordination. Maybe you are looking for cognitive retraining, or improvement or lengthening of attention span, sitting tolerance, or trunk control. Perhaps you want a sense of accomplishment, or a safe way to allow the person to be competitive. Possibly you set the patient up to play with another patient, so that they have a structured way of beginning to interact with each other. Maybe the game, which you know the person can win at, is a symbolic gesture, reflective of the process of figuring out the "next moves" that will be necessary to "win" in the process of rehabilitation. Perhaps a "jump" or a "double jump" is symbolic of a recent accomplishment and affirms that more progress is possible. Any of these "reasons" or "in-order-to" motives may also spark some intentional state that has become dormant as a result of the illness or injury.

Most casual observers of occupational therapy do not have multiple interpretations of the purpose of a given activity. They tend to interpret the activity at face value. To them playing checkers is simply playing checkers. This is especially frustrating to therapists. First, because to them the multiple meanings and purposes of activities are essential to their type of treatment, their implicit philosophy, and therefore the complexity of their reasoning. Secondly, the activities therapists do are everyday activities—dressing, grooming, recreational activities—and the very ordinariness of these activities makes the treatment appear rather simplistic. There is little technological sophistication apparent in this treatment, and therefore little social status accrues to the therapist in the technologically oriented hospital hierarchy.

Therapists are generally not able to convey in words *why everyday activities are important*, or why it is important that the treatment be *individualized*, or why the patient should *direct* the treatment. They do not have an articulated theory or philosophy of intentionality that is universally shared and easily conveyed to the intelligent consumer. However, they do have a strong shared implicit sense of the importance of activity and choice making, and the role these play in rekindling intentionality.

Patients' interpretations of the reasons for the activities seem, on the surface, to fall between the two extremes. They often recognize quite quickly the central importance of activities such as dressing, eating, and grooming to their rehabilitation. Those are activities in which we all want to function independently. Patients seem to "rest" a while in the sick role and then become willing to return to participating in or becoming responsible for their own self-care. Occupational therapists are usually the people who motivate and assist this transition. Therapists seem to have a clear notion of the tasks that their patients can and should relearn. In their minds, experienced therapists have relatively precise timetables regarding when these can be accomplished. Often the therapist has what could be regarded as higher expectations for the rehabilitation process than does the patient. Eventually, though, the therapist is able to convey expectations, encourage participation,, and teach the new tasks. Patients usually are willing to participate, and many will think up new activities, or practice prescribed activities on their own and proudly show the therapist these accomplishments at the next visit. So for some activities, especially valued self-care tasks, the importance of the activity is clear to the patient. The patient, seeing the essential nature of these tasks, does not demean them as do some of the other hospital staff.

Developing Habits and Having Meaningful Experience

HABITS AND MEANING

One early concept of occupational therapy was "habit training." Reconstruction aides felt that if they could train or retrain the veterans with whom they worked to have good habits, these men could not only be employed, but would be physically and mentally improved as well. Physical and mental health were thought to be closely tied to good habits of living. This term is not used much today, probably because of its old-fashioned tone, but the concept is central to occupational therapy practice. Occupational therapists are very sure that they want their patients to acquire habits of various sorts. New habits of self-care, habits useful to school performance, habits of structuring their environment, all are established so that patients can function more easily in the commonplace world to which they will return. Therapists often make comments like "It hasn't become a habit yet," or "Good, I can see you did that automatically," or "It has to become part of the person, otherwise it wouldn't work." Their concept of habit training is very strong. They use it in a wide range of applications. They use it narrowly, in the sense of planning and executing motor patterns, or broadly, in the sense that habits are ways of conducting one's everyday life. Occupational therapists have a strong sense of how habits are essential in providing the substrate for the structure of the conduct of everyday life activities. Habits make action consistent, yet flexible; they allow for an automatic function that permits attention to be directed elsewhere; and they form a reassuring background for the conduct of everyday action.

Clearly physical motor habits are valued. Less well articulated, but quite strongly held, is the notion of mental habits as ways of ordering one's experience in the world. The formation or reformation of mental habits may be more predominant in the OT practice in psychiatry and work with children, especially those with learning disabilities, but it is also visible in the practice of the physical disabilities therapists. A more elegant notion of the role of habits, that expressed by the phenomenologists, also seems implicit in much of the practice of occu-

pational therapists. The concept is that habits both embody and structure meaning.

PHENOMENOLOGICAL CONCEPT OF HABITS

Simply stated, phenomenologists see habit as the embodiment of
previously apprehended meanings and the structure by which new
meanings may be taken up. Habits are the mental and physical medi-
ators between our world and ourselves. This meaning is not an abstract
cognitive construction, rather it is a meaning that is understood or
apprehended in an immediate way. The meaning is there for us without
being converted to an abstraction or a linguistic statement. This type
of understanding is what the phenomenologists refer to as prereflective
meaning, meaning that has not been consciously examined through a
cognitive process.

Kestenbaum comments "habits are the structures of the organisms'
'silent workings' " (1977, p. 26). Through habits we come to make sense
of our life-world. "Through one's habits, indeterminate phenomena are
transformed into determinate objects; the unity of the object is achieved
by one's pre-objective sense-giving power, a power derived from habit"
(Kestenbaum, 1977, p. 32). Habits then are ways of structuring experience so that it is intelligible to us in a very direct way. Occupational
therapists talk about developing habits through experience. It is also a
major tenet of the profession that experiences should be meaningful to
the individual. Further, therapists are strongly committed to the concept of the development of the self and the self-concept. It is not clear
whether they see the intricate relationship of these three factors: experience, meaning, and habit. Kestenbaum clarifies the phenomenologists' view: "Without habits which provide taken for granted meanings, there would be no self to be in a situation. Without an habitual
self, there can be no experienced situations" (1977, p. 30). So phenomenologists believe that the acquisition of habits enables us to make and
express meaning in the hundreds of everyday activities that comprise
our being in the life-world. These habits and meanings participate in
the construction of the self. This self then participates in the activities
that are interpreted through the habitual meanings incorporated with
them. The activity only becomes experience, something that influences
the self, it it is apprehended through some structure of meaning.

Habits are acquired over time and in that process become infused
with meaning. This is meaning that is "felt" in an implicit way each
time the habitual act or thought occurs. In this way past meaning is
brought to the present situation. As Kestenbaum comments, ". . . the
acquired meanings of the past are immediately present in one's habits"
(1977, p. 33).

It is clear to us that occupational therapists have an overt belief in the importance of habits, both motor and mental. They believe that habits are essential to everyday functioning in the everyday world. This is one of many of the commonsense concepts of their professional philosophy. At a deeper and more tacit level, occupational therapists seem to have a philosophy very akin to phenomenology, at least on this point. Therapists believe that habits embody meaning and that embodied meaning is important to the development and perception of the self. Occupational therapists also believe that habits are important for helping individuals maintain themselves and their self-concept in their everyday life-world. Occupational therapists working in psychiatric settings seem especially attuned to this concept. They see their role as one of "maintaining and developing functional skills." Habits— including behaviors, meaning, and a sense of time and sequence—are all important abilities that therapists hope to maintain, develop, or restore in their patients.

THE DISRUPTION OF HABITS IN ILLNESS OR INJURY

If habits are essentially our accrued experience, our sense of self, and our primary way of making meaning of ourselves and our environment, what happens when habits are disrupted? The sense of devastation and hopelessness and worthlessness that able-bodied individuals experience when they suffer a traumatic loss of physical ability is tremendous. It is not only the tragic physical loss and the loss of a projected future, it is the loss of the very ability to apprehend and express oneself and one's sense of being-in-the-world.

Clearly the disruption of the ability to conduct our lives in the habitual way disrupts the meaning structure of one's life in a way that is so significant that it can disrupt one's entire sense of self. Many patients with traumatic injuries say they are not the same person any more. Many refer to themselves as "a cripple," or "just a cripple," or "a quad." Therapists comment that this pejorative way of referring to oneself often occurs in a "stage" of rehabilitation where the person has realized that her injury is permanent but before she has been able to realize some "function gains." The loss of habits means the loss of a sense of self. Therapists have interpreted this phase of referring to oneself as a cripple, or referring to a nonfunctional arm as "it," as a form of depersonalization. The person has lost a sense of the usual self and has not yet constructed a sense of the new self, so the person feels in a very real sense like a "nobody," "just a cripple sitting in that chair" with "these things that aren't my legs—not legs at all, just a nuisance I have to drag around." Therapists go to considerable lengths to help patients negotiate this phase. "It's a tricky balance," they say, between recognizing the magnitude of the problem and not giving in to depression and despair. Therapists often talk to patients about this, but their usual approach is to take action. Often the action involves getting the person to relearn an important everyday task like eating, dressing, or writing.

This "therapeutic activity" is the re-creation of a habit structure, one which like the old one will embody meaning. This too is a "tricky balance," because therapists hope that by relearning an important task (set of habits) the patient will regain important meanings and meaning-making abilities. But there is always the risk that the plan will "backfire." The activity may remind the person too painfully about what they used to be able to do, or do well, and can now no longer do, or do to their own level of satisfaction. The following is an example from a therapist who recalled her worst experience on her affiliation.

> My supervisor gave me a new patient and I was supposed to evaluate him and make up a treatment plan. Well, he was this good-looking guy, he had just graduated from college. It was difficult for me, we were so similar. I worried and thought a lot about what activities we could do. What could a 20-year-old paraplegic want to do? On my way home, I thought of a brilliant idea. I knew he liked basketball, so I thought I'd rig up a small hoop in his room. I thought it would be good for shoulder strengthening, trunk stability, and all that good stuff. So next day, I went marching into his room with my grand plan. I got less than halfway through my planned speech about what we were going to do and why and he said, "Get the hell out of here!" I stood still in shock. He started swearing at me and telling me to leave. I left—in tears of course! Well, as I was thinking about it later—and I thought about it a lot I can tell you—I realized here was a guy who could run and guard and slam-dunk and now he can't do any of these things. No wonder he was angry with me. I was the one that got "slam-dunked" that day and now I see why.

This is not necessarily a "mistake" on the part of the student, nor is choosing a formerly valued activity necessarily a good or bad idea. Much of the selection of the activity depends upon the individual patient.

CASE EXAMPLE

The following story is by an experienced therapist working in a psychiatric hospital.

Dan's Wallet

by Christine Custer

For the past 7 months, I have been working with a young man named Dan. Dan is in his late twenties and has been treated for chronic mental illness most of his adult life. I see him twice a week in our OT clinic through an outpatient day program; he attends the skills group (craft-based intervention) and is a very steady participant.

When I assumed responsibility for this group and began to learn to know its members, Dan was already involved for a number of months. He sat alone, often mumbling and swearing to himself while working. He chose his projects without interaction with me and proceeded independently but haphazardly; the results were unplanned, sloppy, and dissatisfying to Dan.

Early on, I recall two events that seem to have been turning points in gaining rapport with Dan. One day, I had made a pot of coffee for the session. Dan helped himself to a cup and we began talking about our passion for the stuff. He asked if he could make the coffee next time; so for several weeks, we made coffee together before "getting to work." Around that same time, the OT department was undergoing personnel changes. During one session, Dan called me by another therapist's name . . . rather than the usual reorienting or discussing difficulty with change, I took a risk and joked with him about it (I hadn't seen his sense of humor at that point yet, but felt we had some trust built). So I called him "Herbert" when I answered; he just roared! Since then, it's kind of a private joke between the two of us; sometimes Dan purposefully called me by the wrong name to get my joking response (I think this is very affirming for Dan).

Once we developed rapport, then came the task of tackling behaviors and task performance. I gradually introduced more contact while Dan was working on a project. From session to session, and even minute to minute within a session, I could not predict what Dan's responses would be. It was constantly a new "dance" with Dan. . . . I had to always observe and monitor how much I expected, interacted, supported, confronted, or even smiled. When Dan was at his low points, he could be actively hallucinating and speaking to "that old man in there." His voice became loud and the swearing resumed, creating a chaotic atmosphere in the clinic. Dan almost seemed to ruin his projects at these times, and any feedback was met with hostility. Discussions with the treatment team revealed no past successes in managing Dan's difficult behavior, except for consequences of being restricted to the halfway house. On Dan's best days, he was brighter, began socializing a bit with the other group members, and took responsibility for his work. He could plan a fairly complex task and use creativity and resourcefulness successfully (one time he spent tedious hours measuring and drilling holes to make a cribbage board from scrap wood). At these times, Dan spoke of hopes to live in an apartment on his own again. The team noticed that these better times were concurrent with steadier hours at the sheltered workshop and lessened family contact.

Recently, I felt frustrated with Dan's erratic behavior and little tangible progress to independent living. Dan's goal to live on his own was vague and his idea of goals in therapy were highly concrete (i.e., to make a wallet). The team offered little support: the doctor, in short, told me to "just keep Dan busy." In the meanwhile, Dan was becoming disruptive in the clinic again and rejecting attempts on my part to care about his work, himself, or others in the group.

In one particular session, Dan persisted about making a wallet. My agenda was to have him socialize and work in a responsible manner. Partially out of desperation and partially out of ingenuity, I gave Dan a new assignment: he was to look at the Tandy Leather catalog and "shop" for the projects he wanted. I gave him a budget and a few guidelines. Dan spent the entire hour deciding, writing, and calculating his order; he looked at what was already in the clinic to stretch his dollars and asked for feedback from myself and another member. During this same time frame, we talked more about what living on his own meant to him and how what he does in OT is relevant to his goals.

This was 1 month ago. Dan's supplies arrived and he worked on his wallet for 1 month (the longest he's spent on a project yet!). Dan's work looks professional too . . . even stitches, detailed design, et cetera. Dan says he is willing to try some simple cooking and budgeting activities (starting with something he likes and knows how to do, of course . . . brownies).

I have found that the most successful gains with Dan have been when I carefully listened to what he saw as important and brought this together with what I saw as valuable for him. I have to take a "back door" approach with Dan, since direct approaches are too threatening for him; to ensure his commitment and feelings of security in learning new things, I was the one who had to change and become more concrete! Above all, I continued to believe in Dan.

Just yesterday, Dan completed his wallet. At the end of the session he showed it to the entire group proudly and said, "I like my wallet. It took me a long time to make and I didn't swear when I was doing it!"

SELECTION OF ACTIVITY

Activity selection can result in the development of a new, positive structure of habits and meanings, which in turn will result in a reformulated sense of self. Patients seem to recognize the importance of developing this new habit structure and what it does for their sense of self. The following is a transcript of part of a conversation between a therapist and patient. This conversation took place during their last session together.

Don: By the way, I put my shirt on sitting up this morning. (Liz goes to shake his right arm, the less functional one; he offers her his stronger hand; she pushes away the stronger arm, and deliberately takes the weaker one.)

Liz: Did you really? Was it a struggle to get that hand up?

Don: Yeah.

Liz: That's great, Don.

Don: Almost decided to do it lying down, but then I figured I only have a couple more days that I can brag to you. (They both laugh.)

Liz: That's great. Excellent.

Don: I am getting a lot stronger with this arm, and this is a really nice big blue shirt.

Liz: That really makes all the difference. . . . What's great about what you did with the shirt is you were able to problem-solve.

Occupational therapists and their patients work hard to counteract the loss of self and meaning caused by injury, by regaining habits that, in turn, restructure meaning and help regain a positive self-concept.

Occupational therapists take on both the task of reteaching activities of daily living and restructuring one's habits of being in the world. They do not really talk about "being-in-the-world" the way phenomenologists do. However, their strong commitment to the patient's acting on and interacting with the environment and the notion that a sense of self is reflected in and created by the interaction with the "human and nonhuman environment" can be taken for the same concept.

"HAVING" A MEANINGFUL EXPERIENCE

Occupational therapists stress the importance of "meaningful activities." They feel that an essential part of therapy is selecting, usually with the patient, an activity that will be meaningful to that person. The OT literature is replete with this concept. The occupational therapists we have conversed with frequently use an expression that we think is closely related to this. They talk about wanting to "make the session work." These conversations have led us to believe that therapists view the therapeutic process in a way that is very similar to John Dewey's notion of "having an experience." Dewey's concept of experience is not one of simply being somewhere or doing something. He feels that only those acts or events that we make meaning of constitute experience. It is meaning that makes action "an experience" as Dewey would say. The possibility of making meaning and therefore having an experience is there because of our habit structure. If we have mental habits of attending to or interpreting phenomena in particular ways, then these habits will enable us to "take up" new experiences of similar phenomena in a rapid and meaningful way. This experience is taken up by the self. An external phenomenon becomes part of the experience of the self. So it could be said that it is experience that constitutes the self. But the self is not a static entity in Dewey's view; rather it is an evolving process whereby the self is continually developed and modified by experience. The habit structure is continually modified also in response to meaningful experience. Our physical and mental habits not only bring the self into relation with the world; they further develop the self through the making of an experience.

The nature of such experience is complex and difficult to understand in an abstract way, even though at the practical level we have experiences everyday. Kestenbaum explains Dewey's concept of an experience.

> Any experience which is "an experience" involves . . . habit and self-world integration. When a person has an experience, one marked by wholeness, completeness and unity, habits operate in such a manner that

the experience is integrated within and demarcated in the general stream of experience from other experiences . . . (Dewey 1934, p. 35)

This "forming" of an experience as it moves from inception to close is the forming of a new integration or configuration of organic habits. The experience is an experience, and integrated, unified whole, because in interaction with the world, the habits constituting the self are formed into a new or whole configuration. (Kestenbaum, 1977, p. 28)

We see that habits, meaning, experience, and the self continually evolve. This description of the relationship of habits and experience may sound to the reader like this is a conscious cognitive process, but it is not. It is a phenomenological process that happens as a result of an individual being's living in the life-world, in the context of culture. In this process meanings are not "made" in the cognitive sense, nor are habits behaviors that are developed by rote practice. They are much more intrinsic, dynamic, and tacit. Dewey tries to express this notion by saying that habits are "had" or "felt." In much of his work he speaks of the "lived" experience. Experience is "taken up" immediately, it is had or felt or lived; it is not primarily dependent upon any cognitive or linguistic process. It is meaningful in and of itself, provided one has habits of thought or action that can provide a structure by which the experience is apprehended.

Although they probably would not state it in such a way, it is clear that occupational therapists understand the power of experience in the phenomenological sense. This may account for the observation that occupational therapists seem to need little verbal affirmation from the patient that an activity was worthwhile or "it was a good session." Occupational therapists feel that they can sense some meaning-making on the part of the patient and that this fosters their interest in creating an experience for their patients.

If experience that is an experience is as powerful as Dewey thinks, then creating experiences for patients makes sense. If an experience or a number of experiences can change a person's mental or even motor habits and change the self, then occupational therapists have indeed selected a very powerful strategy for treatment. Occupational therapists have chosen to help patients through experiences in the uncommon world of the clinic, not simply as practice for doing daily tasks in the life-world. They use experience as a way to help patients develop habits through which they can make new meanings of themselves and their worlds. Since patients often need to very drastically restructure their sense of self, it makes sense that occupational therapists give them the tools to do that. Habits are those tools, and they are created through "lived" experience. Occupational therapists help the person live or feel an experience in the clinic in order to be able to live in the everyday world.

Consider the story of Ben (told earlier in this chapter). The therapist took him on a "trip" down the halls of the hospital to practice following directions because he had sustained brain damage that had interfered with his pathfinding abilities. But it was also conducted in order to give Ben the experience (occupational therapists call them "success experiences") of finding his way. This experience could be the kind of felt experience that would restructure not only his habits of finding his way in space but also himself, a person who was capable of negotiating his way through the streets of his home city. Through an experience in the hospital Ben may have developed new habits of being-in-the-world.

CASE EXAMPLE

The following is a story where the therapist and patient had worked on developing new habits and a new sense of self. The patient seems to have felt he needed just a bit more help, and fortunately the therapist was perceptive enough to see that too.

The Old Jim and the New Leg

by Brenda Head

I had been seeing Jim on a regular basis for the past couple of months and I perceived that our relationship was coming to an end as he prepared to start his new job at the fish plant. Today's session would focus on a discussion of how the work orientation session went at the plant and any last-minute changes that needed to be made before Jim took on his new job with his old employer.

As I sat at my desk finalizing Jim's vocational evaluation, I marvelled at how well Jim had done compared to others (40-year-old, unilateral lower-limb amputation) whom I had known in a similar situation medically. It had only been a year since his accident, he was back living at home with his wife Susan and their two preschool age children, and was about to go back to work full-time. How fortunate for Jim and his family that his employer was prepared to accommodate him in an alternate job with similar pay.

It was getting late and I wondered what had happened to Jim. This was so unlike him, not to call, or to be late. I was about to call his home, but just at that moment I heard Jim and the elusive squeak in his prosthesis on the stairs. I was glad he had come because I wanted to talk with him and clear things up before he started work. As he entered my office, the phone rang and I answered it. While answering the phone I looked up to acknowledge his presence and to my surprise he looked like someone who had been crying. I remembered hearing from Jim's previous therapist that the rehab team felt he had not allowed himself or his family the time to grieve the loss of his leg. I hung up from the brief incoming phone-call.

I felt the pressure of time, as Jim was a half an hour late and it was just 15 minutes until I had to leave for an appointment.

This was not going to be an easy session, as Jim paced back and forth and seemed unable to sit. Before I could say a word Jim turned around and "shouted" back to me that he would be back in 5 minutes as he was going to the coffee shop to get a drink. I responded by saying I would join him in a minute and we could talk there.

I had not seen Jim like this before; he seemed uneasy. What was going on? As I gathered my coat and briefcase, I picked up Jim's file and laid it back in the filing cabinet, and I remember thinking I would not need it this afternoon.

Upon entering the coffee shop I picked up a coffee and was about to take a seat when I noticed Jim sitting way over on the other side in the smoking section. I sat down next to him and opened with, "Jim I never knew you smoked." That seemed to be the opener he needed, as he quickly replied, "There are a lot of things people don't know about me." "What sort of things?" I asked. "Oh, you know, how things have changed," Jim said.

We talked. Jim talked. He talked about how he, his family, and his friends were having difficulty connecting with the old Jim and the new leg. As Jim finished his coffee we both shared how we had to go somewhere else but that there was a need to meet again. And we did....

Case Discussion

Creating experiences for people that will be "taken up" as an experience is not easy. It requires careful consideration of the person, an understanding of their current habit structure, and a great intuitive sense of what might help in this particular situation to "make the session work." Merleau-Ponty says "habit expresses our power of dilating our being in the world or changing our existence by appropriate fresh instruments" (1962, p. 327). The fresh instruments therapists help patients acquire are a new way of perceiving themselves, and their ways of being in the world. In the above story Brenda helped Jim start this process by understanding how difficult it was for Jim and his family and friends to perceive the "old Jim" with his "new leg."

Meaning and Metaphor

Occupational therapists use activities and their meanings as a way of helping the person gain or regain a sense of self, a self comprised of an image that is structured by acquired habits and the meaning embedded in them. While the meanings embedded in habit are important, some therapists offer patients an opportunity to explore deeper meaning through therapeutic activities and the conversations surrounding the activities. Some therapists and patients can interact very directly and can discuss the meaning of the disability for the patient in a very direct way. For example, Liz and Don discussed his situation on his last day in the hospital.

Liz: [Why do] you say that you are not that critical a case? How critical is that right arm to you?

Don: It's very critical—

Liz: Yeah. Yeah. So don't minimize your feelings about that, this is really important to you.

Don: Yeah, well I remember early on when I was beginning to appreciate the fact that I was going to be able to walk again, and that my left arm was working well enough that I was going to be able to manipulate the environment, that I was thinking that I was going to consider myself lucky if I got out of here with my right arm in a sling for the rest of my life. I would be very lucky.

Liz: Wow, uh . . .

Don: But I guess the more you get, the more you want.

Liz: Right, I was just going to say, right.

Don: Now I really want this right arm to be as good as this left arm is now. And I want the left arm to be perfect. And I guess I want a 50-pound grip compared to, I don't know, the 100-pound grip that I used to have. It has roughly, let's say fifty percent at this point. I know it's got a long way to go still. It's, I don't know, all like a vanishing point on the horizon, you know what I mean, the more you get to it, the more you want.

Liz: (moves closer to him) I think that (pause) you are very clearly describing your feelings about that.

Don: I really want this *arm*, because at this point, it's almost like if I had a choice between more return in my legs or more return in my arms, I think I would go for the return in my arms right now. I am more handicapped by the arms right now than the legs. I can reasonably maneuver around the household situation, you know. I can walk up and down the corridors three or four times without getting that tired. It's easy to see that I'm going to gain more strength in those legs, and stuff, the arm is not so easy to see, it is difficult to imagine what I'm going to have to do to get it (pause)

Liz: . . . better . . .

Don: . . . better. The doctor seems pretty confident when I see him.

Liz: What does he say about it?

Don: He . . . you know I started moving the finger and he said, "Wow, great, great." He says in a year you won't believe it. He is talking like it's going to be slow. And that doesn't scare me, to think in a year, that's fine. If I can keep it up in the air in 3 or 4 months, I will be very happy. If I don't have to have it in a sling or something when I walk or something, if I can have it as strong as this in 6 or 7 months, (indicates his stronger left arm—patient was right-handed) that will be great.

Liz: What happens if you can't?

Don: I'll manage and . . . still consider myself lucky. I want more but I'll consider myself lucky. There's no question that I am lucky.

Liz: It's just interesting, when we have talked about this, you want to call yourself lucky. Yet this is one of the worst things that has ever happened to you and it really stinks.

Don: It is definitely the worst thing that has ever happened to me in 40 years or 35 (Don is rolling back and forth in his wheelchair), but, uhh . . .

Liz: Relatively speaking.

Don: Yeah, mmm, uh . . .

Liz: You can't use your right arm. You can't use it to be (not clear) to be a touch typist . . .

Don: . . . a guitar player, piano, volleyball . . .

Liz: I mean, I am not trying to rub your nose . . .

Don: No, no. I know, it's there and it bothers me (Don appears jittery).

Liz: There's a perspective, you think about what could have happened. But, don't sell yourself short about the loss.

Don: I think it's going to come back, I really . . .

Liz: (whispers) Go for it.

Don: I really have almost no doubts at all, I am soorrry . . .

Liz: "Almost no doubts." (laughs, warmly) That's a little close to having . . .

Don: Yeah, well, you've got to be realistic about the thing, I am just mad that it is so much work.

Liz: Well, one thing is, you know . . . is that nobody knows.

Don: Yeah.

Liz: Nobody knows.

Many activities seem to be designed specifically as metaphors for complex actions and meanings—meanings that the patient may value but does not have the physical or linguistic skill to express. We saw many examples where keys or key chains were used as metaphors for "keys to the future," or "keys to the problem," or "keys to understanding." Games such as checkers and backgammon were full of words like "block," "move," "home," "beat-it," which often led to discussions or simply "knowing looks" between therapist and patient; and it was clear that "home" in the game held some meaning relative to the patient going home—an event usually fraught with meaning and a lot of anxiety. In the discussion between Kathy and Ed about the cars in the auto magazine, Ed drew parallels between himself and cars. He said his accident resulted in his breakdown and now he was in the shop for repairs and a new set of wheels.

Therapists varied widely, as did patients, in their use of metaphor. It seemed to us that therapists often chose activities specifically because they would have meaning for the patient. Yet when patients began to explore these meanings in depth, some therapists immediately "backed off and stuck to the procedural," whereas others were more willing and able to participate in deeper discussions. Some therapists consciously planned activities that would offer the opportunity for meaning-making at deep levels and were facile with interpreting the patients' metaphors. Others interpreted meaningful activity as actions that are inherently meaningful like eating and dressing.

PHENOMENOLOGICAL SENSE OF ACTION AND MEANING

Some therapists seem to think, as do many phenomenologists, that the very participation in the activity conveys meaning. There is an assumption on the part of some therapists that action is always a metaphor for a more inexpressible meaning. It is not deemed necessary that the patient be able to reflect on or discuss this meaning. It is assumed it is there for the person at the level she or he is able to apprehend it. Activities seem to be offered to patients, and they can make the choice of the level at which they choose to interpret them.

This was especially clear on a tape of a therapist working in a psychiatric hospital with a very difficult older woman with Beinswanger disease, a very rare syndrome. The task is stringing beads to make a necklace. In the 30-minute session the conversation, which is almost nonexistent in the beginning, shifts from one focused on the size, color, and attractiveness of the beads to a discussion of who will get the necklace and what it is worth. The patient increases her estimate of the value of the necklace as the session and the necklace progress. This change and progress are also reflected in the depth of the conversation, which evolves from a very superficial one to one discussing her place and role in her family, and finally her desire and hope to be able to control her behavior, see herself as able to plan and direct her day, and be recognized as an important family member. Here, a patient who was almost nonverbal became articulate about the deeper meaning of making the necklace and the remaking of her life. However, as stated earlier, therapists are also content to believe that the meanings do come across, even if the person cannot talk about them.

FORMULATING MEANINGS

If we assume that everyday actions take on and express meanings at both personal and social levels for people in the everyday life-world, then the same must be true for those who have suffered an impairment. We may also assume that most of these meanings come fairly directly in a taken-for-granted manner. The meanings are absorbed along with the actions or, said another way, the action and the meaning are the same. When a person's everyday activities are disrupted, so are their meanings. With injury the person's activity pattern and meaning structure are disrupted. Therapists seem to have a strong sense of this disruption. They work on the manifest problem—relearning everyday activities—and the patients usually participate willingly. Therapists seldom speak to the patients about the deeper meaning of this, and if they do, it is often after they have developed a good trusting relationship with the patient. It is not uncommon to see therapists in early interactions with patients say very little to the patient. They have a quiet professional presence. This is not simply because of the newness of the relationship. It has to do with the therapist's belief that if the patient goes through the actions, the meanings will eventually be understood. Therapists say you just keep doing the activity and eventually the patient "gets the message."

Deep levels of meaning or the metaphoric message contained in some activities may or may not be grasped by the patient. To the therapist, a simple act of combing one's hair may be both a new physical accomplishment and a symbol of one's readiness to become "presentable," to present oneself to society. The willingness to comb one's hair may be a metaphor for the willingness to reenter society, or even present one's new, altered, but still significant self to the world. Patients vary in their levels of interpretation of the possible multiple meanings of activities.

One phenomenon seems to be clear. That is, that the patients often seem to "absorb" these multiple meanings fairly early on in the therapeutic process, and, if they can articulate them, often do so very much later. These are often stated as indications of particular turning points or breakthrough points in therapy. Therapists, too, seem to keep quite complete mental logs of these events and meanings. It is not uncommon for therapists and patients to recall these events together in the context of a discussion around a new goal or challenge. It is a frequent type of discussion of discharge.

It appears that not only are there multiple reasons for doing a particular activity, there are also multiple levels of meaning that the activity may convey. The activity then becomes more than just itself, it becomes an identifiable milestone, and a metaphor for some larger and more difficult process of transition. The meaning of the transition is apprehended through the action that stands for it. It may be that the meaning is absorbed directly as part of the action, and that only after repeated action or reflection, or both, can the patient raise this level of meaning to the linguistic level.

Therapists seem quite attuned to this necessity of conveying meanings through actions. They are also aware that the patient may or may not be ready to deal with meanings at a deeper level. A therapist may spend a good deal of time in a sort of medical care mode, or appear more like a nurse or physical therapist—dealing with and determining levels of involvement or impairment. The manifest message here is "I will take care of you until you are ready to start getting better on your own." Conversely she or he may spend time discussing and acting out, in either a direct or metaphoric way, the sense of loss, or anger, or depression the person feels. Often therapists operate at several levels at once. While it seems that even in experienced therapists the manifest purpose—the rehabilitation procedure per se—is the dominant mode, it is not uncommon for them to abandon direct treatment rather quickly when the metaphoric message or the social meaning of something becomes more important.

Therapists sometimes are willing to temporarily sacrifice the procedural purpose for the metaphoric message, if they feel it is essential to meeting the long-term goals. In one tape a young therapist is working with an older lady who looks strikingly like the actress Ruth Gordon. What appears to be happening on the tape is that the therapist is asking the lady to go through various motions presumably to increase or improve or maintain her range of motion in her upper extremities. The lady is very cooperative and cheerful, calls the therapist "Suzie" and talks with the camera person as well. The lady frequently compliments herself and says, "I'm doin' good," "That's great isn't it," and so on. The therapist is only mildly reassuring and encourages her to try this, or do it like this.

In discussing the tape it turns out that this was not a good session at all in the mind of the therapist. The lady did not do the motions in a way that would have helped develop or maintain range. She could not remember the instructions and, as an exercise session, it was generally a disaster. However, the therapist also said that she realized that it was very important for this lady to see herself as productive, "doing good," and being independent. The therapist thought it best to not destroy that self-image, of which "doing good" in therapy was a part. She reasoned that it would be best to work gradually over the next few days to improve on the exercise program rather than to correct the lady at that time and risk possible loss of self-esteem or hope for improvement in her condition.

Putting It All Together: Treating the Whole Person

The therapists often used two phrases to describe their treatment. They were "putting it all together" and "treating the whole person."

Treating the whole person did not mean that the therapists were in charge of the patient's whole medical and psychological treatment. In fact, in the traditional medical sense of the word "treatment," occupational therapists are quite peripheral to the treatment of the patient. The phrase is intended to convey the feeling that therapists concern themselves with the patient as a person, an individual with many facets and interests and concerns. By saying that they treat the whole person, therapists meant that they treat the person as a whole, not a sum of ill and healthy parts. This need to view people as a whole required that they attend to many different aspects of the person, in light of their past and their potential future. This required many forms of reasoning. The disparate forms of reasoning and the different processes and bodies of knowledge forced the therapists to integrate them in some reasonable whole that would guide and monitor therapeutic practice. We propose that conditional reasoning is their method of achieving this integration.

The phrase "putting it all together" seemed to mean that while therapists often had to think only about the disability, or only of the individual patient, at a given moment, they were concerned that they should eventually think about and do something about the patient as a whole person: that is, an amalgam of person, illness, and condition. Although they used several types of reasoning and addressed several different types of concerns, therapists always wanted their reasoning to track back to making a better life for the patient as a person. Their ultimate goal was to use as many strategies as necessary to improve, as they say, "the individual functional performance of the person." Since functional performance requires intentionality, physical action, and social meaning, it is not surprising that individuals who concern themselves with enabling function would have to address problems of the individual's sense of self and future, the physical body, and meanings and social and cultural contexts, contexts in which actions are taken and meanings are made. Since these areas of inquiry are typically guided by different types of thinking, it seems necessary that therapists become facile in thinking about different aspects of human beings, using various styles of reasoning. Perhaps these multiple ways of thinking guide the therapists in accomplishing and evaluating the mysterious process that they often refer to as "putting it all together" for the person. This putting it all together for the whole person to function as a new self in the future seemed to be guided by a complex, but not clearly identified, form of reasoning that was both directed and conditional in every sense of the word.

CASE EXAMPLE

The following is a clinical story written by an experienced therapist, who typically used all three ways of reasoning effectively.

Sharing the Healing Experience

by Madelyn O'Reilly

The facility is abuzz with rumors of a new patient who will arrive on Monday for admission to the Head Injury Unit . . . a doctor, rumor has it, who has suffered a stroke. The new "admission" would be unlike the usual head injured patient; not the victim of a violent crime or a motor vehicle accident; not recruited from New York's inner-city streets; but a physician, practicing right here in Boston. Seldom is a resident admitted to the head injury unit after CVA. These clients go to the skilled nursing or geriatric units. What is different about this patient? Why the intensive rehabilitation program provided by the head injury specialty team? As the OT on the team, I know only that I shall be seeing this physician-client twice daily Monday through Friday, and once on alternate Saturdays.

No amount of rumor, no chart review, no case conference could have prepared me for the experience of meeting Peter. The stroke, it turns out, is the result of a cerebral arteriovenous malformation; and Peter is not a senior citizen, approaching retirement from the medical profession, but a strikingly handsome young man, a graduate of Harvard Medical School, and chief resident in orthopedic surgery at a Boston hospital, about to embark on a medical career.

As is my usual practice, I read only the brief admission summary, rather than the entire history, before meeting a new client. This seems to insure that I do not stereotype clients, but meet each as a unique individual, not another temporal lobe lesion, et cetera. Contrasts and comparisons will come later.

I am unprepared for the struggle to hold back tears as I enter Peter's room to see his lovely wife tediously placing pictures of herself, their toddler son, other family members, and of Peter himself, around the room. Peter's father is removing clothing from a suitcase as Peter carefully places books on the headboard shelf. He pauses and stares briefly at a volume of *Gray's Anatomy* before placing it with the other books. I quickly introduce myself, first to Peter, whose handshake feels warm, genuine, and much stronger than I would have expected, given the admission report that cited right hemiparesis. "We'll be working together on things that you'd like to do," I say to Peter, and turn. "You must be Mrs. _____ . It's nice to see you." Peter's dad introduces himself. I repeat that I shall be seeing Peter twice daily and that they are welcome to come to OT sessions anytime, with Peter's permission. "See you later, Kiddo," Peter says as I leave. Was that an immediate congenial familiarity or had he forgotten my name in the few minutes that had ensued since my introduction? . . . I wonder if his records have arrived . . . I'll read them . . . maybe at lunch time. I walk from Peter's room resisting the urge to run away crying. Why am I so overcome with sadness for this patient? Why do I want to cry more for this patient than for others? I learn quickly that I shall cry often, not only for Peter, but with him; not only tears of sadness and frustration, but tears of joy and accomplishment as well. Laughter, too, will become a part of our story as we struggle together to find a common ground for treatment and a means for communication.

His records do describe right hemiparesis, and a remarkably successful treatment program during which he has recovered nearly all active upper and lower extremity range and strength. Most devastating, however, is the accompanying diagnosis of global aphasia. Peter has lost the functional use of verbal language. He has knowledge, ideas, and concepts with which he had made sense of the world, his world, but has lost the words with which to express his thoughts and feelings and to understand the other people in his world! My treatment priorities, however, are dictated, not by medical diagnosis, but by the very first words I read: "Pt. to be placed on suicide precautions." Peter, it seems, wants to get out of the story he is in, but has not yet found an alternative or strategies to create a new story. Peter needs a motive, a vision, hope. Somehow, these must be incorporated into his treatment program, but what program? ADL training? . . . Certainly not the usual . . . Peter is completely independent in self-care . . . meticulously groomed and dressed. . . . Meal planning? Cooking? Shopping? Upper extremity strengthening? Cognitive retraining? Will these be meaningful to Peter? Will he be expected to perform these tasks on discharge? Which of these tasks were meaningful to Peter in the past? What does he need to learn? I have many questions to ask Peter and his folks.

Initially, Peter's evaluation and treatment sessions are a series of "stuck points." Every day, twice a day, I go to his room intending to bring him to "therapy" only to find him lying on his bed gazing at the ceiling, refusing to accompany me to "therapy." For several days, I respect his wishes and leave, documenting, "patient refusal." It does not take long, however, to realize that I must not give up on Peter—so "If Mohammed won't come to the mountain . . . ." Now, I visit with Peter in his room, asking questions about his family, the pictures in his room, his books, his life. Pantomime, gesture, facial expressions, and body language are continuous while we "talk." Peter even laughs, at times, at my clumsy attempts to verify what he's said or to find ways in which to respond. One morning, I find Peter staring at a diagram of the brain, tracing veins and arteries with his finger as if following a road map. I ask him if he is trying to understand what has happened inside his head (pointing first to the diagram, then to his head as I speak). Peter nods. I gesture for him to wait, and run to the nurses station, pull his chart, flip to the acute care report, jot down the exact lesion site and hurry back to Peter to talk, point, and trace that information. Peter takes a pen and retraces the "map" in his book, shaking his head and saying, "Bad, Kiddo, very very bad!" I cannot be certain that Peter fully comprehends the impact and long-term implications of his injury, but I know now that he wants to "talk" about it, and he wants someone to discuss his injury *with* him. Experience tells me it is very likely that medical professionals have talked *about* him even in his presence. How many believe that without language, Peter cannot understand communication?

Peter continues to remain in his room for the next week, but now I find him pouring over diagrams of the brain and extremities. Sessions during this period consist of "discussion" of his disabilities, and Peter agrees to work with a rubber ball and theraplast to strengthen his right hand, as he looks at the diagrams as we talk. Occasionally, Peter prefers to talk of his wife and son. During these sessions, he cries, says, ". . . very bad for her . . . ." He asks about my family, and even indicates that I look young to have children as old as mine. Peter now has a friend for life, and these sessions are documented "cognitive retraining."

Today, several weeks after his arrival, Peter appears to be in good spirits. He is looking out the window when I arrive. He has not been outside the building since his admission. He agrees that some fresh air would be good for him, and gestures that walking would be good for his leg. Finally, we leave this tiny room. Our stroll took us through the OT/PT area, where I point out the various treatments going on. Peter looks from one resident to the next, all in wheelchairs, all quite young. As he shakes his head, his eyes say, "Sad, Kiddo, very, very sad." As we reach outside and walk around the grounds, Peter smiles, and his gait becomes brisk and strong. He even teases about my obvious difficulty keeping up with his stride. We reenter the facility, passing through the dining room, where Peter observes two residents playing chess. "Good, Kiddo, very good," he remarks. He knows; he is beginning to value activity, participation in life. Will we find "activity" that will be valuable to him?

Now, Peter regularly accompanies me to a small treatment room adjoining the larger one, always looking intently at the clients and therapists as we pass. As we begin our session of cognitive retraining, sequencing tasks, and so on, Peter is bored and frustrated by most of the traditional exercises. These are usually abandoned for conversation about his family, school et cetera. Almost always, Peter has a question about a resident that we've passed on our way to "therapy."

One day while wiping my brow, and remarking about the heat, Peter attempts to ask me something about the summer. As I apologetically tell him how dense I am with a finger to my temple, Peter takes my pen and paper. He draws a picture of a house near a body of water. At the water's edge there is a small boy. Peter points to the sun in the picture, mimics driving a car, swimming, says, ". . . every day, no, week, no YEAR . . . ." Peter was telling me that as a child, he had gone to a lake for summer vacations, and I finally understand. More importantly, though, I know now that Peter can draw! He can draw anything, accurately, descriptively. Now Peter can communicate. Now we can truly talk and plan together! I must remember to supply him with plenty of pencils and paper, and to alert the team.

The team . . . this seems an appropriate point at which to relate the tone of team meetings when Peter's case is discussed. Physical therapy reports that treatment goals of improvement of gait pattern and dynamic balance are being accomplished. The therapist, however, impatiently repeats at each meeting that Peter is noncompliant, refuses to complete sessions, and ". . . continues to cry during almost every goddamned session . . . ." Speech and language reports that Peter is uncooperative, labile, perseverates on verbalizations about his wife, and doesn't demonstrate motivation to improve. In fact, he seldom attempts to name objects on picture cards when presented . . . ." Counselling has difficulty communicating with Peter, but reports on his unrealistic expectations for full recovery. I think, ". . . not a hundred percent yet, Kiddo, maybe later a hundred percent . . . ." I report on Peter's improved motivation, increased strength and dexterity, and fill the team in on Peter's artistic talents. All agree that drawing will facilitate communication, but will also be very time-consuming. The program director encourages the use of drawings if Peter chooses the method, and reminds everyone that he must be seen and charged as scheduled whether or not he is cooperative. I leave each meeting wondering if we are seeing neurologically based lability or normal human sadness, anger, and despair. Is he noncompliant, or does he believe that the therapy is meaningless? OT sessions with Peter continue, as described, for about a week, On occasion, we walk outside. I learn that Peter is a Red Sox fan . . . one more timely topic for our discussions.

We even walk to a nearby football stadium, jog around the track, and toss a softball. Peter is more relaxed now, and appears almost pleased to attend OT. . . . Still, the treatment feels haphazard, disconnected . . . I don't know where we are going . . . to what end are we working? What do we expect Peter to do after discharge? Is anyone else considering discharge or long-term goals? Certainly, Peter frequently speaks of home and someday.

Each time we walk through the large therapy area now, Peter hesitates a bit longer; he watches more intently. I think, "of course this must be interesting to him, relevant. After all, he is an orthopedic surgeon." His world was filled with scenes like this one. One day, after our session, I gesture to Peter that I'm late and do not have time to escort him upstairs . . . "Would you mind waiting while I see my next client. . . . You know Terry." As I begin passive range of motion on the client and employ techniques that are somewhat slovenly, Peter watches with a scowl. Finally, he jumps up, "Kiddo," gesturing for me to stop. Through mime and demonstration, on his own arm and mine, Peter points out the flaws in my technique and accurately describes the proximal to distal sequence that should be used. He cannot articulate the particulars of the treatment. He struggles desperately to "tell" me what to do. However, concern and excitement replace the frustration that has occurred in such situations until now. Peter turns to the client, touches his shoulder and says, "Me, Okay?" Terry, knowing that Peter is a doctor, and realizing how isolated he has been, smilingly gives his consent.

Peter, then, with the expertise of a skilled clinician, performs relaxation and inhibition techniques on Terry's upper extremities. He then gently stretches them to nearly full range. When he is finished, Terry's hands lay relaxed in his lap. He is grinning, saying how good it feels. Peter is looking at him with understanding and satisfaction. I am laughing and crying all at once for Terry, for Peter, for me. I call for the PTs and other OTs to come and look, run to fetch the program director, grab a counsellor as he walks by. Other residents wheel over to see what all the excitement is about. Everyone agrees that Terry's arms have never looked so loose, so relaxed!

My mind is racing. Peter has connected with another resident in the way that is familiar, automatic, meaningful to him. Of course, Peter, the physician. . . . back in his room, Peter and I discuss what he had done. He accurately, and more quickly than I can, indicates the location and function of the radial, median, and ulnar nerves. He asks about Terry and his injury. I remind him of confidentiality and encourage him to ask Terry. Before leaving for the evening, I visit the rehab director with a "plan." "I want Peter to assist me with treatment on a regular basis. We've all seen what he can do. I have at least four clients whose plans include passive range of motion and stretching . . . ." I list residents with whom I am very familiar and whose compassion for fellow residents is clear. We talk at length about the possibilities of such a plan: tapping into what is automatic for Peter, meaningful activity, establishing relationships, a reason for leaving his room. The director calls a special team meeting for the next morning.

I believe that I am prepared to respond to challenges regarding the nontraditional treatment proposal. It is not the first time that OT's plan or vision is incongruent with the overall plan. As is anticipated, no one is excited. Peter's counsellor, although interested, fears that I shall encourage Peter's unrealistic expectations. Speech pathologist does not argue strongly, but states that she is unsure of the appropriateness of the plan. "After all, he is a patient, not a staff member." PT is most vehemently opposed. "We don't know how well he remembers techniques" (accompanied by comments about what Peter's intellect has become). All agree that I might be encouraging Peter's fantasy, instilling false hope, intimating to him that he will practice medicine again. "We've all been complaining about a lack of motivation. Peter is motivated to help other residents," I say, attempting to hide my irritation. The executive director asks about the usual OT treatment protocol in cases like Peter's. I list ADLs, upper extremity function, cognitive retraining, and social interaction skills, all of which, I argue, will be addressed by my treatment as proposed. She makes no decision, promises to consider all the team's concerns and await input from the consulting psychiatrist who is to review Peter's progress on Friday.

Friday finally arrives. I give a synopsis of Peter's progress, and relate the event in the clinic and present my plan. The psychiatrist is not only in agreement, but is visibly enthusiastic. We expand the potential of the program. Perhaps Peter can, someday, become an OT aide. Certainly prevocational training is reimbursable treatment! Team members hold fast to their contention that I am unrealistic. My God, they are stuck in the here and now! My rebuttal, not devoid of emotion, is swift, "Reality does not mean the absence of hope! It does not need to hit him between the eyes. I honestly believe that, over time, Peter will come to understand that he will not be a surgeon, but can't we allow this reality to come to him gradually in the midst of a program that has some meaning for him? Please let me give him a reason for being here, a reason to get out of the damn bed in the morning."

After some talk of liability, and so on, the executive director agrees that, with written permission from clients, Peter may assist me with treatments, as long as I am with him at all times and am willing to take full responsibility for his performance. Once again . . . tears and laughter for Peter. I prepare a consent form and choose four residents as potential patients for Peter and me. They all agree and are excited by the prospect of being treated by one of their peers and, most of all, by having the opportunity to help Peter.

During the ensuing weeks, Peter and I see clients together. I learn from him and marvel at the skill, gentility, and empathy with which he performs his OT tasks. Residents look forward to his coming. Although Peter cannot remember room numbers and names, he certainly remembers the people and the problems. At the close of each session, he asks, " . . . How long? Born like this? . . . " We "discuss" diagnoses and histories through *Gray's Anatomy*. Peter eats in the dining room now. He joins other residents in the lounge. The team cites improved motivation, decreased lability and perseveration.

As I think ahead to Peter's vocation, I realize that I shall not always be a physical reminder to him regarding a schedule; nor shall I be with him to escort him on his rounds. He will not be provided with a guide to prevent his getting lost, and he cannot read, his concept of time is severely impaired. I set to work creating a schedule without words: at the top a polaroid picture of me indicating OT; under that, a picture of each of our patients with a digital time printed under it. The time may not have meaning, but he can match it to the time on his watch. Later, I'll add a map to each client's room.

Peter's enthusiasm never wanes. He continues to use Gray's templates to ask questions and ponder the conditions he is seeing, always lamenting the residents' youth and the permanency of their disabilities, lauding their perseverance, and always indicating how lucky he is to have regained the use of his extremities. Peter's enthusiasm is matched by the team's skepticism. Most still believe that Peter will never work again, or will be able to do assembly or rote work only. How foreign that would be to Peter. He could rather not work at all; perhaps he would rather even rather not live at all!

Did Peter continue to believe that he would again be a practicing physician? I cannot be sure, but I think not. I believe that he had begun to understand what this "therapy" business was all about. During the course of his treatment, both the rehab director and I left the facility. The OT who was assigned to Peter's case informed me that at the very first team meeting after my resignation, the team had decided to discontinue the peer-treatment program and employ a more traditional approach, that is, cooking groups, cognitive retraining computer programs, exercise, and so on. After the first few sessions, Peter, again refused to leave his room. Eventually, he refused to eat or drink, was diagnosed with a major depressive episode and placed, again, on suicide precautions. Administration recommended his transfer to a sister facility out-of-state. However, deeply discouraged by his son's regression, Peter's father had him discharged to his home, where he would take care of him and help him to "get on with his life."

Case Discussion

The above story, compelling and dramatic, is told by an experienced therapist. It illustrates her struggle with constructing a possible future for Peter, her incredible ability to understand Peter's meanings, and her skill at finding meaning-making opportunities for him. However, one does not need such a dramatic case or as much experience as Madelyn had to be sensitive to the habits and meanings that can help a person toward a new life.

CASE EXAMPLE

The following is a story written by a student who was earning an entry-level degree in OT. It is about a patient with whom he worked on his second affiliation.

John

by Mark Budgen

I met John while I was on my level II psych affiliation. John is a divorced man in his fifties who attended the Day Hospital program. John suffered from depression and at times had been suicidal. He is also a recovering alcoholic. Despite counseling, medication, and ECT [electroconvulsive therapy], John was unable to free himself for an extended period of time from his depression. John had been out of work on disability relating to his depression for many months.

I worked with John in the OT clinic group. The people who attend this group have a variety of activities to choose from: ceramics, woodworking, stained glass painting, needlework projects, and so on. John looked through some of the art supplies and became interested in drawing and painting. There were a few old art books around, which, over time, he used for tips to improve his skills. John's drawings were well done, especially for a beginner. It was obvious he had some natural ability and was eager to learn.

Oftentimes, I would experience frustration with some of the people in the clinic group, and John was no exception. Through the clinic group many people find they enjoy a particular activity and since they are only at Day

Hospital for a limited time, I would encourage them to work on these activities at home or take an adult education class. Many of the people in the clinic group suffer from depression and would benefit from an enjoyable, low-stress leisure activity. Participation in a group would also increase their social interactions, as well as provide needed structure in their lives. I did not always succeed, nor did I always fail.

John's interest in drawing continued to grow. On weekends he began to visit a few art stores and he also began to draw at home. At this point he was still not interested in signing up for a class. Despite the progress, I was concerned that John would not continue to draw once he left our program, and he was scheduled to be discharged soon. On his last day we arranged, with support from my supervisor, to leave the OT clinic early and spend our lunchtime checking out art supplies at a discount art supply store. John and I climbed into his car, one of those old Continentals that look more like a ship. He made a few jokes about his car and off we went.

On the way to Art Supply Warehouse, we stopped to see an art exhibit and a friend of mine, Carol, who was working in her studio adjacent to the exhibit. The gallery was closed. However, Carol had a key and gave us a private tour. John was interested in the works of many of the artists involved in the show and later asked Carol several questions in her studio. Carol's husband Robin is a well-known local artist who teaches at Rhode Island School of Design. Robin also gives affordable, group drawing lessons and I had previously attempted to motivate John to contact him. I had explored a variety of avenues with John, hoping one of them would lead to his continuing to paint and draw upon discharge. While we were at the gallery, John agreed to give Robin a call. They spoke for a few minutes and though John did not plan to sign up right away for a class, he learned of another opportunity and expressed interest in a class once he gained additional experience and confidence.

John and I finally said good-bye to Carol and drove up the street to the art store. John was thrilled to see the prices as they were considerably less than the supply prices he encountered at the malls. One of the staff took John around the store and they picked out a variety of brushes, paper, and paints to get him started on his own. John was visibly excited as we carried his supplies out to his car. It was a successful lunch hour. I began to believe John would continue his new love/hobby upon discharge. A month or so after he left the hospital, John stopped by for a visit and he looked great. John had lost weight and appeared rejuvenated. He was full of energy and possessed a special sparkle as he told us of the many hours he devotes to painting and how it has opened up a whole new world. John also brought along a nice surprise to show us, his first painting, which he had proudly framed!

Summary

Conditional reasoning is a form of complex social reasoning through which therapists attempt to understand the patient as a person in the context of his or her life-world. Through conditional reasoning therapists form an image of future life possibilities for the person. They enlist the person in the construction of the image and in the activities that will help make those possibilities come about. The activities that therapists and patients engage in necessitate the rekindling of intentionality, the development of new habits and their embedded meanings, and the taking up of significant symbolic meanings that will assist in the reconstruction of the self.

■ P A R T ■
IV

Narrative Reasoning:
Negotiating the Future

■

The Narrative Nature of Clinical Reasoning

■ CHERYL MATTINGLY

Introduction

In each new clinical situation, the therapist must answer the question: What story am I in? To give an answer is to make some initial sense of the situation, a sense on which the therapist can act. Discovering the story sometimes is helped through analogy. Therapists might say to themselves, "How is this situation like others I have been in?" Or, put narratively, "How could I retell, in a new way, an old story?"

Stories help frame practical decisions about what to do. They give an account of what has happened, and this, in turn, suggests a view of which actions make sense as appropriate next steps. Therapists often made stories to describe contexts, in terms of which they decided what to do next. Stories place events within a temporal context, and in order to know how to act, therapists often needed a historical sense that located them in relation to some past and some anticipated future.

Creating Narrative Images

This need for narrative framing as a guide to practice is suggested by a nurse quoted in Benner's study of clinical reasoning in nursing (1984). This nurse, who works in an intensive care nursery, describes what she considers the most essential kind of thinking she wants her newly graduated students to evince at the end of their 3-month affiliation with her.

To my mind, moving the child from Point A to Point B is what nursing is all about. You have to perform tasks along the way to make that happen, but performing the task isn't nursing. . . . I wanted to see a light going on—that OK, here's this baby, this is where this baby is at, and here's where I want this baby to be in 6 weeks. What can I do today to make this baby go along the road to end up being better? It's that kind of thing that's just happening now. They're [her student nurses] just starting to see the whole thing as a picture and not as a list of tasks to do. (Benner, 1984, p. 28)

The process of treatment encourages, perhaps even compels, therapists to reason in a narrative mode. They must reason about how to guide their therapy with particular patients by using images of where this patient is at now, and where this patient might be at some future time when the patient will be discharged. It is not enough for the therapist to know how to do a set of tasks that have an abstract order. Therapists need to be able to picture a larger temporal whole, one that captures what they can see in a particular patient in the present and what they can imaginatively anticipate seeing sometime in the future. This picturing process gives them a basis for organizing tasks.

The nurse quoted above is interesting because she emphasizes both the imagistic character of what the clinician needs to know, contrasting it with the knowledge of tasks, and the context-specific nature of those images. The therapists in this study spoke in a similar language about picturing the patient, and especially about having "future images" of who the patient could be. They felt that what they often held most vividly in mind when treating patients were not plans or objectives, but quite concrete pictures of the potential patient, the future patient. For instance, one of the pediatric therapists said, "You know, when I treat that 18-month-old child, I see the child at 3, then I see the child at 6, learning to hold a pencil. I have all these pictures in my head." They described their difficulty when the patients or their families held different images of the future, and their own dilemma about the extent to which they should give patients or families their own pictures, which were often more pessimistic. (Therapists were often in the difficult position of trying to give hope to a patient, while also gradually letting the patient know a very dark probable future. Patients and families were often already extremely depressed about conditions that were worse than they imagined.) Therapists spoke of these images as necessary but dangerous—necessary because therapist and patient needed some guiding pictures; dangerous because these could blind therapist or patient to what was realistically possible.

Therapists in the study were also, like Benner's nurse, conscious of the need to create quite specific images that were appropriate to a particular patient. General treatment goals devised from general knowledge of functional deficits and developmental possibilities were insufficient guides to practice, in the therapists' view. They worked with much more concrete guide-images, and stories that were the "wholes" that allowed them to selectively choose what aspects of their knowledge base were appropriate to the situation. These images were organized temporally, teleologically, giving the therapists a sense of an ending for which they could strive.

Even if the therapists' general goals remained fairly constant from patient to patient, or from session to session with the same patient (e.g., increase range of motion in a hand patient or improve trunk balance in a stroke patient), the concrete embodiment or playing out of those goals depended on the context. To pick an extremely simple case, increasing range of motion for a working-class young male hand patient who had a good relationship with the therapist did not necessarily translate into the same set of therapeutic actions as increasing range of motion for a hand patient who was a worried middle-aged physician and who was not sure the therapist knew what she was doing. The therapist was much more likely to be aggressive in her therapy with the first than she was with the second. The nature of the injury itself might be quite similar in the two cases, but if the patients' interpretations of the nature of their injury and their views about the role of therapy in treating that injury were different, therapists modified their interventions accordingly.

Although these images of the future were often not formulated in words—unless there was some need to communicate them explicitly to others—they were part of what we are calling a "prospective treatment story." In this prospective story, the therapists "see" a possible and desirable future for the patient and imagine how they might guide treatment to bring such a future about. This "treatment story" is, in turn, part of a larger life story of the patient. Therapists can imagine where to go with a particular patient, and how to get from A to B, as Benner's nurse put it, based on what they observe and infer about the patient's larger life history, both past and future. The therapeutic story that therapists imagine takes on its power and plausibility as part of a larger historical context, one that includes a past that began before therapy started and, generally, a future that extends once therapy is over. In our study, it appeared that expert therapists were much more able to see their treatment as part of these larger wholes than novice therapists, who were often still focused in the very immediate treatment present. It is important to distinguish therapists' stories about "who" a patient is from medical histories. Medical histories are also organized temporally and also provide therapists with a larger temporal context of past and future in which to locate their interventions. What is different about the "prospective stories" I am describing is that they are organized not only around the history and prognosis of the physiologic body as medical histories are, but around the life history of the patient who experiences, and in some way has to deal with, that disabled body.

The treatment approaches and treatment paths therapists tried to follow were often guided by such stories. These stories, derived from past particular experiences and stereotypical (collectivized) scenarios, were projected onto new clinical situations in order to help therapists make sense of what story they were in and where they might go with particular patients. Therapists then attempted to enact their projected stories in the new clinical situations, working improvisationally to narratively pull in and build on whatever happened in a clinical session so that it added to the story's plot. Therapists "saw" a possible story that they recognized as clinically meaningful, and they tried to make that story come true by taking the individual episodes of their clinical encounters and treating them as parts of a larger, narratively unfolding whole.

The Changing Shape of Prospective Stories

The story that therapists first saw in developing a treatment scenario to guide their work with the patient was generally not the story that actually unfolded as treatment progressed. "Prospective stories" were useful not because they were completely accurate predictions of what would happen, but because they were plausible enough to give therapists a starting point. The prospective stories that therapists created provided them with narrative expectations that often ran into conflict with their experience of working with a patient. Perhaps it would be most accurate to say that their prospective story was confronted by the story they would tell in retrospect about what had actually happened in therapy. When this confrontation became acute enough, and at those times when therapists allowed themselves to be open to it, to "feel" the acuteness of the misfit, they would revise the story accordingly, redirecting therapeutic interventions so that they were more in line with what was actually unfolding. In our study, expert and novice therapists appeared to differ in their capacity to make revisions as therapy progressed. Expert therapists were much more attentive to misfits between their prospective stories and what was happening in therapy. And they were often more attentive in those particular areas where they had the greatest expertise. Expert therapists were also much more willing to abandon their anticipated narrative path when it ran into serious trouble and much more adept at improvising, by reorganizing their interventions so that the main story line could be preserved as far as possible.

The clinical stories therapists projected onto new situations often ran into trouble because the new situation was often resistant to the mold. Clinical practice is idiosyncratic enough and illness experiences are contextually specific enough that stories created from other times and for other patients often fall short in providing ideal guides to new situations. While clinical stories are rarely ever applied wholesale—the therapist is always tinkering, always improvising, to make the fit appropriate—this constant improvisational work is often not enough to carry things along. When it is not, therapists experience the anxiety and frustration of falling out of the story, of losing their way. When the story no longer makes sense, they lose faith in their strategies and plans for the patient because the outcomes are too far afield from ones they consider desirable.

The stories therapists told about these troubled times of getting lost portray their extreme discomfort at losing their way and their repeated attempts to "fix" the story or to find one that is more appropriate. If therapists were never able to find their way, never able to locate and enact a story they considered clinically meaningful, the stories they told retrospectively were often explorations or justifications for who was to blame. When things go wrong in therapy, as they do in large and small ways all the time, therapists are no longer narrators with their images of the ending well in tow. Through difficult and unexpected turns in the therapeutic process, therapists become readers of the story, which appears to unfold in front of their eyes as though of its own making. Having lost their place in the story they were trying to play out, they struggle to understand what has gone wrong and, sometimes, what another story might be that could substitute for the one they have had to abandon. Here we see the clinical situation presenting puzzles, dilemmas, impasses, from which there is no graceful exit. Often things are just muddled.

Sometimes things stay muddled. No meaningful sense can be made, except some unsatisfactory, uneasy, and ad hoc stigmatizing of patient, family, or "the system." But sometimes the therapist's confrontation with the puzzling clinical situation provokes a revision of therapeutic perspective. In this case, the collision between the therapist's prospective story and the clinical experience that actually unfolds leads the therapist to a deep reconsideration of values that have implications beyond the particular clinical experience that first triggered the revision. At other times, a more modest revision of the initial story allows therapists and patients to find a therapeutic story they can both be committed to.

Structure of Treatment

The structure of treatment as "doing with" the patient—where the patient is needed to work as an active partner with the therapist—often prompted therapists to revise their clinical stories. This revision often took a particularly narrative form because it was so often created by a surprising patient response that required the therapist to interpret patient motivations from the patient response. Therapists were constantly interpreting the intentions of their patients. In an obvious case, a patient resisted working on an activity the therapist had planned, and the therapist had hypothesized about the intentions of the patient leading to the particular resistance she was facing. Such hypothesizing about patient motives was necessary in order for the therapist to assess and weigh alternative approaches to draw the patient into the process. Take an example from field notes about a very everyday kind of clinical trouble: a therapist brings a chronic respiratory patient into the treatment room. The patient is on a ventilator. The patient becomes extremely upset and says she wants to go back to her room. The therapist must hypothesize what the patient means by this. Is she becoming anxious about her breathing? Is she uninterested in the therapy sessions they have been having? Is she angry at the therapist for not taking her to chapel the day before when she requested it? Is she asking that more attention be paid to her? The interpretation the therapist makes of what the patient is intending by saying, "I want to go back to my room," will directly bear on the intervention she makes with the patient.

In the session I just cited, the therapist made a series of interventions to try to calm the patient down. When she discussed these later in an interview, she described how different interventions were based on different interpretations of what was creating anxiety in the patient. As the therapist described these interpretations in the interview, she often gave different bits of a longer story she had constructed about this patient's anxiety attacks on coming to therapy. The therapist drew on aspects of this longer treatment story of her several months' acquaintance with this patient in trying to assess the immediate intentions "behind" the patient's responses in this particular session.

Schön's (1983, 1987) notion of expert reasoning as a form of "reflection-in-action" is helpful in understanding this process of "conversation," in which each "move" the therapist makes results in a new situation (produced here by moves from the patient), and successive therapeutic moves must take account of the new situation that has been created. On-the-spot reasoning is particularly necessary when earlier moves yield some surprising result, as when the patient responds differently than the therapist anticipated. The surprise necessitates an immediate reflection about what to do next, since any earlier plan will not have considered the surprising response. The therapist who faithfully follows an earlier treatment plan in the face of surprising results will be unlikely to provide effective treatment.

NARRATIVE AND THE CREATION OF SIGNIFICANT TREATMENT EXPERIENCES

One reason we speak here of prospective stories rather than treatment goals and plans is that therapists are often concerned not simply with reaching a set of objectives, but are concerned that the whole process of therapy should unfold in such a way that patients are given powerful experiences of successfully met challenges, successes which can give patients the confidence to actively create a maximally independent life for themselves. Often it was not reaching the final goal per se that measured the success of therapy, but the therapeutic experiences along the way, where patients developed increasing confidence and commitment to take on challenges. The whole treatment story mattered.

Therapists also worked to create significant experiences for their patients—ones worth telling stories about—because if therapy was to be effective, therapists had to find a way to make the therapeutic process matter to the patient, to make it meaningful to that patient. Each therapist faced the problem of constructing therapeutic activities that were meaningful enough to elicit the patient's active cooperation.

The patient had to see something at stake in therapy. Why should he or she bother to try? If the patient did not try, therapy did not work. Partly, this was because therapists required patients to do things in therapy that patients did not necessarily feel ready to do or did not believe were worth the effort. But, more importantly, the patient had to develop a stake in the therapeutic activities in order to take them up. Therapists were with patients only a short time, often a few weeks or less. They might teach a few skills or improve the patient's strength a bit, but generally their effectiveness depended on using therapy as a catalyst to help patients begin to see how they might "do for themselves" even when the therapist was no longer there.

An example of this was a therapist who was working with a spinal cord patient and teaching him to move checker pieces using a mouthstick. It was not enough for this patient to learn to move these checkers pieces for the therapy to be successful. He must also take up a point of view that comes with being committed to the tremendous concentration it takes to perform this trivial task—trivial, that is, if you are not a spinal cord patient. He must absorb a vision as well as a few new skills. The therapeutic time together itself had to provide a kind of existential picture of how he might live his life in the future with his disability. The therapy will not ultimately work, not in any catalytic way that the patient will take home when he leaves the hospital, if he is not strongly committed to the process. Without experiencing his treatment activities from a committed stance, he will not see any future in them. He will not see the point.

If the patient is to become committed to the therapeutic process, both patient and therapist must share a view about why engaging in any particular set of treatment activities makes sense. Coming to share such a view requires the therapist and patient to see how these treatment activities are going to move the patient toward some future she or he can care about. Such a view is not reducible to a general prognosis or even to a shared understanding of a treatment plan. Therapist and patient must come to share a story about the therapeutic process, must come to see themselves as "in the same story." This is a kind of future story, a story of what has not yet happened, or has only partly happened, an as-yet-unfinished story.

How is such a story constructed? Generally not through any explicit storytelling. Rather, it is constructed through sharing powerful therapeutic experiences that point to a prospective story—a path therapy will take. Clinical reasoning involves seeing possibilities for creating significant experiences in which the patient will become committed, making moves to act on these possibilities, responding to the moves the patient makes in return, and, if the therapist is lucky and can get something started—can get the patient "in"—building on the experience by showing the patient a future in which this therapeutic experience becomes one building block. Or, in the language of narrative, the experience becomes one episode in a much longer story. The therapist tells the story not in words, but in actions that create an experience the patient can care about.

The clinician's narrative task is to take the episodes of action within the clinical encounter and structure them into a coherent plot. A plot is what gives unity to an otherwise meaningless succession of one thing after another. Quite simply, "emplotment is the operation that draws a configuration out of a simple succession," (Ricoeur, 1984, p. 65). What we call a story is just this rendering and ordering of a succession of events (say, a series of treatment activities), into parts that belong to a larger narrative whole. When a therapeutic process has been successfully emplotted, it goes somewhere, it is driven and shaped by a "sense of an ending" (Kermode, 1966). To have a (single) story is to have made a whole out of a succession of actions. Those actions then take their meaning by belonging to, and contributing to, the story as a whole. A story, Ricoeur writes, "must be more than just an enumeration of events in serial order: it must organize them into an intelligible whole, of a sort such that we can always ask what is the 'thought' of this story. (1984, p. 65)

Narratives give meaningful structure to life through time. The told narrative builds, to borrow from Ricoeur's argument, on action understood as an as-yet-untold story. Or, in his provocative phrase, "action is in quest of narrative" (p. 74), which therapists use in their quest to transform their actions and the actions of their patients into (as yet) untold stories.

This can be translated into more familiar clinical language through a narrativized reading of treatment goals. When an occupational therapist makes an assessment of the patient, the outcome is a set of treatment goals. Goals, to follow Ricoeur (1984), are not predictions of what will happen, but express the actors' intentions of what they prefer to have happen and intend to try and bring about. These goals express a therapeutic commitment. They capture what the therapist intends to

accomplish over the course of therapy. Treatment goals are an expression of what the therapist has committed himself to care about with a
particular patient.

As occupational therapists have argued (Rogers and Masagatani,
1982; Rogers, 1983; Rogers and Kielhofner, 1983), a primary task of
clinical reasoning is the individualization of treatment goals. To speak
narratively, individualization involves constructing a particular story
of the treatment process rather than relying on a generic line of action
that strings together standard goals and activities.

In the case given below, things go well for the therapist. Things do
not get muddled. But there is nothing rote about the clinical encounters
described in this case. The case illustrates a common form of reasoning
in the clinical situation. Therapists are constantly on the move, looking
for opportunities, building on whatever happens to lead the session in
a direction they believe is meaningful. When things go well, therapists
look like artful shapers of clinical time, creating therapeutically meaningful events out of clinical activities. Most therapists that we studied
worked to create therapeutically meaningful experiences for the patient.
From the therapist's point of view, experiences were significant not
only when they provided the patient time to develop skills but when
they carried rhetorical force, when the therapist had conveyed important messages through the therapeutic effort, such as the need to strive
for independence and the rewards that can result from the hard work
that therapy often requires.

The following example illustrates the narrative reasoning of an
occupational therapist emplotting a set of actions, weaving them into
a meaningful sequence. The session is especially striking because of
the difference between the first half of the session, in which treatment
is a mere succession of events, just one thing after another, and the
second half, in which this succession is transformed by the two occupational therapists into a narratively structured set of actions.

The shift is from a series of interactions in which therapeutic time
is treated as a mere succession of activities, as a procedural movement
ungrounded in context or in a picture of the patient, to narrative shaping
of the therapeutic interaction, in which therapeutic time has been emplotted by the clinician's picture of how to create a significant therapeutic experience for a patient. It is important to note here that this
meaningful sequence which they construct is not the carrying out of
any treatment plan formed prior to the session. The "untold story" that
emerges is structured from unanticipated responses by the patient to
their interventions.

The Tour

The session involves a 20-year-old man suffering from a brain stem
contusion sustained in a car accident 1 to 2 months before. The patient

has undergone surgery and has recently come out of a coma. He cannot talk but communicates through signalling and writing. The therapist has seen this patient only twice before, very briefly.

As the second occupational therapist comes into his room, she finds the physical therapist and a nurse transferring the patient from his bed to a wheelchair. This is the first time he has been out of bed since the accident.*

When the session begins, the patient is lying in bed surrounded by four medical professionals, one nurse, one physical therapist, and two occupational therapists. During the first several minutes the patient is simultaneously treated by each of these professionals: (1) he is given a shot; (2) he is introduced to a new occupational therapist who puts on his sneakers; (3) he has his lungs listened to by the physical therapist; and (4) he is asked questions about his height by the second occupational therapist.

The occupational therapists, nurse, and physical therapist have previously decided that he needs to stand up and then spend an hour sitting in a wheelchair. They are all there at the same time to help in transferring him from bed to wheelchair. The patient cannot speak but he is given a pad and marker and writes notes to them. One of the occupational therapists and the physical therapist tell him they realize he does not want to get out of bed. When given a pad and marker, he writes "Be careful of my back." All four medical professionals work together to stand him up. They give him instructions about how to help, for example, "Don't forget to put your elbow down and lean," or "Lift up your head. Straighten up your knee. Bring the right foot up." Two of the professionals congratulate him on how well he has done, the physical therapist does some more checking of his breathing, while one of the occupational therapists tries to help him get more comfortable in the chair and asks him questions about pain. (Most of the questions directed to him are yes or no questions, to which he simply puts thumbs-up for yes, thumbs-down for no.) The nurse and physical therapist then leave the room, while the two occupational therapists stay behind.

The initial medical checking of the patient and the transferring to the wheelchair form a sequence of actions with little narrative integrity. This is most evident during the first minutes of medical check, where each professional is doing something different, paying as little attention as possible to what the others are doing. The patient is treated primarily as a patient, that is, as an injured body, and is often referred to as "he" when the medical professionals talk among themselves, as in, "He is writing with his right hand. Was he a lefty? That's good writing." These health professionals are primarily doing "to" the patient rather than

---

*This session was observed by a research assistant on the project, Terry Sperber. Her field notes form the data for the interpretation that follows.

"with" him. Minimal cooperation is required on his part during this phase. Neither do the professionals need much cooperation from one another, since the tasks they are carrying out are quite discrete and distinct from one another. They make no effort to build on what the others are doing because accomplishing their task does not require cooperative action. They are quite simply carrying out a preplanned set of fairly isolated activities. Their tasks are certainly not meaningless, and the physical therapist in a minimal sense "emplots" her actions by informing the group, including the patient, that he is improving in his breathing capacity and in his ability to help transfer himself to the wheelchair. She says to him, once he is seated, "That was so much better than yesterday, excellent." And, when instructing him to breathe she says, "Yes, good breathing. A little more. That's better than yesterday. We want to get up this high. To the red line. See how close you can get. Two more times. Good."

But this bare chronicling can be contrasted with the more fully narrative emplotting that occurs in the next phase of the session, between one of the occupational therapists and the patient. When the nurse and physical therapist leave, the following dialogue ensues between a very expert occupational therapist and the patient. (The second occupational therapist is very new, and, while she stays during the interaction, she does not say anything.)

The expert occupational therapist helps in the transfer, and when the physical therapist and nurse leave, she hands the patient a comb and says "Try to comb your hair." He does not want to do it and hands her back the comb. She then tells him this will help him improve balance; it's a kind of exercise. She says, "It's good for balance practice." At this medical explanation, he combs, but with great effort. When he stops, the therapist points to places he has missed. "Try here," she says, "Nurses can't do back here when you're lying down." As she touches spots on the back of his head for him to comb she says, "I'll guide you a little bit." She compliments him several times as he is combing. "Great job," "Nice," "Great."

Finally, they are done. The patient motions for paper. He writes, "Mirror." The therapist gets a mirror and sets it up on a table so he can see, correcting the angle just right. She asks him jokingly, "Going to make yourself look good for your girlfriend?" He signals for paper again. This time he writes, "Want to go for a ride." The therapist agrees enthusiastically, "Great! You want to check out your new place." Their tour begins. She takes him directly to the main occupational therapy room and she wheels him in. "This is the OT room. You will be spending a lot of time here," she tells him. She points to the mat and tells him that they will be working together here. She says, "You will learn to strengthen your trunk."

As they are about to leave, the patient expresses discomfort and the therapist stops to investigate. He indicates that he has pain in his left shoulder when he moves his head. The therapist supports his arm and begins moving it. She explains the movements she is doing, asking him to hold and then let his arm go again. She notes, "Your left shoulder seems OK but that pain makes you not want to move it. But moving it is good. Moving will get it stronger and reduce the spasm."

They leave the occupational therapy treatment room, and the patient writes, "I want more of a tour before I go back to bed." The therapist says, "You've got it. This is Boston University Hospital." As they wheel down the hospital corridors the therapist says. "Today is Friday. Saturday and Sunday I'm not here. But as you get stronger, your family will take you out.

They come to a large window looking out over the city. The therapist stops to let him look out. She says, "Do you recognize the Prudential?" He motions for paper and writes, "Open window." She explains that the windows cannot be opened, which she also demonstrates to him by going over to the window. She takes him past the nursing station and looks around to find any nurses who know him. The patient writes, "Is Beth here?" Beth comes out and they have a quick, warm conversation. The nurse tells him she is glad he is up. He writes down, "Please visit," on a note to her. Then the occupational therapist and the patient proceed on their tour for a few more minutes. The therapist asks him if he is getting tired. He indicates yes, thumbs-up. As they return to his room the therapist asks, "Do you remember which is your room?" The patient indicates thumbs-up when they reach his room. And that is the session.

This story was familiar in the practice of the occupational therapists we studied. It is an everyday example of how the therapist makes a series of decisions that lead to the creation of a significant experience for the patient, and of how a therapist uses that significant experience to sketch out to the patient a larger therapeutic story, a whole therapeutic process, they might carry out together.

The "OT" session opens after the wheelchair transfer, when the therapist asks the patient to comb his hair. He does not want to do it. She persists, giving him a medical rationale—improving balance—that he buys into enough to agree. When he finishes, she urges him to continue combing, pointing out missed spots. In pointing out spots, she subtly changes the meaning of the task from a balance activity to a self-care activity by telling him that "Nurses can't do back here when you are lying down." It may be more accurate to say she adds a meaning, giving the activity a polysemous character. Hair combing becomes both a balance support exercise and self-care. And she decides to push him along so that by the end he has not just carried out an exercise, he has combed his hair. By the end of this activity, he seems to accept this meaning of the task, for he asks for a mirror to see himself, as one might do after combing one's hair but not after doing an exercise for balance practice. The therapist builds on his request in not only getting him a mirror but in carefully adjusting it for better viewing, while simultaneously joking to him about fixing himself up for his girlfriend.

The therapist "emplots" his action by defining it as part of a therapeutic story she wants to carry out. The meaning of combing his hair as preparation for being seen by others, a meaning he acknowledges by asking for a mirror, is reinforced by the therapist's joke. If you are able to comb your hair, her joke implies, you can feel ready to be seen by people you care about.

The patient initiates the next phase of the session by requesting to go for a ride. Again the therapist not only agrees but builds on his request by telling him the meaning of his request. She tells him he wants to check out his new place. She thereby turns a ride, which might have meant going up and down the hall into a chance to see his new surroundings, a chance to see and to be seen.

You could say that this whole session is about reentry into the public world. The therapist builds on her success at getting the patient to comb his hair, which succeeds not only in that he does it, but in that he then asks in succession to see a mirror and to go for a ride. In her response to both his requests, she not only enthusiastically agrees, but explicitly marks them as requests to move out into the world. She "reads" them as moves within a story of reentry, and does so aloud, so that the patient hears her interpretation. To his request for a mirror she replies by joking about his girlfriend, signifying that he is getting ready to be seen. She interprets his second request for a ride as his wanting to see, and in seeing, to take ownership, to "check out his new place." She "emplots" his requests with a plausible but strong reading of the desires motivating them.

And she emplots his requests through her actions, not only bringing him a mirror but adjusting it, not only taking him for a ride but giving him a tour that includes stopping by the occupational therapy treatment room and stopping at the nurse's station to find a nurse he is friends with. She is personalizing the hospital. She is showing him "his" particular version of the hospital, the version that includes a visit to a friend and the occupational therapy room where he will be working with this therapist to get stronger.

She also uses his request for a ride to give herself the possibility of showing him what he will be doing with her. In her stop at the OT room, while both stare at one of the mats, she quite literally points to a future story. She sketches, in the barest phrase, what kind of story they are in. In this prospective story they work together and he becomes stronger. She reiterates this same prospective story when he complains about his shoulder. She says that working, even working in pain, will make him stronger: "That pain makes you not want to move it. But moving it is good, will get it stronger and reduce the spasm." Working, and working through body movement, will make him stronger.

She uses his requests as places of possibility to tell a second story in which work—work that will take time, will involve movement, and will cause pain—will finally make him stronger. She links the two stories, the subplots, into a more complex causal chain. First there is work, work that may even be unpleasant, work he may not want to do; but then there is strength, and along with strength, there is the possibility of seeing and being seen, of reentering what Arendt (1958) describes as the "public world of appearing."

The figure of the session itself, which opens with the patient combing his hair against his own wishes, and ends with a hospital tour, reinforces this story. By the end of the session, everything that has happened, from the initial taking of the comb to the end of the tour, becomes an extension or elaboration of this story of making oneself presentable and thus reentering the public world. And by doing the tour after he combs his hair, the therapist also extends the meaning of the hair combing. What can look trivial to him becomes the very thing that makes it emotionally possible for him to leave his room for the first time.

One thing after another becomes, in narrative logic, one thing because of another. In what Kenneth Burke (1945) calls a "temporizing of essence," earlier events become the causes of later events. Because the session links one small activity, hair combing, to another activity that the patient requests and clearly cares about—leaving his room for the first time—the session becomes an argument in story form about why occupational therapy activities should matter to this patient. The therapist is saying, through the experience, that something that might seem to him a small reward for a large amount of effort on his part is really worth the effort, because it makes it emotionally possible for him to feel presentable and to go out in the more public world of hospital hallways. She gives him an experience of the importance of occupational therapy.

This 20-year-old man would be unlikely to attach any significant commitment to relearning how to comb his hair as an activity in itself. But the therapist finds a task she believes he will succeed at and uses his success at this ordinary task, a success that leads him to want to see himself and then to want to leave his room. The session itself links the occupational therapy task to a possibility he cares about, moving out into the world. The therapist creates significance out of his reluctant willingness to make the effort to comb his hair in the name of a motor exercise. She then uses this tour, his reentry into this more public world and his pleasure at the tour to show him the occupational therapy treatment room and paint a picture of their future work together. In sketching this prospective story in which she tells him how he will be getting stronger as they work together, she is also, then, placing the experience of hair combing, which led to the experience of the tour—a significant and desirable experience for him—within a future story of how he will be working with her and becoming gradually stronger so that he can reenter the real world outside the hospital.

The powerful experience of the tour, which was initiated by hair combing, is thus emplotted by the therapist as early episodes of an as-yet-unlived story that will eventually lead to his reentry into the outside world. She emplots this therapy session for the patient and shows how the things they did that day are just early episodes of a larger whole, a larger story, which is yet to come. She makes it easier for him to believe in this future story and therefore to have a stake in doing his part, to make it come true, because he has just had the experience, in a partial but powerful way, of reentry into the public world and of succeeding at one task that helped make that partial reentry possible.

Five Elements of Emplotment

Therapy does not always resemble an unfolding story. Sometimes it is experienced by both therapist and client as a series of discrete activities, skill-building exercises, which have no particular meaning to therapist or patient, which carry no drama or excitement, and which are forgotten as soon as therapy is done. When therapists are able to collaborate with patients to create a story out of therapeutic time, that is, when they are able to create a plot in therapy, several elements are present. Using the case given above, the following section of this chapter enumerates five features of narrative time associated with story and examines how these are played out in the interaction between the therapist and this head-injured patient.

The principles of this pentad are as follows:

1. Action and motive are key structuring devices. Narrative time is human time, one might say, time in which human actions are represented as central causes for the outcome of events. Multiple actors with multiple motives are operating upon the same stage, and through their interactions, narrative time is created.
2. Narrative time is organized within a gap, a place of desire where one is not where one wants to be, where one longs to be elsewhere. Another way of saying this is that movement toward ending(s) dominates the experience of time.
3. Narratives show how things (and people) change over time. While change is central, not all change is narrative. In narrative, the movement from one time to the next is not linear; it is full of tricks and reversals.

4. Narrative time is dramatic. Conflict is omnipresent. There are obstacles to be overcome in reaching one's desired object. Enemies must be faced, risks taken. One almost never hears the story of how things went without a hitch from beginning to end, just as planned. Stories are told about difficult, even frightening situations. Desire must be strong because danger is also present, and one faces danger only when one wants something badly. In this time marked by conflict, there is an implicit dialogue of points of view played out by the key actors or even by the same actor when the narrative scene moves inward.

5. Endings are uncertain. Narrative time is marked by suspense, by surprise, by the recognition that things may turn out differently than one wants or anticipates.

HUMAN TIME AND THE CENTRALITY OF MOTIVE

Story time is human time rather than physical time; it is shaped by motive and intention. To see myself as in a story, or a series of stories, is to see my life in time as stretching out toward possiblities (both hopeful and fearful) that I have some influence in bringing about. Even in serious illness, constrained by a physical body largely out of my control, my illness story concerns how I and the other actors who surround me respond to the physical press of disease and deformity. Narrative time differs from biomedical time because it is actor-centered rather than disease-centered. While from a purely physical or biomedical perspective, the "main character" in illness is the pathology, from a narrative perspective the main character is the person with the pathology (Sacks, 1987).

Stories need not provide complex psychological accounts of intentions, but they do emphasize the role of intending, purposeful agents in explaining why things have come about in a certain way. Stories are about acts. Kenneth Burke, whose seminal work is a study of the centrality of the notion of act to narrative (or drama) wrote: "As for 'act,' any verb, no matter how specific or how general, that has connotations of consciousness or purpose falls under this category" (Burke, 1945, p. 14). Stories are investigations of events as actions; they are, to use Burke's vocabulary, "dramatistic" investigations. Drama stands for the paradigm of action in its full sense, as distinct from motion, for which the paradigm is the machine.

Emplotted time, then, is a time of social doings, shaped by the actions of oneself and others. In the therapeutic interaction described above, Donna's first task is to turn the patient into an actor rather than a mere "body" that is acted upon by others. She quite directly asks Steven to do something, to comb his hair, an undramatic habitual action, but an action nonetheless. The interactional play between the two is marked. Donna not only acknowledges but structures her own therapeutic actions in response to his. This gives a dialogic quality to their time together; it also, notably, means that carrying out a completely prescribed treatment plan is antithetical to emplotting a therapeutic narrative. How could one plan, for instance, that the patient would ask for a mirror, or, more important, for a ride? And yet it was the request for a ride that structured the entire session and that allowed a reentry story to unfold.

TIME GOVERNED BY DESIRE

The actions that form the central core, the causal nexus, of the narrative, are not motivated in some trivial sense, as when we are moved to make a cup of coffee or pick up the morning paper; they are driven forward by desire. A story is governed, the folklorist Vladimir Propp tells us (1968), by a "lack" or a need that must be addressed. This lack may be caused by some kind of "insufficiency" (p. 34), or created in response to the action of a villain who "disturb[s] the peace" (p. 27). In either case, it is set in motion either by the hero's desire to attain something he does not have, or to right some wrong. The presence of desire brings with it a readiness to suffer. Our desire causes us to take risks (or pay a price when we fail to take risks) and this in itself causes suffering. Often our object will not be attained, or, when attained, it will not give us what we hoped for; and these things also cause pain. Our desire for something we do not yet have strongly organizes the meaning of the present, and makes us vulnerable to a disjuncture between what we wish for and what actually unfolds.

Desire is even a central feature of our response, as listeners, to the well-told story. The essential place of desire in a narrative mode is particularly striking when we realize that not only the story hero but even the story listener is drawn to desire certain story outcomes and fear others. This point has been well discussed in reader response theory, particularly by the remarkable work of Iser (1978). When a story is told, if that story telling is successful, it creates in the listener a hope that some endings (generally the endings the hero also cares about) will transpire. When we listen to an engaging story, we wonder what will happen next because we have come to care about what will happen next. In their studies of story telling among inner city black youths, Labov and Waletzky (1967) have pointed out that the most important narrative question the storyteller's narrative must answer, and in fact must answer so well the question is never explicitly raised, is "So what?" A failed story is one that leaves the audience wondering why anyone bothered to tell it. A story may be well formed from a purely structural point of view, and may have a clear "point," but if the audience does not know why the point matters to them, if the events in the story never touch them, the story does not work.

The parallel between the told story and lived time is easily drawn if life in time is characterized, following Heidegger (1962), as a present located between past and future. Our orientation in time, as Heidegger tells us, is an orientation toward a future. The meaning of the present is always a temporal situatedness between a past and a future that we await. We are not passive in this waiting, however. Desire in the face of an uncertain future plays a central structuring role. We hope for certain endings; others we dread. We act in order to bring certain endings about, to realize certain futures, and to avoid others. While we may not be (often are not) successful, we act nonetheless, striving as far as we can to make some stories come true and thwart others. In so acting, we may come to decide that endings we thought we desired are not so desirable after all and to shift our teleological orientation in favor of a different future. But always we are situated with an eye to the future, and that future saturates each present moment with meaning. This is what Heidegger means when he describes us as always in the process of becoming, organized around Care. It is not merely that the agent somehow "pictures" a future state, which she or he then tries to attain. The future belongs to the present because we are, as Heidegger says, "thrown forward" in a stance of commitment, of care, toward a future. We are always, in Heidegger's wonderful phrase, "ahead of ourselves" (1962). M. J. Good's work on the central place of hope in the practice of oncology provides an important perspective on the need for both clinician and patient to find something to hope for (Good et al., 1990).

Returning to the case given above, the therapist attempts to shift the patient into narrative time by inviting the patient to be "ahead of himself." They take a tour into the future, both the future of therapeutic encounters and the future that matters, the one that leads out from the hospital back home. The therapy room to which she takes him represents a temporary station, a purgatory, which, if endured and even embraced, offers a path to the outside, or at least that is the narrative the therapist hopes will shape their clinical time together.

In this therapeutic interaction the therapist's concern to generate desire for therapy is evident in many of the actions she takes, including how she interprets the meaning to be made of the patient's own actions. When the therapist asks the patient to comb his hair, he does not at first cooperate. Perhaps her fundamental task in this initial encounter is to create in him a desire to act and, quite specifically, a desire to act in therapy. Since there is no story where there is no desire, much of this initial session with the therapist can be seen as her effort to make therapy a place where there is something to care about. She begins to sketch out possible "endings" that she presumes the patient does, or will, desire—especially becoming free of his role as patient and reconnecting to those he cares about (family, girlfriend) outside the confines of the clinic.

TIME OF TRANSFORMATION—TIME DOMINATED BY THE ENDING

In a story, time is structured by a movement from one state of affairs (a beginning) to a transformed state of affairs (an ending). In story time, things are different in the end. The structure of beginning-middle-end presumes, of course, that time is marked by anticipation of some end, one that, to make another obvious point, does not exist at the beginning. So narrative time is marked by change, or by the attempt at change. It is time characterized by an effort at transformation. Things may be changed in an outward, public way, or there may be an inward difference. People may come to think and feel differently. But it is important that in the time of plot, the agency that most matters in creating change is human agency. Even if other factors are more determinant—physical and even structural conditions—these form the background, the setting in which human actors take center stage.

When Donna and Steven take their tour of the hospital, the possibility of transformation is at the heart of the drama they are playing out. At first take, this point is so obvious that it goes without saying. If therapy is not about change, what could it be about? What is powerful in examining the 30-minute interaction between therapist and client is how the topic of transformation figures centrally, and the sort of transformation that is emplotted.

Steven has awakened to a body horrifyingly transformed. Some further bodily transformations will occur as part of a natural healing process, apart from his own actions. And some will occur because of what others do to him. But none of these changes form the core of the plot being sketched by Donna. This is not a narrative of passive awakening; there is no miracle cure and no magician healer. The plot is both more prosaic and more wrenching for it centers on the body transformation that Steven can directly affect through painstaking effort. Perhaps the greatest part of the pain will be Steven's growing acquaintance with his injured body, and his emerging recognition of the limits imposed upon him by that body. Through trying to heal himself, he will discover time and again the limits he must live with, and he will have to reckon with the loss of possibilities no longer available to him. This reckoning will precipitate inner transformations, changes of personal identity, perhaps even changes of character.

TROUBLED TIME

The very drama of narrative is based, in a sense, on the experience of suffering. Even the happy story, the one which ends well, takes us through a drama of plight—a lack or need that sets the story in motion, that propels the protagonist in a quest to obtain his or her goal through the overcoming of a series of obstacles. The process of overcoming, however fortuitous the result, almost inevitably engenders periods of suffering for the story's heroes and heroines. This is such a pervasive feature of the structure of narrative that Propp made it central to his analysis of folktales (1968). Later narratives expanded it to include many other kinds of narratives. And Arendt (1958) used it to characterize one moment in a dialectical treatment of the nature of human action.

Narratives are about acting and suffering, Arendt has said. They are about doing something (acting) and what happens as a result (suffering). Suffering is one name for experience. "Because the actor always moves among and in relation to other acting beings, he is never merely a 'doer,' but always and at the same time a sufferer. To do and to suffer are like opposite sides of the same coin, and the story that an act starts is composed of its consequent deeds and sufferings (Arendt, 1958, p. 190).

The "trouble" that marks narrative time is the necessary counterpoint, a required antithesis, to a causal structure dominated by the concept of human agency. Actions may be the central cause within narrative structure, but their causal efficacy is anything but sure. Nothing is guaranteed in the realm of human action. We do what we can but—in the narrative at least—there are always impediments.

The importance of trouble and suffering in the narrative is due to the sort of actions narratives recount, actions in which desire is strong and in which there is a significant gap between "where I now am" and "where I want to be." If narrative plots turned on the everyday easy-to-accomplish actions that form habitual life ("raising my arm to scratch my head," "putting up my umbrella in the rain," heating a can of soup for dinner) suffering would not need to enter. The strength of our desire comes in part from the length of the reach required to attain what we want. Most stories we choose to tell feature difficult passages toward precarious destinations, journeys fraught with enemies who may defeat us at any moment. Upon examination, it is surprising how regularly everyday stories carry this plot structure; even tales of victory are set against this implicit backdrop of what might have gone wrong.

In attempting to set a therapeutic story in motion, the occupational therapist need not, of course, invent troubles or obstacles for the patient. These come with chronic disability. Suffering is paramount; adversaries are everywhere. The difficult task for the therapist is locating a space for action at all. The problem is how to offer sufficient hope to the patient that the struggle to overcome obstacles becomes meaningful and bearable (Good et al., 1990). Occupational therapists speak often of their need to transform "passive patients" into "active patients." What they mean is that their patients are organized in the hospital to suffer, to wait, to be "done to," as they say. When Donna takes Steven for a tour, she is inviting him into a story in which he will not only suffer passively, as a victim of his injury, but in which he goes out to battle, so to speak, actively incurring more suffering (certainly more physical pain) in a fight to overcome, where he can, the damage that has been done to his body. Within the therapeutic plot Donna hopes to initiate, the patient becomes an aggressor of a sort, engaging adversaries in an effort to become healed, and treating the therapist as a valued ally and trusted guide in this enterprise. Physicians often see themselves as engaged in a dramatic fight with disease—waging war against cancer cells, for example (Hunt, 1992; Good et al., in press; Good et al., 1990); but in the occupational therapist's emplotment, it is the patient, in alliance with the therapist, who is designated as the narrative hero, the one who must wage the war.

SUSPENSEFUL TIME—TIME OF THE UNKNOWN ENDING

The presence of powerful enemies, and of dangers and obstacles, means that narrative time is a time of uncertainty. Our desire for an ending may be strong, but if our enemies are equally strong, or danger is prevalent, there is no telling what will finally unfold. Hence, the fifth characteristic of narrative time is that it is marked by doubt, by what Bruner (1986) speaks of as "subjunctivity." This theme is wonderfully developed by Good (1990) in his discussion of illness narratives. If lived experience positions us in a fluid space between a past and a future, then what we experience is strongly marked by the possible. Meaning itself, from this perspective, is always in suspense. If the meaning of the present, and even of the past, is contingent on what unfolds in the future, then what is happening and what has happened is not a matter of facts, but of interpretive possibilities that are vulnerable to an unknown future.

Life in time is a place of possibility; it is this structure that narrative imitates. For narrative does not tell us that what happened was necessary, but that it was possible, displaying a reality in which things might have been otherwise (Barthes, 1979). Endings, in action and in story, are not logically necessary, but possible; and seen from the end and looking backwards, plausible. Ricoeur writes,

"To follow a story is to move forward in the midst of contingencies and peripeteia under the guidance of an expectation that finds its fulfillment in the "conclusion" of the story. This conclusion is not logically implied by some previous premises. It gives the story an "end point," which, in turn, furnishes the point of view from which the story can be perceived as forming a whole. To understand the story is to understand how and why the successive episodes led to this conclusion, which, far from being foreseeable, must finally be accepted, as congruent with the episodes brought together by the story. (1984, pp. 66–67)

Story time is not, at least in any simple or linear sense, about progress. It is not about building one thing onto another in some steady movement toward a defined goal. Time is characterized by suspense, not only the suspense of not knowing whether a desired ending will come about, but even the suspense of not knowing whether the ending one pictures is the one that will still be desired or possible as the story unfolds.

In the therapeutic plot Donna enacts with Steven, the sense of uncertainty about the future is minimized. If there is one place where therapeutic emplotment in this case diverges from narrative time in the told story, it is over the issue of certainty. For Donna seems pointed toward vivid and predictable endings. When they look out toward the Prudential, she speaks confidently of Steven's return home to family and friends. When they look into the door of the therapy room, she speaks of the gains he will make by working through pain. She does not raise doubts about what he will be able to accomplish, or what life he will return to. Her intent appears to be to offer him a hopeful ending, a set of desirable images, to which he might be able to attach himself. And yet, given the despair many patients feel over their ability to transform themselves and their lives upon awakening from a coma or serious operation, her cheerful certainty is set against the bleak, nearly silent uncertainty of a patient who, at the beginning of the session, did not even want to get out of bed. Her brisk assertions can be seen as a kind of whistling in the dark, an attempt to put a brave (or blind) face on a future that is anything but sure, one where things will never be the same.

CASE EXAMPLE

The following story illustrates how one therapist began with a head injury group in which therapy was experienced very much in this way. Group participants were carrying out their exercises, in a half-hearted sort of way, but "nothing"—certainly from a narrative point of view—was happening. In this case, the therapist is able to turn a group with no narrative coherence into one that contained all the elements of a good story: drama, suspense, desire. Sometimes therapists tell stories in which the moral of their story is about creating a story in therapy. The following case is a story about making a story, about therapeutic emplotment. It is written by an occupational therapist about a memorable experience working with a head-injured group of patients in a chronic-care facility. It illustrates the essential elements of a good story: dramatic events that lead in unpredictable directions, an interplay of characters with different points of view, suspense, and interweavings of an "inner landscape" of thoughts and feelings with the outer world of public action.

The New York Subway

by Madelyn O'Reilly

Monday, 9:00 A.M.

I want you to take over the Upper Extremity Group that meets on Mondays and Wednesdays. It's a disaster . . . lots of absenteeism. . . . Why don't you observe it today and let me know what you think. . . . " These words came from the rehab program director, in what was called a nursing and rehabilitative facility, but which, for most, was a long-term, chronic-care facility from which few individuals had been discharged in recent years. My first thought is, "That title has to go." It conjures up pictures of all these little arms coming to group without any people attached! I checked OT treatment cards to find that the group consisted of five or six young adults, all head-injured, all several years posttrauma and long-time residents, some of whom participate in an independent living skills program and one-on-one OT, and all of whom I have noted to be cooperative and enthusiastic, or at least feisty, during other activities.

Monday, 1:30 P.M.

I enter the large OT/PT treatment area where I see several residents scattered about at tables and exercise equipment. I think, "This looks like PT . . . where is the group? At one table, a resident diligently puts small pegs into a pegboard. At the far end of the same table, the OT sits writing, and occasionally looks up to observe or give instructions, ". . . try that once more. . . ." Most memorable is the silence. Except for the clang of the pulley weights, a dropped peg, or the therapist's quiet voice, there is not a sound in this room. I ask, "Where are Mike and Bobby?" The OT replies, "They didn't show up again."

Having observed the session for several minutes, I go in search of the missing members. Perhaps they need a reminder. Mike, a handsome, red-haired and bearded young man responds to my inquiry about OT group, "That f—— group is a waste of time." Bobby, even younger, and usually quiet and compliant states, "It's boring." I let these fellows know that I'll be joining the group on Wednesday, and would really appreciate their help in finding a way to make it less boring. They agree half-heartedly to come and to think about it. I leave wondering, what do I know about these folks beyond their diagnoses? Mike loves to talk. He has a terrific sense of humor . . . was into TV production before the accident. Bobby is so young, so handsome, so quiet . . . often wears his college hockey shirt and sweats. Nancy is talkative, loves to socialize, talks mostly about home, family, jobs she had in the past. Eileen appears to be out of touch with reality most of the time, never complains about the pain of severe arthritis, is pretty hung-up on the Beatles music. "Wow!! What a group. Maybe I'll rearrange the furniture, get people closer together. How about music? Maybe games that require upper extremity exercise . . . checkers for fine motor . . . ball for gross . . . simon for speed and coordination . . . Will this infantize them? *I'm stuck!"*

Wednesday, 1:30 P.M.

Only Nancy and Eileen come to group. Nancy comments on the radio that's playing, does a little dance in her chair. Eileen mentions the Beatles. I tell her that perhaps she could bring a Beatles album to group sometime, and ask if they have seen Mike and Bobby. "They're on C ward," says Nancy, "They never come to exercise group anymore."

The two women play checkers. I decide not to fetch the men. It is their responsibility to come, and their choice not to come. However, that does not change the treatment plan that says, "O.T. 2X's weekly in small group."

Later Wednesday and During Every Spare Moment Thursday and Friday:

I wonder, "What is wrong with this group?" I make mental lists:
1. The name—I'll talk to the residents about that.
2. The activities—no meaning, no purpose, no life-related goals, no goals that belong to the clients. . . .
3. There is no interaction—among members, with therapist.
4. Nobody is having fun—the residents are bored—the therapist is bored—(and boring).
5. Is there any progress that the residents experience?
6. What are the reasons for attending or not attending? And there is no direction—no theme. . . .

THEME! THE GROUP NEEDS A THEME! A THEME ABOUT PEOPLE—NOT ARMS—NOT EXTREMITIES—NOT EXERCISE. I think about the *people.* What do they want? What do they need? They are all so young—so far from home. They want to get out. They want to go home. HOME! They're all from New York. That is it! NEW YORK! I have a theme with which to begin, but I don't know a thing about New York. The program director is from New York . . . I dash to her office. "New York," I blurt. "The Upper Extremity Group . . . They're all from New York. . . . Tell me something about New York . . . anything, everything. . . ." She lists, "Empire State Building, Statue of Liberty, Long Island Ferry, the subway. . . ." Laughingly, "You could have a New York Subway Group." I replay, "We could be *on the subway.* They can take me to New York. What does it look like . . . is there graffiti? We can graffiti . . . I need a new room, away from the big treatment room . . . can we use the small meeting room?" The program director replies yes and adds that she has a map of the New York subway and will bring it in. "I'll be the conductor . . . I have a blue blazer." She says, "I think I have a funny little hat that will pass for a conductor's hat." We laugh through all the possibilities of this activity. This is going to be FUN!

Monday, 9:00 A.M.

I go straight to Mike's room and ask him to make sure everyone comes to group today. "I have a different type of activity planned, and I'd really like to talk to everyone so that we can make some plans together." Mike states that he hates the d—— group. I tell him that I understand that and that perhaps he could gather everyone for me, and come for awhile. "Then, if you are really unhappy with the activity, you can leave." He agrees. I hand him a small bag containing poker chips and ask him to give one to each member on the attached list and have them bring the chips to group. "Okay, but what the h—— are these for?" "It's a surprise. See you at one-thirty."

Monday, 1:00 P.M.

In the room next to the OT/PT treatment area, I tape white paper to three of the walls, labeling various spots with street names and subway stops found on the subway map, which I hang on the fourth wall. I put out materials, don my conductor's uniform, and stand outside the door, on which a sign reads "New York this way."

As I await the passengers, my stomach churns with anxiety and excitement, and I wonder where this ride will take us.

Monday, 1:30 P.M.

As the members arrive, escorted by Mike, I take their tokens, explaining that it is commuter fare for a ride on the New York subway. Nancy grins; Eileen looks puzzled; Bobby shrugs. Mike says with a great laugh, "You are crazy." As these travelers enter the room, I hear snickers, queries like, "What the h—— is she doing . . . ?" and comments like, "It's better than the other room." Then . . . snickers, laughter, and recognition. They go from stop to stop, reading, commenting . . . all smiling!

Bobby asks, "What's going on?" "Well," I explain, "You're all from New York, right? This is a New York subway station. You've all ridden on the subway, right? M. tells me that there's graffiti, words, and pictures on the walls, in the subway. We're going to do graffiti. You do remember graffiti, don't you?" "Yeah," laughs Mike, "but nothing I could write HERE!!"

With that, I close the door, and say, "You can draw or write anything you want in this room. The only rule is that you use the tools I give you." I distribute materials: large colored pencils and wrist weights for Mike who has a tremor, but brush and paint for Bobby who's working on gross motor skills, crayons to Nancy who needs to strengthen wrists and fingers, markers for Eileen who can't tolerate resistance.

Eileen asks, "Where are we supposed to be?"

"Anywhere you'd like to be, and when you finish working at one place you can move to another. It's up to you."

Nancy starts: "This is neat . . . just like when I was a kid. . . ."

We're off!

From this point, drawing, writing, conversation and laughter are continuous. So much activity fills this room that it is difficult to remember details. Words, pictures, memories, and feelings cover the walls: . . . "This place sucks" . . . "My ass is stuck in Mass" . . . "Home sweet Home" . . . and on and on. . . . I go from one participant to another, asking about their work or just watching. After 35 minutes, I ask the group to finish up their art work so that we can talk a bit and plan for our next group session. Stickball wins unanimously. Since, I admit, I know nothing about stickball, I ask the group to write out rules and equipment we'll need and get it to me on Tuesday. They agree, and, in fact, begin to work immediately. As I leave to see my next client, I tell the group, "You guys can hang out here for a while. Just be sure to take your words and pictures with you when you leave." Thinking . . . cleanup can wait.

Epilogue

The New York Gang, as they came to call themselves met every Monday and Wednesday, and informally, on alternate Saturdays for an OT brunch. Other New Yorkers joined the group. Our activities included making giant pretzels and cooking hot dogs to sell from a makeshift push-cart, a trip to a simulated Central Park, filling of a photo album with pictures of the group, home, drawings, postcards, *New York Times* clippings . . . An unwritten rule, of course, was that every member tease me, at least once, about my ignorance regarding New York and my funny Boston accent!

Case Discussion

This therapist began a plot that spawned additional episodes. The single session upon which this case centers not only had a coherent plot—a beginning, middle, and end (making graffiti or recreating a New York subway scene)—but, because of her success, that session then became just one episode in an unfolding therapeutic story in which clients became a case of characters in the "New York Gang." Specific biomechanical interventions were integrated in a meaningful way as activities that allowed group members to act their part in this drama and the task, writing things on the wall, allowed each person to express an individual voice as well.

Narratively speaking, the shift from the Upper Extremity Group to the New York Gang represents a shift from a series of interactions in which therapeutic time is treated as a mere succession of activities, as a procedural movement ungrounded in context or in a picture of the patient, to narrative shaping of the therapeutic interaction, in which therapeutic time has been emplotted by the clinician's picture of how to create a significant therapeutic experience for the clients.

The story depicts a process of overcoming obstacles. Will the influential residential members (Bobby and Mike) come to the group? Will they find her idea ridiculous or allow themselves to be drawn into the activity? Will colleagues find her too ridiculous?

Action-Centered (Rather than Disease- or Dysfunction-Centered) Therapy

O'Reilly presents a situation where she is asked to take over an on-going head injury group that was being very poorly attended by group members. The first thing that bothered her was its name—the "Upper Extremity Group." Her description of her first visit to the group emphasizes its antinarrative character—it is a group geared to extremities but not to human actors with needs and desires.

Not surprisingly, O'Reilly finds that several members of the group are no longer coming, and she then begins to ask herself what is wrong with the group. Besides the "inhuman" and biomedically oriented name, the activities themselves have "no meaning, no purpose, no life-related goals, no goals that belong to the clients." People are bored, there is "no direction, no theme." While O'Reilly is not using the language of story to describe the problems she notices, this list could easily be restated in narrative terms. When O'Reilly says the group has no direction and no theme, one could recast this and say that there is no plot to this group; there is no story that the group members are in. The group is not going anywhere, narratively speaking. Any particular group activity is not an episode in an unfolding story that members share. The activities of the group are focused on "broken body parts," as the group name "Upper Extremity") implies. While the exercises may help improve body functioning, they carry no intrinsic meaning to the group members, because the group activities are in no sense a "short story" in the larger life story of the clients.

A Focus on Desire

You cannot have a story if you do not have desire. For a therapeutic story to be set in motion, both therapists and clients must have something they desire. Or, as therapists say, clients must be motivated. They must want something from therapy. In the case above, this is the key problem the therapist faces—she has a group of clients who have no desire for therapy. In fact, these clients probably have lost much of their desire for anything, and their lack of interest in therapy is part of a larger problem. The therapist ponders what to do by beginning to think about the group members. Her mode of puzzling represents a shift from a biomechanic framing of the members' disabilities, to seeing the illness experiences of their disabilities and the personal meaning these have in their lives. She describes her reasoning in this way: "I think about the people. What do they want? What do they need? They are all so young; so far from home. They want to get out. They want to go home. HOME! They're all from New York. That's it! NEW YORK! I have a theme with which to begin."

This therapist is reasoning in narrative terms. She is beginning to *envision a prospective story* that all the members of the group could be a part of. She is going to invent some kind of therapy group built around a New York theme. Notably, this not only locates therapy in the relevant past of these clients, it also locates it within the future they desire. These clients not only come from New York. They are young people in a chronic, long-term care facility in Massachusetts, one that residents rarely ever leave. These clients want to go home.

The therapist invents the ingenious idea of turning a therapy room into a New York Subway. The very way that she introduces her idea builds interest in group participants. She goes to each member of the group and tells them there will be a change in the usual group. She does not tell them what that change will be but hands out poker chips to each one and tells them they must present their poker chips to get into the group. When they look at her with astonishment, she tells them they will find out soon enough what the tokens are for. (Notably, she even introduces a key narrative element critical to any good story—the element of suspense.) When the day of the group arrives, she lines three walls of the therapy room with blank white paper. She labels spots with street names and subway stops and hangs a subway map on the fourth wall.

Just as the group is scheduled to begin, she stands outside the door in a subway conductor's uniform (trying not to feel too foolish in front of other surprised hospital colleagues) and waits for group members to arrive. She describes the following scene: "As the members arrive, escorted by Mike, I take their tokens, explaining that it's commuter fare for a ride on the New York subway. Nancy grins; Eileen looks puzzled; Bobby shrugs. Mike says, with a great laugh, 'You are crazy!' As these travelers enter the room, I hear snickers, queries like, 'What the h—— is she doing?' and comments like, 'It's better than the other room.' Then snickers, laughter, recognition. They go from stop to stop, reading, commenting, all smiling!" Desire builds among the members as they begin to imagine themselves back in a scene which at one time was home for them.

This is now the group activity. She closes the door and tells them "You can draw or write anything you want in this room. The only rule is that you use the tools that I give you." These tools have been chosen with particular concern for the motor deficits of individual clients. "Large colored pencils and wrist weights for Mike who has a tremor, but brush and paint for Bobby who's working on gross motor skills. . . ." Thus she embeds these motor activities within a narrative context, one that prompts group participants to experience the desire for home, because desire is necessary for any therapeutic changes to occur.

Transformation

Stories depict lives in time and in doing so they emphasize change. They are eventful. They highlight human experience not as a timeless unaltered truth but as located in a time of before and after, where things were once different than they now are and where they will be different again in the future. Narratives are intimately connected to time because everything moves in a story. Stories are built from events. In stories, people do things and as a result things change; or things happen to people and as a result they change. Events in a story are construed as a passage, a movement from some initial situation, through various twists and turns, to some final situation. Stories are about experience as a movement through time.

A story has the peculiar quality of not being deducible—it gives surprises—while having a plausible direction. The ending cannot be predicted with certainty beforehand and yet carries a sense of rightness or even inevitability when it is reached. This is because narratives concern action. Though narratives present a succession of actions that have a certain direction, they are also unpredictable or at least not determined from what has come before (Ricoeur, 1978, p. 163). Stories always show what happens as action, so that even if fate seems to prescribe a certain direction of the plot, the specific events that occur are always subscribed to the intentional actions of the characters. And intentional behavior is purposeful but not necessary (Arendt, 1958). Because there is no necessity in the connection of elements, narrative is not guided by logical reasoning in the sense that abstract argument is. The rules of story development are not logical rules because narrative connects contingent events. (Burrell & Hauerwas, 1977).

The drama of any story rests on transformation. There are several transformations at work in this case. The therapist transforms her traditional role, though doing this creates a risk for her because she becomes anxious about how she will be perceived by colleagues. The physical environment is transformed—even the room is changed. In all these ways the therapist is preparing her patients to experience themselves as in a therapeutic situation, where it is not clear what will happen but it is clear that whatever it is will be different. She sets the stage (both literally and metaphorically) for the transformations she hopes therapy will make in their lives. She also demonstrates, through her own behavior, what is involved in transformation: namely, personal investment, risk, fun, challenge, drama, excitement, fear, suspense. Her tactics work. The group becomes an instrument of transformation. Most important, the guidance of this transformative process is gradually taken on by group members themselves. O'Reilly works to involve group members in the process, which happens as they go on to plan other "New York" events, such as creating a simulated Central Park, making giant New York–style pretzels, and the like.

The end result of the therapist's therapeutic intervention was the beginning of the "New York Gang" as they came to call themselves. They met not only twice a week but also informally on the weekends, where they planned a series of events and activities. Their ventures included making giant pretzels, cooking hot dogs to sell from a makeshift push-cart, and taking a trip to a simulated Central Park.

The most significant transformations on which this story turns are not concerned with outward behavior or measurable skill development but with a change of heart, so to speak, with a change in the patients' view of therapy. For this story not only recounts actions, but an internal domain of thoughts and feelings that accompany action. The story is especially rich in emotional language. Upon first encountering the group, the therapist is dismayed and puzzled at the deadly treatment activities and the lackluster quality of group participation. Her dismay takes a turn for the worse after talking to group members and hearing such pronouncements as "That f—— group is a waste of time." "I'm stuck!" the storyteller declares, more than once, as she sets out to solve the problem of how to create an interesting treatment approach that will appeal to members and help them improve upper body strength. The shift from frustration to enthusiasm is clearly signaled, both in straightforward declarations of feelings, and in vivid contrast between a "before" treatment group and the "after" group that she is gradually able to create. Her anxiousness about carrying off an unorthodox treatment gives narrative suspense to the unfolding story and points, in an emotionally explicit way, to this key turning point in the story. The story teller accompanies every description of action with an inner conversation of wonderings, surprises, feelings, puzzlings, so that we become privy to an inner movement that parallels the visible plane of observable action.

While this inner dialogue is much sketchier on the patient's side, here too we have some cues about the changing experiential scene as group members make the journey from boredom to surprise, pleasure, and enthusiasm. Notably, the story also conveys a sense of collective experience as it carries us from an experience of estrangement and alienation to one of commitment, hope, and participation.

Trouble

The obstacles to successful therapy with a group of head-injured patients who have resided several years in a chronic-care facility cannot be overestimated. This story begins with trouble. Trouble arises invariably because there is a gap between what is going on in therapy and what the supervising therapist (and later O'Reilly) wants to see happen. More trouble arises as O'Reilly tries to restructure the group, failing in her first attempts. Notice that troubles multiply as hope, desire, and commitment grow. Because O'Reilly really cares about changing things, she asks more from the patients and from herself. The story depicts a process of overcoming obstacles. Will the key house members come to the group? Will they find her idea ridiculous or allow themselves to be drawn into the activity? Will colleagues find her too ridiculous? This care reveals how much the very drama of narrative is based on the experience of suffering. Even the happy story, the one which ends well, takes us through a drama of plight—a lack or need that sets the story in motion and propels the protagonist in a quest to obtain a goal through the overcoming of a series of obstacles. The process of overcoming, however fortuitous the result, is almost inevitably an experience of suffering for the story's heroes and heroines. This is such a pervasive feature of the structure of narrative that Propp (1968) made it central to his analysis of folktales, and later narrativists expanded it to include many other kinds of narratives.

Suspenseful Time

This story, like the case presented earlier in this chapter, reveals the vulnerability associated with therapy. The capacity to create a powerful and potentially transformative therapeutic experience depends upon the cooperation of many actors. Risks run high because it is so easy to fail. Will the therapist be able to create an experience that captivates her clients? This cannot be her creation alone, after all. It must be cocreated with group members if it is to work. Will clients be willing to risk getting involved, and thereby allow themselves to express their own hopes and desires? The risk is higher on both sides, and so, too, the potential for trouble.

Summary

Narrative thinking is central in providing therapists with a way to consider disability in the phenomenologic terms of injured lives. Narrative thinking, especially, guides therapists when they treat the phenomenologic body; that is, when they are concerned with their patients' illness experience and how the disability is affecting their lives. In this book we have drawn upon many stories therapists have told or written about their experiences working with clients. It is not surprising that we have relied so heavily upon stories in conveying the essential phenomenological elements of occupational therapy practice.

Because narratives are predominantly about human actions, they provide a particular vantage point from which one can view the nature of clinical practice and pose clinical problems. The stories therapists tell portray disability from an actor-centered point of view. They are personal, even individualistic, and built on the structure of actors acting. Disability itself shifts from a physiologic event to a personally meaningful one, that is, to an illness experience. General physiologic conditions fall back into the shadow as background context. What is brought to center stage are the ways that particular actors, with their own motivations and commitments, have done things for which they could be praised or blamed.

In this chapter we have emphasized how narrative thinking occurs through story making, or emplotment, which involves the creation rather than the telling of stories. Telling stories is always *retrospective*—a way of considering past events—whereas story making is largely *prospective*, playing out images that therapists have of what they would like to happen in therapy. Story making concerns the way therapists work to structure therapy, as a coherent plot, as an *event* and not just a series of treatment activities, thus creating dramatic therapeutic events that connect therapy to a patient's life. Often, the search for a meaningful therapeutic story appears to be triggered by resistance or alienation of the patient to the initial therapeutic activities offered, as in the case of the members of the Upper Extremity Group. Whatever the impetus, therapists try to create clinical experiences in which there is a significant occurrence or event for the patient in therapy, one in which the therapy itself is a meaningful short story in the larger life story of the patient.

■

Clinical Revision
Changing the Therapeutic Story in Midstream
■ CHERYL MATTINGLY

Introduction

One of the most critical therapeutic skills is the capacity to change course in the midst of clinical work. It is the rare occasion (and not even necessarily the best practice) when therapy goes as planned. It is far more common for the therapist to be faced with the unexpected. Daily surprises range from the comparatively trivial—for example, the patient is not dressed and therapy must take place in the patient's room rather than in the occupational therapy room, to the highly charged—a patient has attempted suicide over the weekend or refuses treatment. Whether large or small, expert practice involves a constant ability to adapt to the changing circumstances of treating an individual patient who is in the midst of change herself and does not present a static picture from one day to the next.

Many therapists we have studied or interviewed have stated that if they had to single out the key ingredient to a successful therapist, it was the therapist's capacity to respond flexibly enough to deal with different types of patients, and that this was even more essential than having a firm basis of theoretical knowledge. As one experienced clinician, whose practice was quite theoretically oriented, said: "If I have to choose between student therapists—one who is flexible and able to deal with different kinds of patients and be responsive to them, versus one who is grounded in theory and has a solid knowledge base—I'd rather have the first. I figure that any therapist who is able to work well on an interactional level with patients can pick up the knowledge base and can function while still learning that. But I don't think it works so well the other way around."

Flexibility is so highly prized among experienced therapists because effective therapy depends as much on the capacity to modify plans and rethink treatment goals as it does on the capacity to create plans and goals in the first place. In the Clinical Reasoning Study and in our numerous workshops with therapists, we found that the most significant impetus for changing course occurred when the therapist became aware that the hoped-for treatment path and the therapeutic goals set out were not shared by the patient, even if that patient had initially appeared to agree to the plan. Put in narrative terms, revision is required when the therapist's prospective story of therapy runs into conflict with institutional constraints (the patient is suddenly being discharged tomorrow, for instance), the story envisioned by other professional colleagues, or the patient. This chapter focuses on the problem that arises when the therapist's therapeutic story differs from the patient's, and deals with the clinical reasoning problem of revision in the face of a constantly changing clinical scene. More specifically, this chapter considers the constant revision of the therapeutic story that is continually unfolding as therapist and patient work together.

Changing the Prospective Story

Therapists come to each clinical situation with a sense of the "story" they are in with a particular patient. This narrative guide, this "prospective story" is a complex portrait built from past particular experiences and stereotypical images that are "matched up" to the new patient. While this initial narrative fixing of the client and the situation is necessary—after all, one must start somewhere—it is bound to be sketchy, and in some cases, almost completely wrong. Such misfit is caused not by therapeutic error but by the need to individualize therapy to the needs and concerns of a unique client. For if the client is unique, and if this is important to good therapy, then any rules-of-thumb or stereotypical pictures (of the usual "left-hemi" or "quad") are bound to be insufficient and in need of modification as the therapist becomes better acquainted with the patient as a person. In occupational therapy, good practice depends upon recognizing that the new patient in the current situation is not simply a replica of other patients in former situations; that is, what was a good treatment plan for one client, is not necessarily a good treatment plan for another. Sometimes, when the therapist thinks she is in one particular story with a patient (helping a patient go back to her husband and house in the suburbs), the patient may have a very different future scenario in mind (moving out of her suburban house and taking an apartment alone in the city). The following case presents a good example of a therapist coming to recognize that her initial "match" of a new client to an apparently similar previous client turns out to need dramatic modification.

Case Example

The following case story is presented as it was written.

Bob

by Lizbeth Squires

When I try to think about a situation with a patient that "didn't work," the first patient that comes to mind is a guy named Bob. He was 23 years old and from South Boston, married with two children. He drove an ambulance. Bob had a wart on his finger that he bit off. That day he played softball. He noted much pain in the finger. The next day, he woke up with more pain throughout the entire arm. He also noticed a red streak moving up from his finger toward his shoulder. He took himself to the emergency room, assuming he had an infection. This was also the assumption of the physician who treated him—until his blood tests came back. The elevated white blood count of several hundred thousand made it rather clear that he had more than just an infection. As it turned out, he was admitted to the hospital that day and within 24 hours was diagnosed with leukemia. His hospitalization lasted over 2½ months.

Part of my role with patients on the oncology floor was to deal with stress management—instructing patients in various coping strategies, including relaxation techniques, visualization, guided imagery, and so forth. I had worked with several other patients in the same mode, including a 26-year-old leukemic man who had many readmissions for leukemic exacerbations, chemotherapy, and so on. This 26-year-old openly expressed his difficulty coping with these multiple hospitalizations—voicing feelings of "going stir crazy" or "being unable to relax." Paul (the 26-year-old, who was also married with children) was very receptive to any technique I could provide him with that would decrease his anxiety or increase his ability to effectively manage being in the hospital and away from his family. As it turned out, in addition to the more concrete instruction I provided, Paul and I also developed a psychotherapeutic relationship that enabled Paul to begin to discuss his feelings related to his illness—including the fear of death, the perceived loss of his role as a spouse, father, and bread winner.

Now, as I received the consultation request for Bob, I had preconceived notions about how our relationship would progress, and I was very wrong. Unlike Paul, Bob was not eager to incorporate the techniques I gently introduced. So, I let Bob know that I would be available if he changed his mind. I also asked him if it was alright if I stopped by occasionally to see how things were going. He pleasantly and willing agreed. My hope was that by providing consistent, noninvasive contact, perhaps a relationship would develop that would allow Bob to trust and seek me out if needed.

I proceeded to "stop by" every few days. We would "chat" superficially. After several weeks, I again asked Bob (who was obviously having difficulty, e.g., unable to sleep at night, pacing) if he had thought any more about trying some of the things I had mentioned. And once again, he graciously declined. He expressed concern about hurting my feelings and I reassured him that wasn't the case. I again explained that my role was to be there if he needed me, that my treatment was not "mandatory" by any means, and that I certainly appreciated his honesty.

Bob never took me up on my offer. I continued to stop by occasionally, to "chat" and to let him know, in a subtle way, that I valued his decision and would not abandon him.

Case Discussion

Here the therapist uses a set of easily observable cues to match Bob's and Paul's cases as similar. She then tries to carry out with Bob a therapeutic story similar to that which she had experienced with Paul. Her written narrative includes no evidence that she ever was able to develop a new prospective story for her work with Bob. Her account does not focus on revision but simply on the initial experience of realizing that her prospective story was not going to fit the situation at hand when Bob turns out to be unlike Paul in his response to her interventions.

Generally therapists were not this explicit about their attempts to reprise a success story taken from their work with a previous patient, in their encounter with a new patient. Such attempts to derive an expectation of the course of a new case by matching it with a previous one on the basis of similarities was often revealed more indirectly.

CLASHES BETWEEN BIOMEDICALLY AND PHENOMENOLOGICALLY FRAMED PROSPECTIVE STORIES

Sometimes therapists were confronted by a mismatch between prospective stories cast in biomedical terms (generally due to the therapist's need to present her work to other hospital staff as the treatment of a medical condition), and the responses of the patient to the illness experience itself. These clashes between biomedically and phenomenologically framed prospective stories place therapist and patient in different types of worlds.

For instance, one therapist told about an experience working on a burn unit with a patient who had been terribly disfigured.* The therapist described his burns:

Somewhere around 60 percent of his total body surface area was covered with third-degree burns. The burns included almost his total face. His ears were burned off. His eyes were quite heavily burned. His hands were

---

*Interview and analysis of this case was done by Jaime Munoz.

both totally burned . . . circumferential burns on both hands, chest, legs. Just about every part of his body was burned.

The therapist was concerned that the patient needed to do active range of motion with his hands in order to keep as much motion in his hands as possible. There was an urgency in the therapist's concern to get the patient working to range his hand right after the accident because "the longer they [patients] wait, the harder it is to move." Soon after the skin grafting there is still some flexibility, and scar tissue has not yet firmly formed. The therapist was anxious to try to preserve some movement for the patient, but it required the patient's immediate co-operation. The therapist's story focused on a physiologic process that he felt responsible, as a therapist, to try to direct in the best possible way. The therapist's story of his own actions was framed within the biomechanical problems the disability was creating.

> Well actually, after the skin takes, which is only 5 days after the graft, you can do active range of motion. But as the new skin matures, the collagen formation becomes thicker and the skin actually becomes thick-ened and scar tissue forms and you have a decrease in range of motion in the skin, which then limits the joints, if the new graft is over a joint.

While some decrease in motion is inevitable, there is some chance to prevent the development of severe contractures and complete stiff-ening of the hands, which renders them useless. The therapist knew this and for him the issue was getting that patient moving. The patient was in a completely different story. He was a young man in his early twenties who had just been horribly burned and who became extremely depressed and withdrawn, by the therapist's account. The patient wanted to hide and to be angry. The therapist said of him,

> He was in the category of 'leave, like leave me alone, I'll do it when I feel better.' So he had to be . . . motivation was always a problem with him. And initially that was one of the most difficult things to work with, was his . . . just anger, the anger, the self-pity. The idea that, well, he's in pain and, you know, 'leave me alone' kind of thing.

Discussion

In this story there is nothing very removed about the therapist's biomedical account. The therapist's experience of trying to catch and ameliorate the disastrous consequences of the burning, his absolute dependence on mobilizing the patient's commitment if he is to achieve this goal, and his helplessness and frustration at not knowing how to do more for the patient, all come through just underneath the surface of his description of a worsening biomechanic condition:

> Then he developed contractures in the elbows, this, heterotopic ossifi-cation, where the elbows, or many joints—primarily the elbows in the case of burns—begin to develop calcifications right in the muscles, right around the elbows, and uh, there's nothing you can do about that. You

can try to attempt range of motion to prevent that, but once it starts going, then it's a process that will just continue, until, until it stops and then at that point they have to have surgery on it to release it. But because of that, we lost the elbow motions and any hope of him doing self-care kinds of things. Because the hands just went.

The involvement of the therapist, his sense of personal failure and failure of the patient show in those last sentences, which say "we lost" the physiologic battle. The therapist's sense of what this loss of movement and loss of ability to do self-care would mean to the patient is utterly graphic. He stated:

> When he has to go to the bathroom he can't even toilet himself. He was able to pull his pants down and everything, but if he had to have a bowel movement he couldn't even wipe his ass. And he would have to rely on nurses, on therapists to do those kinds of things.

The two examples noted thus far are all cases of mismatch between the therapists' sense of what ought to happen in treatment, particularly what they expected from the patient, and the patient's despair or hiddenness. Each of the patients in these stories is a bitter or too-silent partner, who remains mysterious to the therapist, out of reach. The disability, meanwhile, grows worse without the patient's involvement. In the first example, the therapist abandons her prospective story when she recognizes that the new patient will not work with her, that he was not another Paul after all. In the second example, the therapist does not appear to initially perceive the difficult patient as repetitions of other particular patients treated, but as example of general types of difficult patients whom the therapist contrasts with patients who he has felt more successful treating. The therapist working on the burn unit also makes oblique reference to other patients who do not withdraw in the same way. He describes this particular patient as belonging to "that category of . . . 'leave me alone,'" which implies that there are other categories of patients who do not give this message. He also suggests comparisons with other patients he has treated when he says, "They, different people cope in different ways. Some of them, the best comes out. You know, you see some real amazing kinds of things. You know, other times it's the worst comes out."

Reframing the Therapeutic Role

Sometimes the surprises and frustrations that the patient triggers, the misfits between what the therapist wants to see happen and what actually does occur, provoke a rereading and reframing of that prospective story. Even in those cases that are "the best" from the therapist's point of view, there is a constant tinkering with and modifying of the prospective story. At the other end of the spectrum are the more intractable contradictions between the prospective story and the lived experience of working with a patient. In such cases, the therapist is thrown into a state of confusion and, frequently, of anger as he or she tries to sort things out.

Sometimes this collision between therapist expectations and patient realities is so minor, or the therapist and patient so resourceful, that it can be resolved through small improvisations that do not challenge the boundaries of a therapist's understanding of her or his role. In other cases, the two are at such odds that the confrontation provokes a new way of seeing in the therapist.

Sometimes, responding to the difficult case requires the creation of an individualized role for the therapist as therapist, a theme that occurs again and again in stories therapists tell about difficult cases. Responding effectively to a patient often takes therapists outside of preconceived role boundaries. Often the "difficult case" turns out to to be the patient who triggers change in the therapist's own view of his or her role or of what good therapy should look like. When therapists recount such incidents, the recurrent moral is that they learned to step outside the confines of their preconceptions about the required treatment.

In the following case a psychiatric therapist faces a recalcitrant patient who remains passive in the face of her attempts to get him actively involved, to take responsibility for his rehabilitation. She comes to the clinical encounter with a story that she wants the patient to realize with her and grows increasingly frustrated at his unwillingness to play his part. This account more clearly involves reframing of the initial story line than the previous examples. It is a case of collision between her expectations and her experience that provokes an experience in the "emphatic sense," one which involves a revision of her own assessment of herself as a therapist. She tells a story about her efforts with this patient.

The therapist introduced her story by saying, "I'll begin by giving an example of one patient who has clearly changed my way of thinking." This patient, a man in his mid-forties, had a diagnosis of depression. He was readmitted about every 6 months to the acute care hospital where she worked. Upon discharge he would appear to the staff to have improved somewhat during the course of his hospitalization, and yet he would be back to his previous condition upon his next readmission. "When this guy left, always I think in the back of our heads we thought, 'Well, in a few months he'll return,' but we always tried to do the best we could."

Readmitted chronic cases, whether physically or mentally disabled, often frustrate therapists who feel a sense of failure at not have been able to effect significant improvement. They often feel angry at the patients, especially in cases where it appears that if the patient had cooperated properly during the course of the therapy, readmission would not be necessary later, or at least there would be a noticeable improvement in their condition, even if further hospitalization was necessary. Patients are also often angry to find themselves back in the hospital, caught in a cycle they cannot get out of, and frustrated with medical professionals for not being more helpful.

The last time the therapist saw this patient the chronic stalemate between them shifted, for a moment at least, in a way that she felt changed her practice. This experience threw into doubt her assumptions about patients taking responsibility for working on their own rehabilitation. She outlined these beliefs at the beginning of her story.

> This gentleman came back one time, the last time I had worked with him before I left, and, you know, as usual, in the groups we would really encourage people to take a look at themselves, to help them to identify their strengths, and how to use those strengths to overcome certain problems . . . look at different ways to cope. We really focused on taking responsibility for yourself. And, you know, 'You're responsible for your actions, for your own decisions, and so on. And knowing that, what can you do about it? Let's make a plan.' So along with stressing certain points, we're very concrete, saying, 'You have this knowledge. Now what can you do with it?'

The patient's response was an unusually direct resistance to these messages about the possibilities of individual responsibility and efficacy for one's own destiny. The therapist described an instance of direct confrontation between herself and the patient that made her anxious.

> He said, 'It's not up to me, Mary.' He'd say, 'It's up to God.' He had these delusions of religiosity—not real articulated, not real verbalized—but it would definitely come out when he was confronted with what responsibilities he could take for his life. But this guy was adamant about just resisting the whole idea of taking responsibility, of doing anything to change his life. He felt like a victim. A helpless, innocent victim that, what happened, was a result of fate, or a result of God. And he just refused any idea. And at that point in time I had always been real firm on taking responsibility for your own actions, for your own beliefs, for your own thoughts, for your own feelings. And when this guy resisted so much, inside I would, I would get like this turmoil and as a result I confronted him with it.

The therapist described the escalation of increasingly direct and hostile confrontation between herself and the patient, confrontation in which the patient would leave the room and the therapist would find herself getting angrier and angrier.

He had been in the system, he had heard all of this before, and I felt perfectly safe confronting him about it. So I would do so and frequently during this hospitalization he couldn't handle it. He'd get up and he'd walk out of the room saying, "There's nothing I can do about it." And it would infuriate me. Because I thought, Mister, you know, you've been through this, you know, not that I want you to repeat what I'm telling you, but to help him . . . really believe deep down, that he had a responsibility.

When this escalation came to a head the most important result is that the therapist finally came to see the patient as foreign, as not easily amenable to her previous ways of understanding depressed clients. She had an experience of confronting someone strange, someone whom she could not judge and understand in familiar terms. This is the way she described that experience.

Anyway, one particular day, you know, I was becoming somewhat confused as to what to do about this at this point. I made a comment to him one session in which he couldn't handle it and he left the room. And I thought, this can't go on. I don't want this guy to think that I'm threatening him. I mean, if anything, I want to be supportive and I want to help him to realize that he has potential, just how to actualize it. So I went to talk with him. . . . So anyway, I went into the room to talk to him and . . . then he, talking with him definitely gave me a better understanding of him, and of, and of what I was projecting upon him. I honestly felt that this guy was sincere in that he did not think that there was anything that he could do. Prior to that, I felt that he was denying any type of responsibility, just plain denial. But I actually felt that he was sincere. The reasoning being, he had been in several times before and all of this information he had learned before. Somehow or another he couldn't follow through or it didn't work, and it resulted in the same thing, him coming back. He went into God—that's the only thing that he had—to hang onto, and his family. And he went on. I don't remember the specifics of the story but I remembered at that point I stopped and I said, 'Mary, who the hell are you to say, "Hey, these are my values, these are my beliefs, and you should follow them." And it just, it just changed my whole treatment, my everyday treatment from that point on. And at the end I told him, I said, 'Listen, I want to thank you. You've really shown me a new perspective and I've learned a lot from you.' At that point I left. It's amazing, because (sigh) it's so easy as a therapist to impose, you know, like I said, your values and your beliefs on others. And it's not always the case. I think that a lot of people have a potential and they may not see that potential. And I think by reflecting some of your values and beliefs may help them to see alternatives. But I think there's also cases like his where it doesn't matter. You know, that they have a different set of standards. And I think that recognizing that makes all the difference, all the difference in effective treatment.

Discussion

This is an account of the revision of a story about her therapeutic work with this client. Her earlier story, which is abandoned in her final confrontation with this patient, embodied frustration at his irrespon-

sibility, his unwillingness to take on his proper role in the work of
therapy, a role which could have led to improvement and, ideally, an
ability to function in his job and with his family, and an end to the
repeated hospitalizations. The earlier story affixes blame firmly on the
patient: therapy is not working and it is the patient's fault. Her confrontation with the patient reaches a climax in which she comes to
question the simplicity of her earlier story. Therapy is not working with
this patient but perhaps she is wrong in the story she has told about
who this patient is and why she and the rest of the staff have been so
ineffective. In her revision of the therapeutic story, she comes to see
the patient as holding a set of beliefs that she certainly does not share
and that she finds unfortunate but which nonetheless are real beliefs,
not mere excuses for irresponsibility. Her revised story is that she and
the other staff, who believe that patients should tackle their problems,
were coming into conflict with an equally strong, and equally respect-
able set of beliefs that the patient held.

In this example, the therapist relinquishes the right to blame the
patient for not getting well. In this last case, the reframing of most
consequence is not the therapist's recognition that the patient could be
holding a different set of beliefs rather than acting irresponsibly, but
rather, her recognition that certain preconceptions of her own as to the
kind of therapeutic participation that characterized sincere patients
were her own beliefs, not a universally relevant set of truths. This
discovery is one that anthropologists love to recount: That when you
confront the other, you may come to see that what you previously had
known uncritically as the truth, as simple facts, changes its ontological
status and suddenly appears as belief. What was natural is suddenly
visible as cultural.

Searching for a Story and Getting Lost

Some accounts of trouble in therapy are not about mismatches
between expectations based on previous therapies and the realities of
a present attempt. Instead, they are stories about the difficulties of
attempting to understand a new patient through a story about an "ideal
type" of patient. Such matches offer the therapist a familiar starting
point. In addition to past experiences with other individuals, therapists
relied on a repertoire of patient types, and they often turned to the
diagnostic categories of biomedicine for this kind of help in organizing
the treatment possibilities.

When the diagnostic categorization proved uncertain or when new
evidence arose that suggested another category might be more appropriate, the therapist would often find herself lost between clinical stories. Such diagnostic confusion was rarely the sole problem, though it

was often the one therapists initially cited. Even when therapists who were interviewed initially identified their primary confusion as a diagnostic one, further discussion of their problems nearly always revealed a set of issues that connected their difficulties, not only to an uncertain diagnosis, but also to confusions or conflicts with the patient's interpretation of the meaning of the disability. Confusion over the appropriate diagnosis of the disease tended to be confounded by conflicts and confusion over the meaning of the illness experience.

This is evident in the following case. In each, the initial impetus for the therapist's dissatisfaction is a realization that there are symptoms present that do not fit the treatment approach she has adopted. In some instances, this confusion is exacerbated by the therapists' uncertainty as to the biomedical significance of the symptoms.

A pediatric therapist initially diagnosed a 3-year-old child as having sensory integration dysfunction and began working with the child with that in mind. She later became increasingly unsure about the child's problems, wondering if she was not seeing a head-injured patient instead. When she was interviewed, she at first discussed her confusion in terms of the difficulty of making an accurate biomedical diagnosis.

My impression at the time that I first saw him was that he might have sensory integration dysfunction. He was so opposed to any kind of movement and tactile-defensive that I was looking at him and kind of that was why he is so clumsy. But the other issue was the head injury. They really made . . . the family was making light of that. So physically, I guess it is his diagnostics that are not clear. He now looks more like a head-injured child than anything, and even at the time he did to me. He also had a lot of things that shouldn't . . . that sensory integration dysfunction doesn't have. So I was trying to decide: Should I treat him more like a physically disabled child or try to integrate the information from the environment?

As she continued to recount her problems working with this child and his family, other aspects of the situation were presented as candidates for the "real problem." She admitted that she usually does not have a clear biomedical diagnosis when working with young children, a situation that is typical for pediatric occupational therapy in general. Patients are often referred by pediatricians simply as "developmentally delayed," which "doesn't tell me anything," she said. "If I get a referral and it says 'developmental delay' I really don't have any information when the child comes in. I can get information from the medical record, but when they send me the consult often what it says is 'developmental delay.' I don't really know how they will look when they come in." Even though lack of clear biomedical diagnoses was common, we felt especially lost with this child. When pressed by the interviewer, her language shifted and she described the patient as having gotten lost.

Therapist:	I just want to be more clear.
Interviewer:	Do you think that most cases are clear?
Therapist:	I don't think that most cases are clear.
Interviewer:	So why was this case so much more frustrating than others?
Therapist:	I don't know. I think it's because it became kind of lost. I hate it when people get lost.

She never really understood any of the actors involved in this child's illness. It is as though she walked on stage where a play was going on and she didn't know the script. This therapist was new at the hospital and was not yet familiar with how things were done. Her patient's family was Spanish and she didn't speak Spanish. She could talk with the mother through an interpreter when one could come, but she couldn't always get one. The family was not regular in their visits to the clinic so she would go for weeks without seeing him and then when she saw him again, things would look different.

> The thing I feel most frustrated with is he is 3 years and 8 months old and the family is not so good about bringing him in and I see him so infrequently that it is almost like I can't get a handle on him. Every once in a while I'll change my viewpoint but then it is a couple of weeks before I see him again. And just when I think I am getting a handle on him I don't see him for a while.

The mother explained to her, through an interpreter, that the child had been dropped on the head by an uncle, but the mother did not seem especially upset about this or appear to take it very seriously, a circumstance which further confused the therapist. The child had been treated in the hospital for the head injury and yet no one at the hospital had followed him up. The therapist described herself as bewildered at this. "That sort of surprised me that even after he had been to the hospital and the fact that he had been delayed, he hadn't gotten any follow-up except by his pediatrician. This is kind of surprising because to look at the child, he looks very clumsy... very awkward movements."

At the end of the interview she repeated her surprise at the hospital staff's lack of response. "I am really surprised with him after being in the hospital for 4 hours with the head injury at that age, why he never got any follow-up. He definitely doesn't look like a normal child. I mean even if you just saw him you would know it." The importance of the hospital's neglect initially was that it simply added to her confusion about what she was seeing. Neither family nor medical staff had seemed to take the head injury seriously and the child's behavior was ambiguous, so perhaps it was not a problem related to head injury after all. But then she saw increasing signs that this was indeed the problem. But if this was the problem, and the injury happened 2 years prior to her treatment of the child, then a very different scenario should have occurred. The child should have been followed right at the time of the injury and this did not happen. This led her to a whole different kind of conclusion, to a different kind of story, one in which her patient had "gotten lost." "People get lost in the system all the time. That is a very big frustration of mine." She also believed that she had contributed to the child's getting lost for the months she had treated him. The child was not coming in frequently because the family was poor and she was treating him in a private pay clinic. The child really needed to be in a school program that would not charge the family, but she, being new herself, did not know how to go about getting the child into a school program. The therapist summed up her sense of how she had never "found" this child or gotten him to a therapist who could "find" him:

> I started to see him in May and I felt the reason he got lost is the private pay. It is so expensive to the family that I tried to get him into a program real fast. Now I feel kind of bad that it is going to take so long—he is just now into the school system. Part of the problem is that it [seeing this patient] was 6 months after I got here and I didn't know the system well enough. When I first saw him I should have gotten him right into the school system. . . . He really needed more therapy and that is what I feel bad about. They are private pay. They don't want to come in a lot to see me. So they are pretty good about bringing him in but it feels . . . and I can't get a handle on him. I can't get a good feeling of what he can or can't do. I mean, I know I have an OK idea. It is probably pretty good, but with some cases you feel, like you know the child, but with him I don't.

Discussion

The therapist never finds a place in which she can become effective in this story. The patient is lost. He shows symptoms of this, symptoms of that. The family is lost. They are paying for something they cannot afford, and they speak Spanish, so no one is helping them locate good resources for their child. The therapist is lost. As often happens when therapists describe troublesome cases, she narrates a short scenario that conveys her understanding of her proper place in a therapeutic process. Unlike the cases reviewed above, she does not refer to a previous case in constructing her understanding. Instead, she sketches a generic story that sums up a particular aspect of many previous cases.

Changing Stories in Midstream

In the two cases discussed in the preceding section, mismatches occurred when therapists tried to prospectively emplot their work with a particular patient by using a story derived from previous work with another patient. Each of these therapists had serious difficulty in coming to a way of responding to certain aspects of their new patients' behavior. It was as though they could not invent a revision of their initial story that would make their work with these particular patients "go somewhere" in terms of therapeutic productivity. They could not emplot a course of therapy for these particular patients that led to a rehabilitative ending.

The confrontation between story and experience does not always happen in this way. It can also be triggered by changes in the patient. These can be complex, meaning-centered changes, as the patient comes to see herself and her illness differently, or they can be changes in the illness experience that are created by new physiological complications.

In the following example, the therapist had been working successfully along one treatment path until some unexpected and puzzling physiological symptoms occurred. This violation of her prospective emplotment led to an involved exploration and a change in the clinical story.

I've known this client for at least 10 years. He was a student in the school where I was working and he grew up into the adult program. He was verbal and he had some of the problems that are inherent in being severely retarded, you know, poor ADLs [activities of daily living] and things like that. About 6 years ago he developed retinal detachment and he became blind. And I didn't know too much about training blind children, whatever. We got over that hump and he, once again, attained independence for his daily living tasks and vocational tasks, whatever. And then about a year ago, I was still working for the adult program, Joe became very wobbly, poor balance, started to fall. Not tripping over things as if his blindness was getting in the way but like his muscles were losing control. And I was calling the head nurse in the residential facility where he lived and I was telling her these things that I was observing. . . . Well, 2 months later, Joe would fall and not be able to get up. There was no muscle control. Pretty soon he couldn't feel anything. And I was very upset at this point. We ended up, I pushed, got him into a rehab center here—at least for an outpatient evaluation. They found out that he was a T9 paraplegic at that point. And because, what we didn't know, that the neurologist had not even touched him during his assessments these first 4 months after the symptoms were noted. It had gone too far and operations could not help at this point. There was too much nerve involvement at that point. So I had to . . . so this young man is now paraplegic in addition to being severely retarded and blind. So that really made me have to rethink—now what do I do? . . . So I think that's the scenario for how I had to rethink things and really struggle to get him back on his feet, so to speak.

Discussion

In a narrow sense, what was reframed here was the diagnosis as the patient's new symptoms were finally understood and named. The therapist saw her role as helping the patient perform his ADLs, but as new problems arose, this required her to change her approach. The deeper story here, however, the one that she elaborated later in the interview, concerned her sense of uncertainty and impotence, not only about what was happening to Joe, but about what her role should be in trying to get help for him. She was very close to this patient and felt responsible for him. She was the one, according to her story, who was most aggressive in noting symptoms and trying to find out what was going wrong. What she found out in the end was that if he had been diagnosed 4 months earlier, he never would have had to be a paraplegic. This hit her very hard.

There were two vivid narrative moments in this interview. One was where she remembered how Joe talked to her about what had happened to him. "There was a point, it was about 4 or 5 months after the first symptoms happened, where he was saying that his legs were 'gone away.' 'No more legs.' 'All broken.' 'All gone.' And he was sad. He was very depressed. He didn't care. He wasn't eating. You know, he just shut down." He loved music and she had spent time listening to music with him. When he could no longer use his legs he would tell her, "I want to walk. I want to dance."

The other striking moment was when she described what it was like to try to do something for the patient and not be able to find her way through bureaucratic channels, all the while knowing that something was going more and more wrong.

Therapist:	I saw something happening and I was scared. I didn't know what was going on. And especially as it seemed to get in his everyday, in the way of his everyday life, I was afraid. As I tried to take steps to get this situation changed, I, boy, I felt frustrated and angry. Real angry.
Interviewer:	At whom?
Therapist:	Most. Well, I don't know if it's an "at whom" or at the whole situation. But it seemed like every new person we went to talk to, to consult . . . was like running into a brick wall. I felt frustration with the system, quote unquote, working with DD [developmentally delayed] adults to begin with. There's a lot of medical people who don't automatically know how to handle a DD adult in their office. You know, because the person can't talk fluently or can't express the symptoms verbally. It's real hard to diagnose or to treat. And I think I was very frustrated with that situation. And the frustration grew into anger as the problem was not identified."

While this therapist began the interview with a story that centered primarily on how she had to change her treatment approach as this new complication occurred, particularly how she had to call upon her rusty capacities as a physical disabilities therapist (her primary training is in psychiatric occupational therapy), her narrative then shifted to focus on her own frustration and fear at not knowing how to get help for the patient, and her feelings at seeing her patient become paraplegic.

The heart of her revision is not the shift in her patient's diagnosis but the vicissitudes of her own role as therapist. At the beginning of the interview she stressed her role as one who worked on ADLs. But as the interview progressed, she went over and over her fear and frustration at not being able to get the patient diagnosed. She ends the interview by describing her revised sense of what it meant to be a therapist to these kinds of clients. The change that she ultimately emphasizes is not the tragic change in this particular client's mobility, it is the change wrought by the entire episode in the kind of therapeutic story she wants to realize with her retarded patients, particularly in her intensified concern with talking for them to medical professionals who are not used to listening to such people.

This is a much broader story, one that includes more characters, even the entire medical bureaucracy in which she works. And it is less "strictly OT" in its dimensions because it emphasizes her need to listen to patients and then to try to communicate what she sees and hears to others whose help is essential in addressing problems that these patients cannot adequately describe on their own. Her widened conception of the problems involved in treatment is evident in the "moral" she attaches to her case story at the end of the interview.

> I think I feel a little bit more sure of myself in making, yeah, in making decisions for people, for clients that I work with. And I do work with . . . you know, the majority of my people are severely, profoundly handicapped. I feel much more sure of the recommendations I make. The recommendations I have made, I find myself qualifying why I'm making the recommendation and how, if such and such is done or carried out, how this is going to impact that person's life on a daily basis. I think I'm more careful now in putting in more details, so then more people can understand the whole situation when I'm making recommendations for clients. I think it's changed the way that I think about things like advocacy and confidentiality, and even follow-through for somebody who can't talk for themselves, you know, who can't express the feeling or whatever. So it's made me listen with a third ear in a sense.

Reemplotments were often provoked by ambiguities or difficulties in a patient's diagnosis. Accounts of these changes in narrative expectation often took the form of a drama in which shifts in the patient's diagnosis directly provoked shifts in the therapist's view of her role. The following account has many of the qualities of a detective story, in which the therapist is trying to discover the correct diagnosis of a patient. It illustrates particularly well the integration of the two forms of clinical reasoning differentiated in earlier chapters: narrative reasoning, which deals with motive and with developing a coherent story of the illness experience; and propositional reasoning associated with a biomedical approach, which concerns the diagnosis of a disease (and associated dysfunctions) from symptoms and signs.

This therapist's story concerned his treatment of a girl with cerebral palsy (CP) who had been tentatively diagnosed as psychotic. When he heard that she would be arriving on his ward, his first reaction was nervousness about his own ability to deal with someone with a severe physical disability.

I remember feeling apprehensive about it, about going to see her and taking on this case because I felt, 'Oh my God, I don't know anything to do. What am I going to do with this person?' So I went and met her and she was very nice. It kind of allayed some of my fears because at least we had a good rapport from the beginning and that was good.

The medical diagnosis provides therapists with an initial picture of the patient and therapists can have quite strong reactions to that picture even before they meet the patient. Because the patient was in an unfamiliar diagnostic category, the therapist felt at a loss for those particular skills and competencies that physical disabilities occupational therapists accustomed to handling CP patients would have. He was also at a loss for ways to "make sense" of the patient. "What am I going to do with this patient?" he asks himself. He did not have a repertoire of stories about working with such patients. He then turned to puzzling about what is really wrong with her, because he mistrusts the tentative diagnosis of psychosis that has brought her into the hospital.

Her school was sending her to the hospital. They were afraid that she was psychotic, that she was hearing voices and that she was hallucinating more, and things like that. My immediate thought, even before I met her I guess, was that, 'Well, is this psychosis or is this just a retarded person's consciousness talking to them and it's being construed as auditory hallucinations, which sometimes happens?' An MR [mentally retarded] person will get labeled psychotic when that's just the way the [unclear] can express themselves and, when they express it to someone who's not also MR, they start to (unclear). But it's not so weird. It's normal.

His initial response to meeting her, as he narrates it, is relief because "she was very nice." This is an interesting statement, implying that in that first meeting she began to emerge as a person for him, someone more than a member of an unfamiliar medical category. In his story he discovers more and more about her life history and about the particular pressures and stresses that plagued her up until her entrance on his psychiatric ward. This portrays his progression from a biomedical way of seeing to an increasingly phenomenologic one. The therapist himself refers to this theme in conclusion to the account. William Labov (19_ : __) has described oral narratives as tending to conclude with a final evaluation segment, where the storyteller informs the audience about how the story should be interpreted. In this story the narrator gives an extensive final evaluation that returns him to the opening theme of the story, his initial concern with treating a "CP" and his relief to discover that he could see her "as a person."

> So at the end it felt much better because I wasn't seeing her as CP [cerebral palsy] anymore. I was seeing her as another person who came in with a psychiatric problem. . . . What's weird now is since her, I've had two other CPs on the unit. It's kind of neat because now I don't feel so . . . I don't feel like such a (unclear) that I've never had this complication. In fact, we're getting more medically, or dual-diagnosed, patients. It's just another patient with a psychiatric problem, too.

This patient emerges as an individual person only as her therapist is able to recategorize her from an unfamiliar to a familiar medical category. The narrator never leaves his professional categories behind, and his journey as he becomes able to see the patient follows a rather different path than hermeneuticists have described. He confronts a patient who is initially foreign to him, not because of some unassimilable uniqueness but because she represents a member of a medically unfamiliar classification. The story is one where the therapist is gradually able to make her more familiar to himself. This familiarity goes hand in hand with the therapist's growing understanding of the patient's particular life history. She is most stereotyped when she is the strangest to him. As he can assimilate her into familiar ways of seeing and familiar ways of treating, as he is able to see her as "just another patient with a psychiatric problem," he is paradoxically making it possible to see her as a particular individual. Familiar categories are not at war with the ability to experience someone as having a personal identity that comes from a particular life history and illness experience. They serve to help the therapist see the patient in less stereotypical ways.

The drama of this story is the therapist's work to try to make sense of this patient, diagnostically speaking and narratively speaking. He begins his diagnostic search with the question of whether the patient is really psychotic or whether she might be retarded (an MR patient). That was quickly settled: "It turned out that her intelligence was OK. So that wasn't a problem." Having ruled out that possibility, he examines other options, unwilling to settle for psychosis and confronted by another complicating factor that might explain her unusual behavior.

I remember thinking that (unclear) or I wasn't going to believe that she was psychotic unless I had good reasons to believe. I remember another thing that I didn't like about this case. One of the reasons she was coming in was because she had gotten more autonomy away from the school where she was staying and could leave the school and come back. On one of these trips she had met this fellow from a church group and he was kind of, very, oh, I guess the best way to say this is he was kind of a cult church follower. He started putting into her, she started having more and more problems after this relationship because a lot of her hallucinations, or such things, had to do with religiosity. So there was a lot of concern by everyone, all her school teachers and the dorm manager where she was staying, and things like that. So I guess the first way I started approaching her was that, was to find out whether or not she really was psychotic. After I had heard all of these other stories about the religious cult and, I guess I felt less and less confident that she was schizophrenic and just our interactions were also pretty logical.

His attempt to understand her was organized as an attempt to appropriately categorize her, as is evident in his description of his interactions with her as clues favoring various possible diagnoses. His interactions with her gave conflicting evidence about her mental status. At this point, he was trying to decide between two possible categories, psychotic or "just a behavior" probably induced by her association with the cult church leader. While for the most part her interactions with him "were pretty logical" there was some conflicting evidence.

We were setting goals in a group one time and she said her goal was to not live in an imaginary world. And I go, 'Oh my God, she is psychotic!' And, but then she wrote some of her days (unclear) down and some of her steps that she was going to take, which didn't sound so psychotic. But what was weird was that later on that day she came up to me and told me that she shouldn't have told me about living in an imaginary world, that was a mistake and I should just forget it. Then I said, 'Oh (unclear)' [audience laughing, covers storyteller's words on tape]. So then I thought that she was trying to be manipulative with me and wanted to talk about certain things but not other things.

The turning point in the story came when the therapist had a talk with the school social worker, who offered some background information on her. This changed his whole picture of her, because crucial facts about her situation emerged. The girl was graduating from her school in 3 months and was going to have to find a place where she could live on her own for the first time in her life. This led him to become confident that the diagnosis that he had suspected—behavioral rather than psychotic—was the correct one, but it also required changes in the story that he had constructed about why these symptoms had emerged. Rather than believing that her association with the cult church had caused them, he decided that it was her impending departure from the school to live by herself for the first time—an impending loss and a difficult test of self-reliance—that had created the stress that led, both to her wish to join another home (hence the church group), and to her fantasies and hallucinations.

> Then when I talked to her social worker at school there was a whole different picture of her altogether. I started. . . . I think I started reframing it right then. The problem was that she was going to graduate in like 3 months and she didn't have a place to live and she was going to have to find a place to live. The school was going to help her, but that was something that she was going to have to deal with. She had been living at the school for like 3 years or so and she really didn't have a family to speak of. They weren't supportive. They didn't see her that often. I started seeing this attempt to go find this church group as an attempt to find a family. The . . . [thing I] was starting to see was that . . . she was really worried about this change in her role. She was going to have to be on her own, yet she didn't know how to do that. So her response was to forget how to do everything else. She forgot how to get to school on time. She forgot how to clean up her room. She got kicked out of everything that she had been doing before.

The reframing the therapist describes allowed him to choose between the two competing diagnostic categories he had been debating and to assemble a convincing narrative of the patient's history, in which the cause of the patient's symptoms was interpreted as a common psychosocial stress. A biomedical model of clinical reasoning and a narrative model of clinical reasoning go hand in hand here, one reinforcing the other. "Getting a handle on the case" simultaneously means coming to understand the patient's illness experience better, suddenly understanding the stressful and frightening situation she was facing—a young girl with cerebral palsy and little or no family support about to be let loose on the world—and feeling confident about his diagnosis. The therapist goes on to describe how this sudden emplotment of the patient's life entailed a significant revision of the story of the onset of her current symptoms that he had developed earlier, a story that had also diagnosed her problem as behavioral but that attributed the cause to the church group.

> And it was funny because I started, I think, going on a path that it was all a result of meeting this guy and getting into this religious cult. And that certainly was one, I am assuming, one of the major precipitators to her coming to the hospital. But I was going on this path thinking that that's why her other roles got disrupted. She started this church role, and her school and homemaker roles were disrupted as a result. But I think that was just kind of a (unclear) because, eventually, I started thinking that the case was that she was having difficulty with the idea she was losing her family, losing the school.

When the therapist was able to identify the patient as belonging to a familiar category of problems, he was able to draw on his own competencies and therapeutic narratives to emplot her treatment. He was able to act. He was able to create a prospective story that led to a rehabilitative ending. This prospective story is informed by (1) diagnostically relevant concepts from biomedicine and psychiatry, (2) an illness narrative constructed from information gleaned from the social worker and other sources, and (3) theories within occupational therapy, notably role theories from the Model of Human Occupation (a theory of practice in occupational therapy). All of these he utilized in constructing a practical story about how treatment would go with this patient. The "behavioral" category in which her current problems were ultimately classed was given solidity and concreteness by the illness narrative that the therapist constructed, a narrative that explained the onset of her symptoms. Simultaneously, her illness as diagnosed led him, via his knowledge of the principles of treating psychiatric disorders of this type, to a repertoire of narrative fragments, which he then saw as appropriate to draw on in prospectively emplotting a course of treatment.

> So I guess I ended up feeling real good about the case because what I ended up doing was to focus with her on roles and reorganizing her life around activities that support certain roles and how she was going to make plans for the next 3 months between the time she went back to school until the time that she graduated. Although, during the acute hospitalization she wasn't able to set . . . to be realistic with that 3-month period. I think that she did learn some skills in terms of realizing that, I mean, she had a plan for at least the first week when she went back to school, things that she was not going to do and strategies that she was going to use with the team. Her team came in from school, and we had a talk both as a team and I had a talk with her [the social worker] as a leisure (unclear) and felt like we were able to come up with things that were realistic for them [the team] to do in terms of giving her more structure.

This case shares some important features with others in this chapter. The accounts of reemplotting therapeutic expectations given by the pediatric therapist and the psychiatric therapist who worked with MR patients concern difficulties in getting a fix on the patient, both diagnostically and narratively. This lack of a clear diagnostic category appears to leave therapists at a loss for resources out of which to fashion a convincing prospective story, a story which they need in order to identify their role and plan their interventions. The case of the psychiatric therapist with the CP patient concerns the therapist's search for a diagnosis. The closer he gets to a good diagnosis, the closer he gets to the patient's illness experience. His deepening understanding of both diagnosis and illness experience enable him to orient himself with increasing confidence to a particular set of therapeutic plots drawn from his own past experience and training. His initial prospective story is hardly a story at all, giving him no confident ground for action; so he searches for a different story, and chooses to conduct this search via the search for the correct psychiatric diagnosis. He explores different versions of the etiology of her symptoms. When he identifies causes and symptoms that he feels confident about applying to this patient, this allows him to construct a better prospective story, one crafted for this individual patient, but informed by general professional theories.

> And, when I reframed it, I could use the whole idea of roles, from the Model (the Model of Human Occupation) but also psychodynamically, the issue of family, and having a place to live, and how the disruption was a symptom of this psychodynamic issue that she was facing. And she was able to have some insight about it too. She realized what she was looking for, at some level. It was an interesting case.

Summary

At first glance, the need to revise treatment plans and goals en route, so to speak, might seem to betoken an unprepared therapist, or an inadequate assessment. It is clear that planning, goal setting, and initial assessment are integral to effective therapy. At the same time, the Clinical Reasoning Study and subsequent case stories written by therapists show that revision is essential, no matter how prepared the therapist and how thorough the assessment. Revision is not only necessary when things go wrong. There is also an important revision that occurs when the relationship grows between therapist and patient, and allows greater opportunity for challenging treatment goals not available early in the therapeutic relationship. Sometimes things go better than planned. Sometimes the trust that develops with a patient allows for the creation of a therapeutic story that was not imaginable when treatment began.

And yet, however faulty and provisional the therapist's original plan or original prospective story, this original story is what sets therapy in motion. One cannot revise from a blank slate, from no plan at all. Revision requires careful initial thought, the creation of plans and stories that are best seen as hypotheses that will not only be tested, but be revised, based on the data that emerge in an ongoing fashion from subsequent clinical sessions.

Implications for Practice

■

The Underground Practice

■ MAUREEN HAYES FLEMING
■ CHERYL MATTINGLY

Introduction

We have written extensively in this book about the graceful syn-
thesizing therapists sometimes manage, treating both the physical body
(body as machine) and the meanings surrounding disability (the lived
body). We have elaborated multiple modes of reasoning that therapists
rely upon in this complex, interwoven practice. This chapter exposes
a darker side, the dilemmas and frustrations of trying to "treat the whole
person" without offending colleagues by treading upon their professional turf or looking unprofessional because treatments and activities
lack a specialized precision and outcomes are difficult to measure. We
also sensed a deeper dilemma, a conflict between some essential OT
values, such as the importance of the individual and the role of choice
making in constructing a sense of self, and essential medical model
values such as scientific objectivism and the need for control.

"Double Binds" of Good Practice

While conducting several group discussions with the therapists
early in the Clinical Reasoning Study, it became clear that therapists
regularly experienced several dilemmas in their practice, especially
concerning what they could report to colleagues. The phenomenological domain was far and away the one which produced the greatest

tensions. Therapists often speak of the strong sense of "turf" that characterizes the social organization of hospitals and most other institutional settings where they work. In the Clinical Reasoning Study, it became clear that while the therapists had doubts about the legitimacy of the phenomenological side of their practice, it was also what they tended to value most. They often found themselves in "double binds," to borrow Bateson's classic descriptor. Or as therapists sometimes said, therapy was often a "damned if you do, damned if you don't" situation. Their most common problem was this: To be a good professional in the eyes of non–occupational therapy colleagues, and to ensure that services were billable, therapists were driven to narrow the scope of treatment goals and activities along more biomedical lines—to treat the physical body. But to be a good professional in attending to the meaning of disability and to elicit the strong commitment of clients, therapists were drawn to broaden the scope of clinical problems, addressing many "real life" issues that did not yield neat, precise, or measurable outcomes. Many therapists were masterful at understanding patients and the illness experience and helping patients to formulate, either through words or actions, deeper understandings of themselves and their experiences. Because they valued this work, they continued with it. But because it was not "reimbursable" they did not document it. We soon came to call this the "underground practice," a term with which many therapists readily identify. This disjunction between what therapists do and what they report to others can put therapists in a difficult position. Their values concerning action, engagement, and quality of living in the everyday world often bring them into conflict (though often a silent conflict) with the values of the dominant biomedical culture held by other members of the clinic world.

Occupational therapists often find themselves torn between a concern to "treat the whole person" and a concern to be credible within a medical world that pushes the therapist to redefine problems and treatment goals in biomedical terms. Though functional assessments are intended to capture something of the patient's experience of disability, it is often the case, as Joan Rogers and Gladys Masagatani (1982) noted in their earlier study of clinical reasoning in occupational therapy, that therapists can bypass the functional assessment, and select a treatment approach directly on the basis of the medical diagnosis. Rogers and Masagatani have noted that the medical diagnosis was used to organize standard problem lists and that "therapists regarded the medical diagnosis as the most essential information for formulating assessment plans" (p. 213).

Findings from our research indicated neither a rejection of, nor a comfortable accommodation to, the biomechanical model on the part of therapists, but an unease at the heart of their practice. Most therapists were deeply ambivalent about the phenomenological aspect of their practice. This ambivalence appeared both in the way therapists talked and in the structure of the clinical sessions in which they attempted to straddle two very different approaches to their patients. One consequence was that when therapists departed from the medical model during a therapeutic session in order to treat the patient's "lived body"— to treat the disability as it affected the patient's work, relationships, independence or other areas of concern—this was often done more casually, less directly, and was easily relinquished if it interfered with therapeutic exercises intended to improve the biomechanical functioning of the patient.

The Professional Image Dilemma

The institutional context of the hospital is powerfully restrictive of the occupational therapists' practice, funneling therapy into an acceptably biomechanical channel and constraining the sorts of creative alternatives considered. In general, these constraints are maintained by means other than explicit rules and regulations. Where such regulations exist (e.g., regulations concerning what can be reimbursed), they are easy enough to circumvent. The influence of the institutional context is more covert. Medical values and authority structure become internalized in the way therapists view themselves and their ability to treat patients. This internalization is evident in therapists' expressions of concern about how a particular treatment activity might appear to other staff members, about whether a treatment will cross turf boundaries of other professionals, and about whether a treatment will be seen as "professional" by the medical staff.

Clinical reasoning about what would be best for the patient thus becomes inextricably mixed with reasoning about the politics of maintaining respect and not causing trouble for oneself with other members of the staff. This observation is not in itself a criticism of occupational therapy practice, since clinical reasoning does not occur in a vacuum and the therapist who ignores institutional issues will not be able to win battles with more influential staff members. The more serious drawback of the hospital context for occupational therapy is that it is governed by doctors and insurance companies who operate within an almost exclusive biomedical view of the patient. When this frame is internalized by an occupational therapist, as, for instance, when the therapist is concerned with gaining approval from a doctor, that therapist's ability to address the broader experiential aspect of a patient's disability, those aspects beyond the biomechanical problem, is often precluded.

Here are two examples of the way institutional concerns directly enter into clinical decision making:

1. A psychiatric occupational therapist decides not to give a patient a project to work on over the weekend because the request comes from a nurse and the nurse asks in an inappropriate way. The nurse asks, "Why don't you give this person an activity to keep them busy over the weekend?" a request that cues the therapist that the nurse perceives psychiatric occupational therapists as "the fun people." This therapist sees part of her task here as "staff education" of nurses and psychologists who seem to confuse occupational therapists with recreational therapists. She says, "The bottom line is that OT is not a department store, and we don't have the funds also to be just giving things out." In deciding not to give an activity to the patient, she does not consider the particular patient and whether this makes sense. She considers the attitude of the nurse requesting the craft activity and bases her decision on that.

2. A physical disabilities therapist who works with respiratory patients has a patient who continually asks to be taken to chapel during occupational therapy time. In thinking through what to do, she considers her role as an occupational therapist on the floor. She feels that going to chapel would be very beneficial to the patient, who is quite religious, because this patient is extremely depressed, has been in the hospital off and on for 2 years, and has not been able to go to church because of her physical problems. She eventually decides not to take her patient to the chapel, and explains this decision as follows: "I guess I thought in my own mind, is this something that I can do as an OT? . . . I didn't want to set any kind of precedent." She wanted to avoid creating the perception by either the patient or other medical staff on her floor that she does activities requiring no skill, activities that could be done by an aide. It is not the patient's need that determines her action here, for she is clear that going to chapel would be beneficial. Rather it is her professional identity, especially her public identity within the hospital staff community, which she is concerned to preserve and which finally determines her decision not to comply with the patient's request.

What these examples point out is that clinical reasoning is not conducted only with reference to the contact between a patient and therapist. There are other people in the room, so to speak, who have decisive voices in determining what treatment is appropriate and what is not. When occupational therapists decided to act without regard for the institutional environment, as though their reasoning was shaped only by patient needs and their skills, they could pay a heavy penalty in reprimands from influential medical staff. For instance, one therapist told a story about treating one of her spinal cord patients when the doctors came in to examine the patient during rounds. This patient had just left the ICU (intensive care unit) a few days earlier and had been in critical condition. During rounds that morning, the attending physician turned to the patient and asked, "If you go into cardiac arrest again, do you want DNR [do not resuscitate]?" The patient was aghast and, being ventilator-dependent and unable to speak aloud, just looked at the therapist in horror. The therapist reassured the patient that the doctors would do everything to keep him alive and that this did not mean he would go into cardiac arrest again. The chief physiatrist turned to the therapist and said, "Professor, let the doctors do their job and you do yours." The therapist was mortified and later apologized to the chief and the attending physician, although she still felt strongly she had done the right thing as far as the patient's welfare was concerned. Such instances of public ridicule from, or subversion by, a strong authority figure made it difficult for occupational therapists to reason about treatment with only the patient's welfare in mind. While the hospital context discourages a phenomenological approach to treatment, interactions with the patient discourage a strictly biomechanical approach.

The Professional Role Dilemma: To Treat or Not to Treat the Whole Person?

Perhaps the most striking and consistent evidence of a dichotomous practice was the therapists' demarcation of a clinical session into "work" and "non-work." "Non-work" was categorized as "rapport building," "chit chat," or "not strictly OT." When therapists described and analyzed clinical sessions, they nearly always separated certain parts of a session, which they labelled as peripheral (e.g., "getting set up," "building rapport," "distracting the patient," "making the patient comfortable"), from the "work" of the session, which was almost always identified with carrying out particular treatment modalities, most of which had a biomedical rationale. Put simply, among most of the physical disabilities therapists, "therapeutic work" referred to carrying out a treatment activity, while talking with the patient was considered peripheral.

When talking and activity went together, as when the therapist engaged the patient in conversation while the patient was carrying out an activity, the talking was not considered the real work of the session. This view was evidenced both in therapists' descriptions of clinical sessions and in what the therapist paid attention to when working with patients. Even when therapists spoke with patients in a way that clearly encouraged them to discuss feelings about their disability, those therapists would often dismiss this aspect of the treatment in public discourse. For instance, in an intense session that centered on talking, the patient told the therapist he had lost his will to live. The therapist manipulated his hands in hers and they talked about how he felt, about his possible future, and his family and friends. The intense part of the session culminated with him taking the straw into his mouth. This seemed to us to signal a willingness to give life another try. After the session, the therapist was asked to describe what had happened in the session. She replied, "I went in and he wanted some water, so I gave him some water. And I started ranging his right hand because he has (unclear) on his left hand. So we started with that. I tend to say, I ranged his right hand, I ranged his left hand, I scratched his upper lip and that was the end." There was more than a little irony in this description and, when pushed by the interviewer who said, "but so much more happened in the session," the therapist was prompted to tell a much longer, more detailed story of the conversation between herself and the patient. However, at the end of a 10- or 15-minute account of what was said, and the meaning of what was said for the patient's depression, she concluded her story by saying "You know, I pretty much ranged him." The message about what counts as "real therapy" in the public world (if more ambiguously, to this therapist herself) came through clearly.

The power of the biomedical frame is demonstrated most strikingly at those moments when patients directly asked therapists to deal with the difficulties they were having in adjusting to disability. These pleas for help or, sometimes simply for attention, often caused therapists to feel torn between doing what the patient seemed to need and doing what appeared to be the most appropriate professional path of action. When therapists were confronted with a patient asking them to help in working through feelings related to the disability, they generally felt called upon to do something. At such times therapists expressed their own anxiety about such roles in postsession interviews, often worrying aloud that they were "moving beyond OT"—either by crossing professional boundaries, thus trespassing into the domain of social worker or psychiatrist, or by abandoning their professional role altogether and "acting like a peer."

In the following example, the therapist was trying to sort out her role with a patient who had turned to her for help with life problems. She stated, "My responsibilities to him are to get his hand better, and to be very real, very open, very honest because he doesn't get—his doctor's a very closemouthed person." By attempting to be real, honest, and open, the therapist allowed the possibility for the patient to confide problems to her, to reveal himself as a "lived body," to discuss his experience of his illness. Therapists' desire to treat the "whole person" was an ambivalent one. Despite the concern not to neglect the whole patient, that is, to resist a mechanistic reduction of the person to a disease entity, when the patient did develop trust in the therapist and began to confide deep personal problems attending the illness or disability, this often threw therapists into a quandry. They felt they had strayed out of their depth, out of their role as an occupational therapist, and were being called upon to act in a way that they did not feel professionally competent to do. Thus the therapists' concerns to treat the whole patient sometimes led to a level of discussion that therapists rejected as no longer occupational therapy. The therapist quoted above described this dilemma to a researcher (also an occupational therapist) as it arose in her work with one patient:

Interviewer: Do you think that's one capacity of OT, that we go beyond a single hand to try and look at all . . . ?

Therapist: Yes, I think we do. I think it's important to look at the whole dynamics and I think it's not realistic to treat him [a patient being discussed] not looking at all these issues. But I think . . .

Interviewer: But yet you said you felt as though you did step beyond [your boundaries as an OT].

Therapist: Right, because I think that the idea is for him to be seeking psychological and social support from a trained professional. . . . If he wants to share what's going on in those sessions, sort of in a more informal way, that's fine, but I should not be that person. I can't be both roles. I can't be an objective therapist.

Interviewer: An objective occupational therapist knowing . . .

Therapist: Becoming very involved in all the dynamics . . . I know we have a lot of empathy for our patients. As OTs, I think we're like that. But . . . it's a hard time drawing the line. It makes it more complicated to treat. Because rather than knowing he's going to get that support somewhere else and that I can really focus my treatment on that extremity, you find that you do a little work and maybe not as much work as you should have. You are spending time talking and you are still limited in time because you have another patient coming.

This discussion presents the dilemma of working within two different discourses, the examination and treatment of "that extremity," which involves a mechanistic discourse, and a second, very different kind of discourse, in which the patient begins to reveal deep problems raised by his disability. In this case, the therapist outlined these problems as sexual problems with his wife, drinking, and depression. The therapist described her problem as one of having "two roles." The first, treating the extremity, she referred to as "work." She also characterized her role here as being "objective," implying that her treatment of an extremity is a role with credibility. She contrasted work to talk when she noted that she did not get as much work done as she should have because she ended up spending more time talking. Yet she cannot abandon the idea that she is also responsible for initiating and carrying through discussions with the patient, for when the interviewer says, "So the talking part of the treatment is not really the issue at hand. You'd rather be working on the activities?" she replies, "Talking too, and conversation."

In the case of this patient who has come to trust the therapist and to attempt to share personal problems that he has refused to take to a psychologist, the therapist faces the dilemma of feeling wrong no matter which direction she goes, because she has presented herself as someone who is sincerely concerned about the patient as a person and he has responded by beginning to talk out his problems with her. The therapist's response to the patient's request that they discuss his experience of disability and how it has changed his personal world, is to feel uneasy and conflicted. While talk is important she is not, as she says, a "trained psychologist or social worker." Her stated strategy for avoiding the problem of having talk go "too far" is to try to maintain a precarious balance of "superficial personal conversation." She finds herself in difficulty when "the person goes deep into their interpersonal relationships." Perhaps a significant reason for the scattered and nondirective questioning of patients mentioned earlier is precisely to prevent conversation from deepening into serious discussion of the trauma associated with disability or disease.

Even among occupational therapists working in a psychiatric setting, conversations often tended toward a superficial and broad noting of "facts" about the patient's life, rather than an exploration of the patient's concerns and meanings. This was sometimes the case even when patients raised issues that were particularly "occupational" in nature, such as major career changes, or the horror of having to depend on others for self-care. Here, for instance, is an example from an initial evaluation done by the psychiatric occupational therapist. They are discussing a leave of absence the patient took from her regular job, a leave which gave the patient a chance to work in politics, working for the reelection of the mayor. The patient is extremely concerned about her job situation and about what career choices she ought to make, as she reveals at several points during this initial assessment interview with the therapist:

> **Therapist:** Was the 2-year LOA [leave of absence] OK with you?
>
> **Patient:** No, but it was a good opportunity. [Patient is referring to her chance to go into politics and start a new career] I love politics, just love it! Rather than quit, I took LOA, because you never knew if the mayor would be reelected.
>
> **Therapist:** When's the LOA up?
> [The therapist has been discussing the groups the patient will participate in.]
>
> **Patient:** It seems so vague to me. It's like, I know it's important but it's hard to think of getting better.
>
> **Therapist:** I know, you've been in the hospital a long time.
>
> **Patient:** I don't want to build up to something else, because then something comes up, it's like protective devices. I know I have two options, working in the mayor's office or going back to my old school job. I have a difficult major decision. [This is the second time she has raised this in the interview.]
> [The therapist responds by describing in more detail the groups they have, finds out if the patient has schedules for the group.]

Here again the general strategy seems to be a checklist approach to a discussion of the patient's life, even though the main issue this patient raised was one of major career choices. Although occupational therapists are not usually vocational therapists, issues around work are considered central. Yet this therapist does not ask for more detail, nor does she indicate that this will be pursued in more detail at some later time. The first time the issue is raised, the therapist responds by asking a factual question about her work situation and the second time the therapist simply ignores the subject. She does not reflect on or express concern for the patient's feelings, which are expressed quite clearly. In light of how common this therapist's response was among therapists studied, this example indicates an often-used therapeutic strategy of using a "checklist approach" to problems that allowed therapists to stay very near the surface of the patient's life.

The surface orientation was not merely a personal strategy of therapists, but was built into the standardized assessment tools used by therapists to identify salient clinical problems during initial patient evaluations. The surface treatment of problems was guaranteed by a very long list of questions, so that no one subject was dwelt on at any length. Important themes, such as that of work, which was raised repeatedly by the patient in the excerpt above, may not be picked up by the therapist. The superficiality of the initial evaluation in regard to the patient's illness experience and personal concerns is often duplicated in treatment, in the level of conversation the therapist encourages, as in the example of the hand therapist given on pages 298–300.

The Depth Dilemma

Many therapists experience the above-described conflict over whether to treat the whole patient or to "stick to the procedural" and were not clear what aspects of their interaction with patients was "work" or "non-work." Others were quite convinced that interaction was an important part of the therapy. Still others were committed to and facile at assisting patients through the difficult task of personal and social reconstruction. But even they sometimes wondered how deeply involved they should become with helping the person face the tragedy of loss. Part of this quandary is exacerbated by a particular feature of OT practice that many therapists have mentioned. They say that the occupational therapist is often the person, perhaps the only person, who helps the patient through the dreadful process of recognizing *both* the concrete results of the disease or disability and the personal and social meanings it carries. It is not clear to us exactly why therapists are often in this position. Perhaps it is because they spend a great amount of time with their patients involved in intimate activities, such as learning to dress and bathe, and therefore a trusting relationship is built up that forms the basis for trust in other intimate areas, such as one's feelings toward oneself. Therapists have also theorized that the very fact that the person discovers he can no longer do simple daily routines forces a deeper recognition of the whole dramatic life change he has to face. As one therapist said, "You are teaching a person to put on her pants, which is really difficult for quads to do. And you are the one standing there, making her do these things that she used to be able to do and now can't. So you are there when the realization that she will never walk again *hits*. So you have to be ready to talk about it."

Whatever the reason, therapists are faced with helping the person cope with the realization of a tragic physical loss and the loss of one's former self and former life. When a person is traumatically injured, life is forever changed. The new life, it seems, is only possible when the person recognizes the loss of the old life, while simultaneously holding out hope for the possibilities of finding meaning and a sense of self in the new life. Occupational therapists are intimately, even if inadvertently, involved in helping their patients negotiate this process. A critical part of this endeavor seems to be what we have called "claiming the disability and reclaiming the self." (Fleming, 1990) This involves an elaborate form of social interaction, and mutual construction and reconstruction of meanings. A common dilemma created by this intimate level of involvement with patients is that therapists find themselves addressing life issues that reach beyond their level of trained expertise, or beyond what they are comfortable handling, and that may be beyond their scope of experience.

CASE EXAMPLE

The following case illustrates how a therapist, through her close relationship with a client (triggered in part by sharing stories of her own life) finds herself helping the client deal with the difficult emotional issues surrounding her disability. These emotional issues were particularly difficult because of the circumstances surrounding the patient's injury—a suicide attempt in which her husband played a questionable role.

Sarah: "What You See Is Not What You Get"

by Debbie Pinet

The following case story is lacking in details in certain points due to the fact that I assumed the patient's treatment from a departing therapist who focused primarily on the physical aspects of the rehabilitation. Valuable information such as mechanism of injury, acute rehab experiences, and psychological management were omitted from the original history.

Sarah is a white, middle-aged woman, mother of two children—one son, age 16, and a daughter, age 14. Sarah has taught English as a second language to individuals and has been involved in various literary projects. Her husband of 20 years is involved in academia, and their social life had previously revolved around related activities.

Reportedly in January of this year, Sarah learned of her husband's extramarital affair and plans for a divorce. Consequently she attempted suicide. The exact method or manner is unknown to me. The only subjective information relayed included that Sarah was not "found" quickly and that her husband delayed medical intervention (for what reasons I am not sure). There may be some relationship to Sarah's history of alcoholism and the time of year (? was she outside). As a result of the suicide attempt, Sarah lost both legs below the knees, and the DIPs and partial PIPs of the 2nd, 3rd, 4th, and 5th digits of her left, nondominant hand. Sarah was treated initially at a community hospital and then was transferred to a large rehab hospital. During her rehab stay she reportedly participated in an alcoholism recovery program, yet this was said to occur only to defer return to the home situation. There has not been any mention of psychological intervention, during either Sarah's acute stay or long-term rehab.

Sarah came to me via the outpatient setting. She had been participating in twice-weekly occupational and physical therapy for approximately 1 month when I took over. The focus of OT had been on ROM, strengthening, edema control, desensitization, and dexterity of the left hand. I initially continued with the delineated treatment plan, but as I exchanged information about myself during the sessions, the focus began to change. As I talked about my recent return to school, Sarah shared her desire to also further her education and elaborated on the programs she had investigated. Bits and pieces of the person Sarah was, is, and would like to become, began to emerge. An overflow of emotion was brought forth from a woman who on the surface seemed composed and focused. Sarah commented that for the first time "I've realized that this is not just a physical problem." Even though Sarah had done remarkably well in her physical recovery, she had not dealt with the psychological impact of her suicide attempt and had not reclaimed herself to give meaning to her life. She had the physical capacity to perform daily living tasks, yet she had not accepted the fact that things would be different in the performance, meaning, efficiency, and context of these tasks.

My role as occupational therapist was now frightening, overwhelming, and powerful as the interpersonal connections had been made to impact the quality of this woman's life. I quickly decided this was not going to occur in the previous mode of ROM, and so on.

I have only treated Sarah for 3 weeks at this time. My first intervention was to discuss Sarah's current ADLs, what she was doing and not doing, who was performing the tasks and why. (She had returned home with her two children and husband, which was a very stressful situation.) I explored how communication was occurring and learned that her interactions with her husband were minimal, with the divorce proceedings placed on hold. The two children reacted differently to their father: The son was hostile, while the daughter, although recognizing her mother's pain, did not want to lose her father, no matter what he had done. Sarah shared that her feelings toward her husband ranged from anger, bitterness, and sadness, to apathy and denial. Because of the severity of the psychosocial needs, my plan with Sarah was to recommend formal counseling as the complexity of her situation went well beyond my expertise.

The focus of clinic activities has been on actually performing difficult tasks such as typing, driving endurance, cooking, and handling small manipulatives. The purpose was to encourage problem solving and recognition of strengths and deficits. A journal was also recommended to record daily feelings, assessments, and progress when performing tasks that were once routine. Sarah was very excited about the journal activities, probably due to her literary background, but also because of what she explained as her desire to see and deal with her emotional status. The journal activity was started just prior to my attendance at the Clinical Reasoning Institute so the utilization of its contents has not occurred in the clinic.

Sarah was also encouraged to develop a priority list of things she wanted to accomplish this summer. My plan is to use both the journal and the priority list to structure therapy to address the functional, psychosocial, and physical deficits that Sarah and I perceive her to have. Sarah's participation in counseling is also critical. I can assist her in maximizing her abilities; yet what relevance would they have in a dysfunctional home situation? Sarah's ability to also pursue goals outside the home, such as an advanced degree, would consequently be impacted upon by the psychosocial dynamics of her current situation.

This short but meaningful opportunity to work with Sarah has move me emotionally because of the intense level of connectiveness I feel, and my only hope is that this tie will allow her to trust my recommendations and pursue additional guidance in her recovery.

Case Discussion

One dilemma therapists face in this task is how to help a person construct a self, a socially meaningful and personally satisfying self and life, in the midst of a society that makes this very difficult. The therapist and patient have to break and transcend all sorts of cultural values and behavioral norms in order to construct a positive sense of self for the person. The question becomes: Can one function in, see oneself as a part of, and be accepted by a society whose values one is challenging and whose rules one is breaking? Often this does not present a dilemma for the therapist so much as it does for the patient's family.

The Values Dilemma

Seeing possibilities for clients, or being client advocates, can place therapists in conflict with other health professionals. Often the stories that therapists tell about their most successful cases go far beyond their work with an individual patient and involve them in persuading other members of their staff to see the patient differently. Success that depends upon strong patient advocacy sometimes requires high-risk confrontations with staff.

CASE EXAMPLE

The risk and difficulty of this advocacy is heightened, as in the following case, when the staff member one is confronting occupies a higher status position in the institutional system.

Free at Last

by Ruth Atwood

Barbara had a reputation . . . and I should have known she'd end up on my caseload. After all, that's who I treated—the ones with a reputation. When I saw the referral on my desk, everything I had ever heard about her raced through my mind. Barbara was young and had profound mental retardation; no one liked her; she was aggressive, had a reputation of being difficult to work with, was unpleasant to look at, had a diagnosis of atypical psychosis/self-injurious behavior (SIB), and was blind as a result of her SIB. My mind finally stopped running long enough to process what the referral said. Barbara was being referred for modification of her protective equipment. She had learned how to circumvent the equipment and was injuring herself.

I called her psychologist and set up a meeting. In the meantime, I received her chart and internal file. Her SIB had started when she was young, and every treatment that was tried just seemed to increase the frequency and intensity. Her current program called for the use of a padded helmet with face shield and full-length arm air splints. When she engaged in either head hitting or head banging, she was physically manipulated through a meaningless movement protocol that prevented her from hitting or banging her head. It didn't seem to be working.

When Barbara and I first met, it was a sweltering summer day and the air-conditioning was broken. We met in a small treatment room which felt like an oven. Barbara was encased in plastic air splints from her fingertips to her armpits, and was wearing a football helmet with a face shield and chin cup. There was extra padding on the outside of the football helmet. I couldn't believe it. Here was a woman who was blind and she was being deprived of tactile and auditory input by her so-called protective equipment. And that equipment had to be hot and uncomfortable. Her hair was drenched with sweat, and I could see pools of sweat inside the air splints. I wanted to rip the equipment off her.

During my conversation with the psychologist, I discovered that she and I had very different ideas about what to do for Barbara. The psychologist wanted me to design arm splints that prevented Barbara from reaching her head with her hands and prevented her from using her hands to injure any other part of her body as well. I wanted to give Barbara back her senses. It seemed to me that if I was deprived of that much sensory input I sure would be trying to give myself input in any way that I could.

Barbara sat on the edge of the mat table throughout this discussion, occasionally hitting her forehead with the radial side of her wrist, or she would work her fingers through her faceshield and tap on her cheeks. The psychologist and I finally reached a compromise: if I could design splints that provided enough protection from injury but at the same time gave Barbara back hand use and sensory input, I could do it. If I couldn't, then I would have to develop even more restrictive splints in order to prevent further injury.

During the next 2 weeks, I spent every minute I could with Barbara, studying the sequence of her SIB, getting to know her, allowing her to get to know me, and trying different splint ideas. I also did some research on her previous treatment programs. She had only been treated with a behavioral approach. The more time I spent with Barbara, the stronger was my conviction that her SIB was, in large part, an attempt to gain sensory input. She seemed to crave tactile, vestibular, and deep-pressure inputs. I couldn't believe a sensorimotor treatment approach had never been tried.

After several tries, I finally came up with new designs for Barbara's splints and helmet that gave her back hand use, arm motion, and sensory input, while at the same time preventing injury when she engaged in SIB. The new splints and helmet were also designed to minimize the sensory input she received during SIB. I hoped that if I could minimize the input she received during SIB and provide her with input during intensive one-on-one treatment sessions, she would decrease the intensity and frequency of her SIB.

As we worked together over the next several months, Barbara's behavior began to change. When she got her new splints, the frequency of her head hits immediately decreased by 50 percent. She began to use her hands to explore her environment and herself, and to manipulate objects. But she really sparkled during treatment. We spent several hours each week in the pool along with her PTA . . . and Barbara loved it! She played, kicked, jumped, and even learned to splash herself and her therapists! Her favorite activity was being swung from side to side and around in circles for 15 to 20 minutes at a time. Luckily for us, the PTA and I worked out a system of passing Barbara back and forth so that *we* didn't get dizzy. Barbara also loved to swing—indoors or out. She would slowly shake her head from side to side to feel the air flow through her hair. And she smiled!

Barbara began to smile, to reach out to staff, to initiate hugs, and to seek out people's companionship. She was able to remove her protective equipment for 2 to 2½ hours during OT treatment and only hit her head one or two times during that period—and those were light hits. As Barbara became more social and her SIB continued to decrease, other people began to take an interest in her. Eventually we had a core group of direct-care staff who were interested in working with her and willing to carry over much of what we had been doing during treatment sessions.

Barbara blossomed. She was able to go for longer and longer times without her protective equipment. She still engaged in SIB but it was much less frequent and not nearly as severe. When I left, 1½ years after Barbara and I had begun working together, she still had a reputation—she was fun, pretty, social, responsive, and nice to be around.

Yes, Barbara had a reputation—a good one this time.

Case Discussion

Because therapists face a common dilemma of how to work well with clients, advocate on their behalf, and at the same time negotiate their roles in interdisciplinary teams, part of the clinical reasoning skills necessary for effective therapy involve learning how to present oneself to other professionals, or how to deal with their discomfort when appearing to be on the professional territory of another staff person.

CASE EXAMPLE

Louisa

by Susan Merrill

Louisa was a 17-year-old girl with juvenile arthritis (JA) whom I first met when she was admitted for the tenth or eleventh time to the rehabilitation unit of a children's hospital. Louisa had been coming to this hospital since her arthritis had been diagnosed, 11 years earlier. The physicians were the same ones she had been seeing all those years, and many of the other staff—nurses, social workers, physical therapists, occupational therapists—had also known or worked with her through those years. I was new to the facility when the story that I am going to tell you about took place.

Louisa had the classic appearance of a person who has had arthritis since childhood; bone growth and epiphyseal closing are interrupted. As a result, her jaw and chin were quite small (micrognathia). Her shoulders, too, were very narrow and small. She was shorter than average. Her joint deformities, in virtually all joints, resulted in flexion at the elbows, wrists, knees, and (slightly) in her narrow hips. Her gait was waddling and slow. All of this combines to make any person with JA look younger than, in fact, she is (this is not my opinion, it is part of the folklore of working with the population) and this was the case with Louisa.

In addition to these features, Louisa had beautiful honey-colored hair that was long and thick. Her eyes were a beautiful hazel with long eyelashes that matched her hair. Louisa enjoyed wearing the styles popular with teenagers at the time and because of her narrow body, she looked stylish and attractive in them. She took great pride in her appearance and spent considerable time each day getting dressed and putting on makeup. It was not uncommon to find a nursing student painting Louisa's toes and finger nails. What I am trying to convey is that Louisa was a very attractive and appealing, even beautiful, girl despite, or maybe even because of, her JA.

Her family situation is somewhat relevant to the story. Louisa lived with her mother and sister in a small (hot and dusty) town about 1½ hours from the hospital. Her parents were divorced. Her father had remarried and was raising a second family, also far from the hospital. So although one of them always brought her for "tune-up" hospitalizations, neither could visit her often. Her younger sister was not yet old enough to drive, so although the two sisters enjoyed a very close friendship, the sister could not come to visit readily, either. She had a circle of friends (boys and girls) who would come together about once a week to visit. These friends would bring pizza and soda and stay for several hours on a Friday or Saturday. These "parties" were very important to Louisa.

This hospitalization was partly for an annual "tune-up." This consisted of reassessment by OT, PT, SW [social work], Rheumatology, Psychology, and Nursing. Typically, the patient was evaluated for any changes in joint status, medication effectiveness, and functional abilities. In Louisa's case, this was only part of the reason that she had been admitted; she was also being evaluated for surgery. The question was whether to give her a hip replacement (left hip) or to wait a year or so longer. At the time of this story, the technology of hip replacements was not as good as now; typically a hip replacement would have to be replaced in 10 years and the concern for Louisa was that she would have to go through surgery several more times in her life. There was some thought that waiting as long as possible would be better than doing it immediately.

The doctor, Dr. B., told her all of this at the outset and told her that her compliance with therapy and medical procedures during this admission would have an influence on his decision. (She had become less and less compliant during the last several hospitalizations, much to the confusion and annoyance of the staff.)

My intervention with her consisted of reassessing her occupational performance in the areas of self-maintenance, work, and leisure. I modified her wrist splints and, at her request, adapted a razor so that she could shave her legs in the shower. We discussed the "typical" OT treatment activities (crafts, cooking, self-care . . .) and she honestly told me that she felt "too old for those children's activities." So, I asked her what was important to her, what we could work on that would help her at home. We settled on talking about the possibility of her going to community college in the fall.

Our sessions consisted of her figuring out what needed to be done (i.e., call schools for information, including maps, so that she could determine things like admission requirements, and look at parking and getting to class).

Usually we would decide on some "homework" for her to do for the next session and then discuss what she did. For example, she was to gather all the phone numbers of the community and small colleges near her home. When doing this, she found that using a thick phone directory was difficult, so we discussed simplification and conservation concepts around that task. We also discussed some of her favorite leisure activities, and related simplification and conservation to these. She enjoyed the problem-solving sessions, especially when we tried new ways of doing things that had been difficult for her.

I remember one time she told me that she liked to go hiking (this was in a desert, so on flat terrain) with friends and that she accepted that her legs would be sore, but that her wrists and fingers ached from holding on to her friends. We tried several other ways of holding and being held by friends and walked all over the hospital to practice. She would tell anyone who asked that she and I were not really in the hospital but were actually hiking in Joshua Tree National Park. I felt that Louisa and I had developed a close relationship and that she was invested in her OT (something she had not been in a while). I did not, however, realize how this relationship could change Louisa's life.

Although our sessions were going along well, Louisa was not doing well on the rehab unit or with her PT or the nurses. She was generally petulant, if not outright hostile. In PT she often refused treatment and said that she was in too much pain to work on the mats or on walking. With the nurses, she refused to comply with almost everything, from eating meals with the other patients, to taking her meds, to turning her lights out at the designated time.

One day when I went to get Louisa for OT, she was sullen and would not talk to me, except to say that she was no longer interested in OT. When I asked why, the first answer I got was that she was too busy watching her soap opera. When I told her that I did not buy that as an answer, she said she wasn't interested in what I would or wouldn't buy. I told her that she would get discharged from the hospital if she refused to attend her therapies and that I didn't think that was what she really wanted. Her response surprised me. She told me that nobody "at this place knows what I really want. I am tired of being treated like I am the same person I was when I first came here when I was 6 years old. I am different, I am not even the same person I was last time I was here!" I asked her if she could tell me about it and she said, "Dr. B. has been really great to me but he doesn't see that I am not a little girl anymore." I expected her to tell me that she was in love with him or something like that; I did not expect what she told me.

Dr. B. had been in to see her shortly before I arrived and told her that his recommendation was to wait on the surgery, a year or more if possible. Although she understood his reasons, she wanted the surgery but would only tell him that she wanted to walk better. She told me that she could not tell him the real reason. Then she asked me if I had seen Mark, one of her friends that came to visit each week. I told her I had met him and that he seemed like a nice guy. Well, to her he was more than nice: "I'm in love with him and want to be able to have sex with him. I need to be able to get into the position to have sex and right now, with this hip, I can't. I need a normal hip." She wanted to know if I could "tell them, tell him why I need this now, not in a year."

The very next day was the team conference on Louisa. She refused to come (and only I knew why!). Members of her team talked heatedly about her attitude, her anger, and her noncompliance. It was suggested that she be discharged from the hospital since "we can't do anything with her." Someone speculated that something was going on that was making her unhappy. In one of those moments of crystal-clear thinking, I realized that was true. All these years she had been coming to this place; the doctors were like fathers, the nurses like mothers; the therapists perhaps like aunts and uncles. Something was happening in her "family" and that was that the family was not seeing that the child was no longer a child but a young woman with very different needs and issues than she ever had before. Additionally, I realized that she had asked me to help her, to mediate for her, in just the way one might as an older female relative (sister, cousin, or aunt) because telling your parents you want to have sex is an almost impossible thing to do in most families.

Realizing all of this made my task easier, but I was still uncomfortable, not because I was discussing someone's sexuality, but because I was a relative newcomer and did not want to interfere with the good aspects of Louisa's relationship with each member of the team. Some members had grown defensive around me and didn't "understand why she works so well with you." I didn't want them to feel that she had told me because she did not care about them and the history they all had shared when, in fact, I felt that part of the reason she did confide in me was because I was more of an outsider. And so I told them what I had to tell them, why Louisa felt so strongly that the surgery happen on this admission. I speculated out loud that she had told me this because we had been looking toward her future in her OT sessions and that her sexual activity was a very important part of that future for her.

There was surprise and shock on people's faces; some disbelief and then realization. I think it was Dr. B. who spoke first, kind of laughing (at himself), "I guess she is no longer 6 years old!" Immediately, there was discussion about how to help her with responsible sex; who would discuss birth control and possible positions that would take her other joint limitations into account (these discussions were to be held after the surgery). The team decided right then that she should have the surgery on that admission. I was not involved in telling her, but I think it was Dr. B. and the nurse who had been with her the longest (symbolic parents).

I do remember that the next day she came to find me in my office and told me that she was grateful for my help. "Mark will thank you, too. It is going to be a lot of work, the surgery, the therapy afterward and my life after that. But at least now they know that I am not a child anymore. Thanks to you."

Case Discussion

In the examples above, we have two stories about very different patients written by very different therapists; but they share several features. Both therapists had developed a relationship with and empathy for their patients. This empathy led the therapists to understand each patient from the person's own perspective. Both therapists valued the person's wishes and comfort, and championed a campaign to help them get the cooperation of other professionals to achieve these goals. What seemed reasonable to the therapists and their patients did not necessarily seem reasonable or therapeutic or the best decision to others in the institutional hierarchy. But both therapists valued freedom of choice and freedom from the restrictions imposed by their patients' conditions and they valued these patients as people with lives to lead, so they thought attaining that freedom and level of humanity was more important than what might be perceived as medically correct.

In these stories both therapists were experienced and had confidence in themselves as therapists and they attained what they wanted. So the dilemma of what to do, what you think best, or what the medical staff says is not clearly illustrated. Many therapists have told us stories of frustration when the thought that what was morally right for patients was different from what someone in a socially higher capacity thought was right. Many of these stories revolve around medical decisions for patients.

CASE EXAMPLE

Here is a story written by an affiliating student, where she wonders about the wisdom of an administrative decision. Here, you can see her empathy for patients leads her to question the value of safety precautions that seem to be putting patients in a more unsafe situation.

The Fire Alarm

by Susan Hheremans

My clinical story is about a situation I experienced on my summer affiliation. I had been working with a 45-year-old patient named Armond. He was diagnosed with schizophrenia and severe MR [mental retardation]. He was admitted for violent behavior after striking a staff member at his group home. He also had difficulty tolerating loud sounds, especially airplanes flying overhead, and would become extremely anxious, continually repeating that he believed he was going to die.

John, a 35-year-old MR patient also admitted for violent behavior, shared a room with Armand and two other patients. John had been having difficulty controlling his anger during his hospitalization. The previous day he had to be restrained after throwing a large wooden chair across the room. He had become scared and confused after watching another patient being restrained by several staff members because the patient had overturned a dining-room table.

I had been working in Armond's room reviewing an ADL check-list with him when the fire alarm went off. Almost instantly, there was a great deal of confusion. This was my first experience with a fire drill. Procedures had been provided during my orientation. There were three patients in the room; Armond, John, and another patient sleeping. I told Armond and John that we had to go out into the hallway. Both were very scared and overwhelmed by the whole situation. They could not understand that the noise they heard was a fire alarm. I took them both by the arm and led them out of the room.

Unfortunately, the fire alarm was much louder out in the hallway with the speakers located overhead. I went back into the room to get the other patient, who was still sleeping. It took me a few minutes to wake him up and escort him out into the hallway.

At this point, both Armond and John were extremely upset and losing control fast. Armond was crying and rocking back and forth, which was his way of handling anxiety about loud noises. He was repeatedly saying that he was going to die and could not be convinced otherwise.

John was more upset than Armond. He had his hands over his ears to block the sound and was screaming loudly. He began to get more hysterical and backed his way into a corner of the hallway.

As part of the fire drill procedures, patients were required to move to the emergency exit, where John, Armond, and others were now standing. As time passed, more patients gathered at the end of the hallway. Unfortunately, the longer the fire alarm rang, the louder John screamed, and the more upset patients became.

I was pretty scared myself and didn't really know what to do. At one end of the hallway, I saw poor John and Armond, both very much out of control. At the other end, I saw more patients being escorted towards us. I didn't know how we were going to handle more patients in such a small area, especially when things were so disorganized and getting very crowded. But more patients began to accumulate—along with additional staff members, thank goodness.

All of sudden, Richard, a 70-year-old patient suffering from severe dementia, became overwhelmed by John's screams and the fire alarm and lost control. He began to fight the staff members who were trying to help him out of the building. He had to be brought to the floor to be controlled because it was so crowded with several patients nearby.

Of course this brought the anxiety level of the hallway to an all-time high. I really didn't know what to do. I was able to console Armond enough so that he could understand and follow simple directions. Unfortunately, I was at a loss with John. He was so out of control. At this point, his face was flushed from screaming and crying, and he could not hear or understand any comforting statements, let alone simple instructions.

I thought, in my heart, the only way to help John was to gather him up and hold him. To try and help him contain his fears by providing some sort of comforting shell around him. On the other hand, I also remembered that, after watching a patient being restrained, John had thrown a wooden chair the day before. It began to mirror the events that were unfolding at that very moment.

It was painful to see someone so upset and feel unable to help because of my own fears for safety. It's a selfish feeling that torments me to this day. As a more realistic response, I realized that John didn't know me very well, and I wasn't very sure whether he would have welcomed any sort of physical touch from a stranger at a time when he was totally out of control. I also knew that he had a history of violent behavior.

Finally, a social worker that worked well with John rushed in to help him. She put her arm around him and began to console him. This seemed to help John a little and the emergency door was opened so that the patients could be escorted down the stairwell. As we moved down the stairwell the fire alarm got louder and louder and so did John's screams. We all eventually made it out into the parking lot and to our designated area.

It was a hard lesson to learn as an OT student. To listen to what your rational mind says rather than what your heart feels. I guess there are times when you can't help patients the way you would like to.

In retrospect, I probably could have removed Arnold and John from the confusion of the hallway. Perhaps their room might have provided a bit more security and a little less noise. This might have helped the other patients as well.

Case Discussion

Here a student who is mature and sensitive and always shows good judgment and great ethical sensibility is thrown into an impossible situation, one so impossible that it is difficult for her to use her considerable intellectual and interactive skills. She "does the right thing," but her ability to analyze the situation is hampered by the chaos itself, and by the values and rules imposed by the institutional hierarchy. Later, when we discussed the situation in class, none of us could conjure a good reason why this situation should have occurred. Why did the administrators of the hospital believe that a fire drill in a psychiatric hospital should be a surprise like in a public school? Why was extra staff not available? Did they think the patients and staff would learn by this experience? No one could come up with the institutional logic that would have supported such poor treatment of these patients. Fortunately, a social worker as sensitive as Susan was able to help one patient.

Summary

In this chapter we have discussed several concerns, most of which were raised by therapists themselves. Therapists often found themselves in a quandary about treating patients, especially when they considered the phenomenologic aspects of the person and the situation. Conflicts over how involved the therapist should be in the personal life of the patient seemed to arise in a variety of forms and caused discomfort regarding the therapist's role and place in the institutional setting. This was especially difficult for therapists when they felt that their personal or professional values regarding good patient care conflicted with either individual persons or with stated or perceived institutional policies or implicit norms. While the prevalence of the "medical model" and some of its attending norms, values, and restrictions may be blamed for part of this problem, it may also be that individual therapists or the profession itself lacks clarity and confidence in its professional role.

■

Action and Inquiry
Reasoned Action and Active Reasoning

- **MAUREEN HAYES FLEMING**
- **CHERYL MATTINGLY**

Introduction

In this last chapter we discuss three sets of concepts. First, we will comment on the prevalence of the assumption that all good clinical reasoning is guided by a hypothetical-deductive logical style as prescribed by the scientific method. Next, we will highlight some of the features of clinical reasoning that we observed among occupational therapists, and around which we developed the theoretical constructs presented in the earlier chapters. Much of what we found is very different from the data and declarations that are usually found in the general problem-solving literature and in medical decision-making literature. We feel it may be useful here to summarize our concepts, and at the same time contrast them with the more common, above-mentioned assumption about problem solving in general and medical decision making in particular. We will also hazard some guesses as to why we think these differences were present.

We will then introduce a few new concepts drawn mostly from two related branches of philosophy, phenomenology and American pragmatism, to explicate some specific, subtle processes, such as inference making, that we feel are important to attend to in making clinical judgments. We link these especially to the active nature of occupational therapy practice and the judgments in action that guide that practice.

Many professions are organized around at least two levels of abstract knowledge—theoretical propositions and factual information—and two levels of practical knowledge—principles of practice and specific procedures. This sort of structure is also seen in occupational therapy. However, because occupational therapy is so dependent on participation, and because therapists insist on "individualizing" treatment as much as possible, action plays a large part in their clinical reasoning processes. Action and reasoning are inextricably linked in occupational therapy. This is not simply a case of thinking something through and then taking action. It is more complex. Actions are both the basis for and the result of reasoning. Reasoning is often conducted using action as a vehicle. Conversely, actions are often taken in order to test out a reasoned hypothesis.

Clinical Reasoning and the Scientific Method

Health professions tend to identify good thinking with a process that looks rather like the scientific method. This includes the preference for hypothetical-deductive logic as a basis for guiding problem solving. It also presumes that the general truths or laws of science are both accurate and pertinent to all (or at least most) of the particular instances of the general phenomenon. Practice is considered the application of empirically tested abstract knowledge (theories) and generalizable factual knowledge. Therefore, reasoning is presumed to involve recognizing particular instances of behavior in terms of general laws that regulate the relationship between the cause and a resultant state of affairs. The model of scientific reasoning has guided most research on clinical reasoning in the health professions, where clinical reasoning is viewed as applied natural science. This perspective presumes that professional reasoning is a comparatively straightforward application of knowledge and theory. The assumption is that practical clinical action applies scientifically derived knowledge to the particular instance of the problem at hand, which is simply the manifestation of the general disease category.

Scientific reasoning is intended to link the concrete particular with the abstract general, ascending to the general in the mode of logical abstraction (Bruner, 1990). Classically, the physical and biologic sciences have been understood as involving the discovery of general causes (ideally, universal laws), which, being general, can be predicted to produce certain effects. The presence of universally or probabilistically applicable cause-and-effect relations is critical for a strongly predictive practice, where effects of interventions can be anticipated and controlled. This, of course, is the powerful form of explanation most fully developed in the physical sciences. In explaining particular symptoms and signs by referring to an underlying disease, the clinician is explaining the particular by the general, revealing how particular manifestations have been caused by general law-governed physiologic processes.

It is not surprising that this scientific model of explanation, when introduced systematically into medicine during the eighteenth and nineteenth centuries, produced a medical revolution. In medicine, the scientific task for clinical reasoning has been defined as the discovery of causal relations between symptoms and underlying diseases.

Clinical reasoning has primarily been associated with diagnosis in the medical professions because, within medicine, the essential clinical skill for the professional has been the ability to investigate the particular signs of bodily malfunction and symptoms evinced by a patient (which may be felt or experienced in unique ways by different patients) and to treat them as cues to a deeper level of reality, the pathology. This identification allows the professional to select from his or her repertoire of treatment interventions those which have been scientifically proven to be effective in treating the pathology. The concern to link the idiosyncratic particulars with a general law or state of affairs (such as a disease category) is related to a concern for effective intervention. Thus, if professionals can come to recognize general processes underlying particular cases, then general techniques can be designed to change those processes in predictable ways. Certainly some medical interventions work in this way. For example, if the physician learns to recognize a unique set of cues as a fracture of the humerus, then she or he can perform a standardized procedure (immobilizing) with predictable success. This procedure can be learned and applied to a 60-year-old patient in Hong Kong or to a 15-year-old patient in Cincinnati with little variation and similar results, once considerations for age and nutritional status are made. In occupational therapy, there has also been an equating of clinical reasoning with initial assessment, perhaps because this is the clinical task most closely aligned with medical diagnosis. Some aspects of occupational therapy practice can be standardized, since certain aspects of occupational dysfunction can be predicted to follow from particular pathologic conditions. Rogers and Masagatani (1982) found in their research on clinical reasoning in occupational therapy that the medical diagnosis was the most critical factor influencing how therapists assessed their patients. The therapists who were studied in the AOTA/AOTF Clinical Reasoning Study also used the medical diagnosis as an important organizer in developing their treatment plans. They linked medical diagnoses with generally expected dysfunctions, and these dysfunctions, in turn, pointed them toward certain treatment activities and procedures. To know a person's pathology was to be able to predict with high probability what performance difficulties one would encounter. To be able to predict dysfunctions meant that the therapist could also predict which interventions would improve the body or remediate some of the performance problems.

Clinical reasoning, treated as applied natural science, is reasoning directed to the practical problems of prediction and control; it is a type of instrumental reasoning. From an instrumental perspective, it is assumed that the professional's expertise lies in his or her capacity to identify and put to use the best means for achieving given ends, that their professional expertise lies not in identifying those ends or goals (e.g., better health through cure of disease), but rather, in achieving them. The professional is better able to predict what will follow from certain conditions (e.g., the disease process in the presence of certain symptoms) and from particular interventions used to control the future (e.g., the effect of certain medications on the disease process). Instrumental reasoning is considered to be value-neutral concerning the best means for attaining given ends. Ends can be clearly and explicitly given prior to the reasoning process. Although the *ends* are treated as subjective givens (e.g., good health), are identified by the values of the actor, and are not considered something one can reason about (because they are subjective and value-laden), *means* can be strategically and neutrally identified for reaching those given ends. If clinical reasoning is defined as a form of instrumental reasoning, it is presumed to be reasoning about how to best reach explicit ends.

Instrumental rationality is derived from a positivist understanding of practical knowledge (Schön, 1983, 1987). Schön (1987) described this dominant paradigm of professional rationality:

> Technical rationality is an epistemology of practice derived from positivist philosophy . . . [it] holds that practitioners are instrumental problem solvers who select technical means best suited to particular purposes. Rigorous professional practitioners solve well-formed instrumental problems by applying theory and technique derived from systematic, preferably scientific knowledge. (p. 4)

Perhaps the clearest analogy is the reasoning involved in solving a puzzle, which is an analogy that Thomas Kuhn (1962) used in describing the reasoning of physicists. A puzzle presents a simple world with comparatively few features that need to be attended to and with one correct answer that shows itself to be correct once it is found. Clinical reasoning within a biomedical frame is like puzzle solving, in that a clearly identifiable correct answer exists (e.g., a pathology, a cluster of physiologic deficits), and the player's task is to find that answer.

In general, this model of reasoning and view of knowledge suit the practice of Western medicine, particularly in diagnosing and treating acute conditions. However, the model of knowledge widely known as the scientific method leaves out some of the most important aspects of thinking that characterize expert occupational therapy practice. Attention to the meaning-centered nature of much clinical reasoning in occupational therapy reveals the depth of the clinical problems therapists face on a daily basis. Occupational therapy may look trivial from a purely physical point of view. How can teaching someone to feed themselves compare with open-heart surgery? But this is not necessarily trivial from a phenomenologic point of view. Often, health professionals unfamiliar with occupational therapy notice the usual paraphernalia of occupational therapy practice (e.g., backgammon boards, bright plastic balls, oddly shaped forks and spoons) and assume that occupational therapy is a trivial practice. Therapists complain of being called "play ladies," of being seen as versions of physical therapists somehow assigned to the upper extremities, or of being expected to keep patients occupied when they become too bored in institutional worlds. The danger of such characterizations lies not merely in politics involving other professional colleagues, but also in the insidious way in which such identifications can be internalized, and therapists can begin to see themselves in a reductionistic way. Therapists can come to reduce their practice to a manipulation of the physical body, forgetting how much their interventions are directed to a person's life.

In the previous chapter we have discussed some of the conflicts therapists have faced, as professionals, with values that favor the phenomenologic approach to patients in a world ordered according to the medical model. In the next section of this chapter, we repeat some of our findings about the reasoning of occupational therapists and contrast them with the typical assumptions made in the problem-solving and medical decision-making literature.

ACTION, OBSERVATION, AND INTERPRETATION

Therapists often ask patients to produce particular actions. This request may be a verbal command or suggestion. There are many reasons for asking a person to act. The therapist may ask a patient any of the following questions for the following reasons:

Question: "Can you do this? Let me see."
Reason: To determine if the patient is physically able to perform a given task.
Question: "How did you do that?"
Reason: To learn how the person managed to perform a task in a novel way.
Question: "Let's try this . . . how about if we try it this way?"
Reason: To help figure out how a person can perform an action that she has not yet been able to perform.
Question: "Do that for me again."

Reason:	To assess the quality and consistency of a movement.
Question:	"Do this again."
Reason:	To determine if there has been improvement in the amount, degree, or quality of movement.

Therapists request action so that they can observe the patient's motions and make qualitative assessments about their current performance. Therapists assess the quality of action and make inferences about the patient's potential to take other actions and perform functional tasks in the future. Therapists simultaneously observe, assess, and interpret patient's actions.

Therapists ask patients to produce particular actions so that they can observe the patient's performance. But what are they observing? Therapists want to know how—and how well—a person performs particular actions, which therapists assume will ultimately contribute to the ability to accomplish everyday activities. They want to see if a patient can do the activity, and how the person does the activity. But the seeing "if" and "how" are not ends in themselves. They are cues to past or potential accomplishments. Therapists are not looking for a yes-or-no, can-you-or-can't you answer. They look at the quality of the motion. Here, seeing is not simply seeing. It is observation, a step in coming to know more about this patient. This seeing if, or seeing how, is not done with a "naked eye" but with a practiced eye. Patients seem to be very aware of the nature of this clinical gaze and go to considerable lengths in cooperating with the therapist in order to produce the requested action. The therapist observes and interprets the actions.

Observing may take the form of fairly elaborate and precise evaluation procedures conducted according to specific protocols. More frequently, observations are made in the course of doing a therapeutic activity with a patient. Therapists typically refer to this as "ongoing evaluation." They mean that even though they might be engaged in a treatment activity, or even a casual conversation, they are continually making observations. They report that the frequently proffered sequence of *evaluation→interpretation→treatment* does not reflect how they think and act in practice. They say: "It's all right for a classroom exercise. But that's not how it works in practice." "You don't have time to sit around and think about these things, you have to see what you have to do and do it." You have to be on your toes the whole time."

Therapists observe—apparently most of the time—in order to gather information about the patient. These observations inform the therapist about global categories of behavior and specific aspects of the patient's action so that the therapist can quickly interpret it and respond with action. It seems that *action→seeing→observing→interpreting→acting* is a more accurate representation of the reasoning sequence they follow. In experienced therapists, observation, interpretation, and action comprise a fluid process that is more complicated than simple recognition or problem solving.

Therapists make fine observations of movement patterns and sequences. They observe motion as it happens and make judgments about the quality of the motion. These qualitative assessments are often made about a given movement sequence that the therapist then asks the patient to try in a slightly different way. Small variations in the movement pattern and careful observation of the quality of performance allow the therapists to make inferences about why the motion was limited and how the performance could be improved.

Observations are made to acquire *specific* information about this patient. Can he or can't he do a certain task? How well? Is this better or worse than before? Observations become information only if they can be used against a backdrop of prior knowledge. Therapists need general abstract knowledge about body systems, human development, psychologic processes, and so forth in order to direct their observations and interpretations of the state and behavior of this particular patient. And they need to know what normal performance looks like in order to determine if this particular action represents good, bad, or indifferent performance. They need to know how the muscles, nerves, and bones are organized to permit motions. They need to know what diseases and injuries will interfere with motion. With this basic knowledge, therapists can observe patients' actions and compare them against the stock of basic knowledge to determine the quality of this particular action taken by this particular patient. Therapists also need to know what this particular patient's performance was like last week or yesterday, in order to know if the motion was better or worse today. Prior knowledge of action, and of acceptable ranges and degrees of actions, is acquired by the therapist in several ways, including academic and clinical instruction, experience, and inquiry.

THINKING IN ACTION

Experience, as Benner (1984) and others (Dewey, 1929) have noted, is essential to expert practice. Experiential knowledge influences therapists' thoughts and actions all the time. Experienced therapists are able to move from observation to action so quickly that they typically describe their actions—correct and rapid ones—with sentences like "It happened so fast, I didn't have time to think about it, I just did it." Clearly, therapists do think about it, or the action would not be so precisely correct. But prior experience, action, and reflection develop their stock of tacit knowledge so that it need not be brought to consciousness in order to direct and guide action. Current thought and action are so closely linked that the thinking does not seem to take place at all. The thinking is tacit, the action is explicit and often expert.

Therapists have a habit of participating directly with the patient in the treatment. Polanyi (1974) and others have made the observation that many people use familiar tools as extensions of their own bodies. Therapists certainly do this; but more often they do the reverse. They use their bodies as if they were part of their tool kit. This is most obvious in pediatrics. For example, in a videotape made as part of the Clinical Reasoning Study, Cathy literally molds a child, Nicholas, across her lower leg to get him into the proper position. Then, she places him between her feet while they sit on the mat. The baby obligingly holds onto Cathy's socks and toes and sits contentedly. The point is to help Nicholas develop trunk stability. Cathy could have used bolsters to put him in this position, but this simple arrangement is so much more sensible and convenient. It probably made the baby feel more secure. Used in this way, Cathy's body became a kind of therapeutic device or piece of equipment.

Typically, therapists use their hands to manipulate the hands of their patients to "warm them up" for treatment. Their own hands become a sort of device to prepare the patient's hands to move. Often they go through a fixed routine of moving each joint separately. Other times they use more generalized motions. Therapists also use their hands as probes and sensors, noting minute changes in muscle tone or tightness of skin.

Actions are direct ways of sensing and interpreting what is "going on with" the patient's neuromotor system, healing process, arthritic processes, and so on. Therapists note change, for better or worse, from the last similar situation or action. Their fingers—and in Cathy's case even her toes—are highly tuned sensing devices that are always "picking up cues" for the therapists to interpret. A therapist often knows when the patient will fall before the patient does. They know when a child's muscle tone has changed, even before the results of it are visible in his altered posture. Therapists' bodies become tools and gauges. They take precise actions and glean what could be called calibrated information. They are not so much looking for presence or absence of something. They are looking for qualitative information. They mentally ask themselves questions like—How much tone? Is it fluctuating? What is stiffness and what is tonus? Is this weakness or wasting? How smooth is the movement? How directly does she reach the target? How much left-right imbalance is there? Therapists' sensory systems become tools to gain information that can answer these and many more questions.

Experienced therapists glean a lot of information from relatively small bits of action. Conversely, inexperienced therapists require more lengthy evaluation sessions to acquire fairly basic information. Less commonly encountered, though probably equally frequent in occurrence, is the phenomenon we have observed where the fine nuances of actions that the practitioners perform result in their collecting correspondingly nuanced data. New therapists evaluate hand function or muscle strength using routine procedures they learned in school. They tend to evaluate one muscle or joint at a time. Experienced therapists seem to be able to attend to every muscle and tendon in a group and make fine discriminations about what muscle or percent of a muscle is functioning and how well. They can make these evaluations based on a whole action rather than having to isolate each individual motion. For example, one therapist told us that if she wants to make a quick assessment of the range of motion someone has in their right arm she asks them to pretend they are hitchhiking and make the classic motion. Here, assessment of range is usually better than what a novice can discern with the aid of a goniometer. Experienced therapists take less action, but more precise action. They glean greater amounts of information from fewer movements and more subtle sensations as their experience increases.

INTERPRETATION

Interpretation is the mental process of making links between present information and past knowledge. It is the process whereby the therapist imagines possible relationships among cues. Cues are gathered and interpreted as being (or not being) related in some way. Cues may "aggregate" in a pattern that the therapist is familiar with. In such a case, interpretation is simple, rapid, and automatic. In unusual cases, interpretation may be a lengthy and complex enterprise, causing the therapist to hypothesize many possible patterns of relationships among cues. Such interpretations may involve a fairly conscious process of hypothesis generation and testing. Experienced therapists usually make interpretations based on a combination of automatic recognition and complex conscious interpretation. They generally recognize a pattern and quickly interpret it to have a particular meaning, but they usually subject their initial interpretation to further analysis by generating other possible interpretations.

Inquiry

It is often said that problem solving is possible only after one has identified that there *is* a problem, and then decided on the nature of the problem. But, how does one go about problem identification? It seems that casting the whole process as problem identification is not sufficient to understanding the workings of the problem-solving process. Problem solving is a process of *inquiry*. Inquiry is both a process and a mental attitude. The inquiring or curious therapist is almost always in a mental state of inquiry. Therapists continually think about, puzzle over, or mentally or verbally inquire about the numerous tiny details and qualities that comprise the patient's actions, problems, limitations, and abilities. They further inquire, of themselves and others, about the relationship of one small element of an action to another, or how changing one element might make a task easier or more practical for a patient. Thus, inquiry seems to be an essential element of good therapeutic practice. Joan Rogers (1982a,b) suggested the importance of a respect for inquiry by occupational therapists. She used the concept of inquiry to emphasize the need for formal inquiry, in the form of research. We are using inquiry in both the day-to-day sense, of inquiry as a process of thinking about something, and in the sense of inquiry as a "mental attitude" (Dewey, 1929). The process of inquiry is undertaken in order to understand a particular phenomenon. Philosophers refer to this as "intelligibility." As people, we want to understand our environment. We want it to become "intelligible" to us. Therapists make inquiries about their patients' actions so that their performance problems become intelligible to the therapists.

Therapists use very active methods to determine the nature of the perceived problem. They are in essence trying to make meaning of it. They are rendering intelligibility to a perceived object or complex. Intelligibility is the intersection of the meaning-making functions of the individual with objects of interest in the environment. The concept of intelligibility highlights the central importance of the intersection of the individual in and with the world, and dissuades us from falling into the common assumption that there are specific meanings to things in the world and the task of the individual is to unlock or discover them. "Man does not passively inhabit a world of meanings; he is rather a builder of meanings" (Yankelovich and Barrett, 1970, p. 391).

Smith comments that "the total reality includes the world and ourselves plus the fact of intelligible relations obtaining between the two" (Smith, 1971, p. 604). Such relations are modulated by our senses, by symbol systems, and by the ability to analyze and reflect. There is a broad range of sense-making activity aimed at rendering intelligibility. Some of these may seem virtually unconscious, whereas others are often characterized as highly conscious. Two subtle types of intelligibility that seem especially relevant to occupational therapy are "appraisal" and "inference."

Appraisal

The rapid response to the information gleaned through observation and sensation of the patient's and therapist's actions is definitely *reasoned*. But the reasoning is so rapid, so seemingly automatic, that it is clear that it does not fit the narrower notion of reasoning as the application of logic to a problematic situation. An early part of the therapist's reasoning process involves trying to get a "general sense of the situation." Polanyi's term "appraisal" seems most suitable to describe that process. Appraisal is a term we use in everyday language to mean much the same as it does in philosophical terms. Appraisal is a "quick summing up of the situation" (Polanyi, 1966, p. 33). It is not the last word. It is the first best estimate of a complex that presents itself to us in a particular way, in a given context. One determines the likely character of the complex based on the features that seem salient. Appraisal is possible because of one's stock of prior knowledge, both abstract and experiential. Polanyi says, "the act of knowing includes an appraisal: and this personal coefficient, which shapes all factual knowledge, bridges in doing so the distinction between subjectivity and objectivity" (p. 34).

Appraisal is not only quick, it serves to integrate. It is a conscious, dynamic process. Though rapid, it is not automatic. The "inquisitive practitioner" (Rogers, 1982) sees a new situation as being like—but not just like—some other situation. Appraisal moves one quickly to the right general category of a problem, but not necessarily to the specific details. Appraisal is a mental attitude that serves the practitioner well. It helps one to be mindful of both the general and the particulars.

Additionally, appraising a new situation serves to modify—to add to—the therapist's stock of knowledge, if the therapist takes an inquiring attitude toward practice in the first place. Buchler goes so far as to say that "an attitude is an appraisal. . . . It is an estimate of a situation in the context of a history" (1955, p. 10). Appraising is an activity—an act of coming to know—engaged in by the interested practitioner, and serves to simultaneously judge an external situation and contribute to the internal stock of personal knowledge. Through continuous appraisal the therapist improves the ability to "think on your feet," "know what's happening before it happens," "keep a session from getting out of hand," or "stay attuned to the situation." This is not a mysterious process of intuition, or "flying by the seat of the pants." It is a legitimate and valuable intellectual operation, which operates rapidly and effectively.

Appraising a situation accurately, rapidly, skillfully, or not, does not always lead to appropriate action. However, the converse is true. Correct or close enough appraisal is necessary for appropriate action. Experience and confidence are probably important attributes of therapists who appraise well and act with speed and precision. Appraisal is one form of active reasoning.

Some therapists seem to make very finely tuned appraisals and are able to change their actions slightly and quickly to suit the particular situation. Others seem to take nearly the same approach to all patients in a particular category. Appraisal and an inquiring attitude are necessary for the "fine-tuning" process that makes the difference between an adequate therapist and an excellent one. Therapists who were not very inquisitive seem to "know" in a more limited and literal sense what the condition is and what to do about it. In contrast, the more inquisitive therapists hold a more flexible view of diagnostic or procedural knowledge and are more open to identifying fine differences and distinctions among patients with a given condition.

Appraisal is not the total inquiry process, only a beginning. It results not in the last word, but in the first, best guess; an estimate of a complex that presents itself to the therapist in a given context. Therapists often use action, their own and the patient's, as a vehicle for making an appraisal. This may occur in the initial contact with the patient. For example, a therapist may observe a patient's facial expression and appraise it as an indication of a shift in mood. Therapists appraise aspects of the person's mood, posture, or performance many times in a given session.

TACIT APPRAISAL

Appraisal is a form of reasoning or judgment that therapists seem to be engaged in almost continuously. They appraise in the formal evaluation stage and during treatment. They seem to be always in a sort of subconscious appraisal mode, as a part of their general awareness of their surroundings. Incidents like the following are common. Liz and Peter were working on his grip-strength and coordination. Jim came by and asked a question. Jim was still behind Liz and she turned her head to answer him, but was never able to directly face him, due to the room and furniture arrangements. Jim turned his wheelchair to leave and Liz apparently returned her attention to Peter. As Jim was leaving, Liz seemed to catch a glimpse of Jim out of the corner of her eye. She remarked, "Hey Jim, that's not good posture, are you wearing your seat belt?" Thus she made an *observation*, an *appraisal*, and a possible *interpretation* in a few seconds, even though Jim was not the focus of her attention. Buchler comments:

> Every judgment is a tacit appraisal. That is to say it can be expanded to reveal as part of its meaning, some determination, selection or decision; it is extraction from the environment of something specific to the exclusion of something else. (1955, p. 28)

Tacit appraisal is not an appraisal of the entire situation. Liz apparently did not assess everything possible about Jim. It is an appraisal of some aspects of the situation that, because of her particular interests or knowledge, she selected from the broader field of all possibilities and "extracted . . . something specific" to notice and process—to appraise.

Appraisal, in addition to being a process of selection and extraction, can also be a form of comparison. This may be formal comparison, involving any level of careful deliberation, or it may be a fairly simple process of discrimination. Buchler comments, "Comparison and therefore appraisal is present on any level of estimation" (1925, p. 29). For example, therapists often comment that although this person has a given diagnosis, the particular ways she or he performs is not exactly like the usual behavior seen with this diagnosis. Therapists appraise the given situation and compare it to similar situations they have encountered in the past. The inquisitive therapist continually collects new knowledge and thereby modifies, enhances, and nuances old knowledge. The acquisition and modification of a somewhat unique body of knowledge is what Polanyi (1974) refers to as "personal knowledge." This personal knowledge is readily accessible—and ready for action. This readiness accounts for the speed and the smooth automatic quality of the therapist's spontaneous responses to the patient's actions.

Inference

Inquiry is a process of coming to understand something. Further, it is a process through which one not only learns something in the here and now, but also formulates a kind of knowledge that can be saved for future use. The process of inquiry is used to transform daily life interests and events into useful personal knowledge. Through inquiry, raw events become meaningful experience. Dewey (in Buchler, p. 104) stresses

> the contrast between gross, macroscopic, crude subject matters in primary experience and the refined, derived objects of reflection. The distinction is one between what is experienced as a result of minimum incidental reflection and what is experienced as a consequence of continued and regulated reflective inquiry.

If experience is what accounts for smoothness and insight in clinical practice, then inquiry is the key to making raw events into experiences that are "had" in Dewey's sense. Experiences that are "had" or "lived" are ones that are essentially transformed into useful personal knowledge by the inquiring individual. Such experiences seem to be used in a very dynamic way by the therapists. They can recount several instances when they came to a new understanding of something based on an experience with a patient. These may serve to change their whole point of view, or simply modify their current conception. Inquiry is clearly the catalyst that transforms events and actions into experience, and thus personal knowledge.

Inquiry is not a single focused event, but rather an attitude, a way the therapist approaches practice. Bernstein explains Pierce's conception of inquiry as an ongoing process. Pierce held a "view of inquiry as a self-corrective process which has no absolute beginning or end points and in which any claim is subject to further rational criticism" (Bernstein, 1971, p. 175). Action is ongoing, it is one direct way of participating in the world—in this case the world of the patient. Through this action, the therapist creates the opportunity for having an experience. Inquiry transforms mere action into experience.

In most situations encountered in everyday life there are many elements bearing upon a situation that are unknowns. In order to deal with the ambiguity caused by the unknowns, or lack of complete understanding, the individual *appraises* the situation and *infers* the presence of the unknowns. The process of inference is used to "fill in the gaps," where elements contributing to an understanding are not immediately apprehended or directly known. This sort of inference functions in an automatic or natural fashion in our daily lives. It seems to be one of those "silent" functions of mental processes that Dewey describes. Dewey sees inference and inquiry as being closely related to one another. Inference is an informal or "natural" process of "going beyond the assuredly present to an absent" (1916, p. 424). Inquiry is a more formal process of pursuing the unknown and rendering intelligibility to new situations.

Inference is a basic and widely used form of rendering intelligibility in our everyday lives. The same is true for practice. In most ordinary cases, inference may be either the only, or the dominant, mode used to determine the absent, that is, causes or consequences of conditions. In cases where an understanding is less easily achieved, inference leads the way by supplying certain aspects of the missing data, and even some potential conclusions. However, inquiry is required to achieve a dependable level of intelligibility. Dewey feels that inference always, in effect, supplies the unknown and that inquiry is employed as a "system of checks and tests to be used before the conclusion of inference is categorically affirmed" (p. 425). For example, a therapist may appraise a patient's facial expression as a change of mood and then infer that something about the immediate interaction caused that change in mood. Or the therapist may infer that the facial expression indicates that the person is anxious or angry or pleased. Then, further inquiry is needed to confirm or negate those inferences.

However dynamic these processes may be, and however successful in contributing to increased intelligibility, they do not always provide satisfactory understanding. Perceptions and habits are useful, but not absolutely trustworthy. Thus, inference is a rather risky process. "Through inference, men are capable of a kind of success and exposed to a kind of failure not otherwise possible" (p. 423). When the content or conclusion of the natural inference is seen to be incorrect or incomplete, one must take a more careful course toward intelligibility. In this case, one "makes the transition from natural spontaneous performance to a technique or deliberate art of inference" (p. 424).

APPRAISING THE VISIBLE, INFERRING THE INVISIBLE

In addition to making fine observations and rapid appraisals, therapists infer the presence or absence of other aspects of the individual, condition, or both that were not observable. Many inferences are fairly automatic; for example, if a therapist said an individual had "low tone" (meaning the person had low muscle tone), fairly automatic inferences were made about the state of the person's nervous system. If a child was assessed to be "jittery," it was a fairly common inference that he would have a short attention span, need to be handled carefully, and probably exhibit behavior that would fluctuate. Other inferences were more difficult to make and often depended on the therapist's own experience. Experienced therapists in our studies made complicated inferences. They were often interested in encouraging this sort of inference in students as well. Inferences that were automatic to the therapists had ben developed over time, usually in interaction with other therapists and clients. Thus particular cues or parts of the appraisal process often were given simple verbal designations, for example, "low tone," or "tactile defensive," or "flat affect," labels that implied a whole host of possible inferences to the experienced therapist and appeared as meaningless jargon to the outsider.

If inference is an essential quality, perhaps the dynamic core of tacit reasoning, then it is necessary that inference be controlled or guided in some way by some sort of mental structure. If not, meaningful conclusions could not be reached. Pierce (in Bernstein, p. 188) refers to these as guiding principles.

> These guiding principles can be formal principles essential for all reasoning, as well as material principles based on experience. Moreover, these guiding principles are involved in "warranting the transition from premise to conclusions . . ."

Guiding principles both structure and streamline the process of inference. Occupational therapy as a field has several such guiding principles, which range from the strictly experience-based, for example, "it is important to break down a task," to the formal use of developmental principles and stages to structure inference making about the performance capacities of young children. These guiding principles direct the inferences therapists make, and the actions they take in observing, assessing, and interpreting the patient's problems. In many practices, including occupational therapy, formal tests and evaluation procedures are used as a way to carefully assess a patient's condition or skill. These are essentially guides to making inferences regarding present and future performance. In some cases, the inferences are made for the clinician based on standard interpretations of the particular patterns of test results. A few such formal guides are available to occupational therapists, for example; the use of a goniometer to measure the range of motion at a joint. Although many therapists use and value standardized evaluations, many tend to eschew standard measures as being too general, and not specific enough to capture the subtle details of the condition of *this* patient. They also tend to rely on and value their own judgment and inference making over and above standard measures. There is a common tendency to develop individual evaluation activities by which the therapist structures observations of the patient's performance and progress. Some of these are fairly common within a type of clinic. For example, pediatric therapists place a lot of stock in observations of block building, handling of crayons, and stacking cones. Psychiatric therapists tend to use their observations of collage making, self-care, and cooking skills as a basis for appraisal and inference making.

Whether these evaluations are formal or informal, they are sets of actions that the therapist asks the patients to perform. The therapist observes details of the action—such as the sequence or quality of movements, the number of cues or prompts the person needs to complete the task, or the overall quality of the object produced—and uses the observation and appraisals to make inferences about the patient's physical, cognitive, or emotional state or status. This, in turn, is used to make judgments about the patient's present and potential performance. This sort of action, appraisal, and inference making goes by the term "activity analysis." Therapists place a lot of value on their ability to analyze activities. It is not so much the activity that they are analyzing as the patient's performance of that activity. Such analysis is the essence of the problem identification and predictive capabilities of the occupational therapist. Therapists take for granted that they can observe and appraise a person's current actions and can infer and predict potential improvements or problems. A discussion that took place among some therapists working a psychiatric hospital will provide an illustration.

Chris: The other members of the staff want us to evaluate how a person functions. But they sometimes don't

Harriet: seem to believe that we can actually tell how a person will perform on another activity given how they performed on the ones we observed.

Harriet: They seem to think we should be like psychologists, have a different test for every task.

Chris: And we do our evaluations on the spot with everyday activities.

Harriet: And they have to go back to their office for an hour to figure out what the tests mean!

Judgment and Action

Judgments are more conscious than appraisal but are dependent on appraisal. Buchler comments,

> Every judgment is a tacit appraisal. That is to say it can be expanded to reveal as part of its meaning, some determination, selection, or decision; it is extraction from the environment of something specific to the exclusion of something else. (1955, p. 141)

Appraisal, in addition to being a process of selection and extraction, can also be a form of comparison. This may be a formal comparison, involving any level of formal deliberation, or it may be a fairly simple process of discrimination.

> Comparison, and therefore appraisal is present on any level of estimation. Comparison can take the form either of deliberation and criticism on the one hand, or of unmediated discrimination on the other. Both are appraisive, the former through systematic production, the latter merely through production as such. Discrimination or selection from alternatives is present in the simplest products; it helps to explain the product as judgment. (p. 14)

Appraisal may function at several levels of complexity and involve greater or lesser degrees of conceptual focus. Appraisal is an activity that may involve estimation, discrimination, selection, determination, or comparison at many levels of awareness and depth. The dynamics and complexities of these activities will greatly influence any judgment and vary with the particular type of judgment being made.

The notion of action as a method for and process of reasoning was made obvious in the actions and conversations of the therapists who were part of the Clinical Reasoning Study. While this is not a common notion, it has been addressed in studies of the phenomenology of practice by both Dewey (1915) and Buchler (1955). Buchler has enlarged our understanding of judgment with his development of the idea of actions *as* judgments. In Buchler's view, action toward or upon something is a judgment about it, a response to an interpretation of it. This concept easily applies to the actions therapists take, and which, they say, informs their practice. Practice is not simply the result of judgment; it is a process of judging and an act of judgment. Through actions, the clinicians make judgments, and by making such judgments expand their experience. Reflection on that experience creates new meanings, which develop new habits of thought and action.

Experienced clinicians have acquired many skills and meanings. These enable the therapist to make judgments regarding the nature of a situation and immediately generate the appropriate response to it—an action. The knowledge, habits, and skills required to make these active judgments become incorporated in daily judgments and actions so that therapists can operate smoothly and seemingly automatically. The incorporation and repetition of these actions and judgments—active judgment—become part of the clinician's "second nature." Thus, even though the type of knowledge involved in making clinical judgments may be highly specialized, the clinician is able to make these judgments with a great deal of precision, efficacy, efficiency, and speed.

Characteristics of Occupational Therapists' Reasoning Contrasted with Common Assumptions about Decision Making

Most of the literature on clinical reasoning among health professionals focuses on the cognitive aspects of the diagnostic strategies and the decision-making processes of physicians. We were well versed in the medical decision-making literature, and thought about some of the central concepts in that body of literature, and initially wondered if some of them would apply to occupational therapy. Some did, but many did not. Occupational therapy is a practice that, in philosophy, problem-solving style, and professional practice, is very different from clinical medicine. We found many differences between the ways therapists thought about their clients' problems and the ways physicians are encouraged to make medical decisions.

THE BEST WAY TO REASON

Investigators who study how practitioners think often assume that clinicians usually employ one of the three problem-solving strategies proposed by Newell and Simon (1972): "recognition (p. 94), generate-and-test (p. 95), and heuristic search" (p. 96). An implicit goal of many clinical reasoning studies is to identify the "best" way for a particular group of clinicians to think about problems in practice. For example, many studies of medical decision making seek to map the best problem-solving strategy for physicians.

The Clinical Reasoning Study was designed to examine the reasoning strategies of occupational therapists in their day-to-day practice. In this study, actual treatment sessions with real patients and therapists were videotaped and analyzed. It appeared, at first, that reasoning and clinical performance in occupational therapy was considerably more random than suggested by other clinical decision-making literature. Later, we realized that it was not randomness but complexity of thought that we were observing. This necessity for complex thinking seemed to be a result of the type of problems addressed. Occupational therapists insist on focusing on many aspects of the person, rather than specializing in just one system. That approach, of necessity, leads to complexity in both thought and action. The problems therapists addressed were problem complexes rather than the clearly delineated "closed-ended" (Dreyfus, 1972) problems typical of those presented in most clinical decision-making studies. Therapists were dealing with several different types of problems simultaneously. Therefore, they sometimes shifted rapidly from one aspect of the problem to another, or even to a whole different problem. What at first looked like messy practice we later saw as a responsive practice. Attending to "the whole person" resulted in the therapist having to respond to several aspects of the person, either simultaneously or in rapid succession. This, in turn, required a complex set of reasoning strategies.

Meehl (1954), an early advocate of the need to study clinicians' thinking, proposed that psychologists could benefit from the use of statistical (or actuarial) methods to guide their thinking about patients and problems. He also proposed that reasoning based on statistical probabilities might be best suited to some situations, whereas the "clinical" (case study) method might be preferable in others. Statistical methods are used to reduce uncertainty in making a diagnosis or selecting treatment (Raiffa, 1970). However, this does not address the problem of how clinicians categorize information in a way that is useful, before it is subjected to statistical analysis (Cutter, 1979). In the past 10 years, studies of the problem-solving strategies of clinicians, especially physicians, have been analyzed and modeled with the use of an impressive collection of sophisticated methods, such as statistical modeling and the development of expert systems. However, it is still recognized that studies of actual clinicians are very valuable. The so-called descriptive studies of how clinicians think take the naturalistic perspective and study how clinicians think on the spot, without the use of computers. In the Clinical Reasoning Study, the naturalistic or ethnographic approach was selected as the methodology best suited to the object of inquiry. We found that therapists often used some notions of probability in making on-line judgments, but they had little interest in statistical models. The therapists who participated in this study used a great number of problem-solving strategies, including, but not limited to, the strategies identified by Newell and Simon (1972), and Elstein et al. (1978). The clinical problems addressed were significantly more conceptually complex than we had been initially assumed. Further, the complexity of the problems addressed seemed to govern the choice of the reasoning strategy employed. Simple or familiar problems were resolved with simple reasoning strategies such as recognition, recall, and common sense. Complex or unfamiliar problems prompted the therapists to use more complex forms of inquiry. These included inductive and deductive reasoning, active judgment (Buchler, 1955), intuitive reasoning (Hammond, 1988), tacit reasoning (Polanyi, 1966), procedural, interactive, and conditional reasoning (Fleming, 1989), and narrative reasoning (Mattingly, 1989).

CONTINUOUS RATHER THAN SEQUENTIAL REASONING

Clinical decision-making research usually focuses on hypothesizing diagnosis, predicting prognosis, and assessing the probable outcome of available treatments. Each is considered an important decision point. Problem solving for occupational therapists did not take the form of clear-cut decision points or events. It was not time-delineated, with decisions following in an orderly sequence. Nor were diagnosis, prognosis, and treatment selection considered only once, or in that sequence. There were few "one-time" decision-making points or events. Thinking about problems and possible solutions seemed to be more of a continuous stream of small decisions or temporary hypotheses. Reasoning occurred so rapidly that all these processes seemed to be conducted simultaneously. Continuous revision seemed to be the norm. This was not because therapists did not "get it right the first time." It was more a matter of fine-tuning adjustments to the particular person's needs, wishes, body, abilities, and limitations. The simultaneous consideration of, and rapid flow between, what are often seen as separate aspects of thinking led us to describe this problem-solving process as clinical reasoning rather than clinical decision making. Clinical reasoning in occupational therapy was characterized not simply as multiple hypothesis generation (Elstein et al., 1978) but rather as "continuous hypothesis modification" (Fleming, 1991a).

Therapists frequently said that diagnosis is not separate from treatment. They used words like, "You are always evaluating," or "Treatment and evaluation go hand in hand," to express what seemed to be a continuous process of what they call "ongoing evaluation" of the patient. This included the person's abilities, physical and emotional status, preferences, degree of change, progress, and a myriad of other details. What therapists seemed to be referring to when they said that evaluation and treatment go together was a process of nearly continuous hypothesis generation, evaluation, and revision. Therapists were attentive to many cues, in several categories of problems that might affect functional performance. They recognized cues as patterns or potential parts of patterns. These, in turn, prompted hypotheses about the patient's physical or emotional condition. These hypotheses were then evaluated against further observation or subjected to further inquiry. Following this evaluation, the dominant hypothesis was substantiated, negated, revised, or modified. Processes such as attention to cues, pattern recognition, and hypothesis generation and evaluation (Elstein et al., 1978) were used to continually monitor, modify, revise, and refine both the conceptualization of the problem and the process of treatment. This led us to understand the important role that an intense spirit of inquiry plays in the conduct of good occupational therapy practice.

DISCONTINUOUS HYPOTHESIS GENERATION

While reasoning about the problem, therapists were also concerned about the individual client's interests and feelings. Rogers and Masagatani (1982) found that during an evaluation procedure, therapists often moved out of a strictly problem-solving mode to address the immediate concerns of the patient. Later, therapists resumed their logical thinking pattern in a search for definition or resolution of the clinical problem. The same pattern was often seen among therapists in this study. They would be engaged in a stream of hypothetic deductive reasoning concerning the patient's physical or performance problem. They would interrupt that stream when the patient said or did something that caused the therapist to temporarily abandon the focus on the physical problem. Therapists would shift to another form of thinking and address the concerns of the patient as a person. Having addressed such a concern, they would return to the evaluation or therapeutic task and the more directed problem-solving process. This apparent discontinuity was another feature that initially led us to think of the practice as somewhat "messy." Later we realized that because occupational therapists have assigned themselves the task of "attending to the whole person," they have to be quite facile at addressing many aspects of the person almost simultaneously. Many observers of the videotapes have commented that good occupational therapy looks like good parenting. This simultaneous focus on several levels of concern seems to be present in both practices—occupational therapy and parenting.

FOCUS ON FUTURE FUNCTION RATHER THAN PAST HISTORY

Most studies of clinical decision making focus on diagnosis, because it is often seen as the most critical aspect of decision making and practice. Prognosis is a second important factor. It usually influences the selection of treatment procedures. Treatment selection is often seen as the end of the formal reasoning process (Feinstein, 1973a,b; 1974). The occupational therapists involved in the Clinical Reasoning Study found diagnosis interesting or necessary, but they were far more interested in treatment. Patients came to therapy with a medical diagnosis. The therapist's task was to know how that diagnostic condition would influence present and future function. The primary concern was about what a person could do now and might be able to do in the future. The therapists considered etiology important, but it was in the background rather than the foreground of their thinking. Therapists conducted careful evaluations and made very fine-grained observations of current functional performance. Here they employed strategies that Rogers and Holm refer to as "diagnostic reasoning [which] encompasses problem sensing and problem definition" (1991, p. 1045). They made accurate predictions of possible gains in functional levels. They were concerned about what those gains would mean to the patient's eventual performance level and what that would mean to her or his future.

Prognosis was considered to be a relatively likely outcome, but not a fact or a fate. Possibilities for the future and progress toward it were the main concerns. In other words, the clinician's thinking primarily focused not so much on the disability and the present treatment, as on the possibilities for the person's functioning in the future. Treatment selection, rather than being an end point, was close to the beginning of the therapists' reasoning process.

Therapists helped people learn or relearn common everyday activities such as bathing, dressing, and working. To do this they had to discover what the functional problem was and how the person could develop strategies for accomplishing desired tasks in the most efficient or effective way, given the limitations of the disability. How a person would conduct and manage everyday life tasks was the primary problem complex that occupational therapists addressed. This aspect of reasoning is probably important to occupational therapists because their risk is not to treat the illness or disability per se. It is to help remediate the limitations placed on the person's function as a result of the disease or disability. Further, the therapist's role is to help the person move out of the position of being a patient in the hospital and to return to the community. So the focus on future function may influence the therapist to think more about current treatment and future performance than diagnosis or evaluation.

INDIVIDUALIZATION RATHER THAN GENERALIZATION

Central to the OT approach to reasoning was the notion that treatment success was very dependent upon a process that the therapists referred to as "individualization." Individualizing meant tailoring the treatment to the particular skills, needs, and interests of the patients. The notion that a treatment is specific to a particular patient runs counter to the common assumption that all people with a given disease or disability can be treated with the same solution. This assumption has its foundation in scientific notions that true knowledge is generalizable and that scientific knowledge can be converted into law statements (Bunge, 1967). This promotes the view that, as physical bodies, patients and their diseases are all predictably the same. That set of assumptions is usually called the disease-centered approach. It is often contrasted with the person-centered approach. Another way of illustrating this difference is to speak of the "disease" versus the "illness experience" (Kleinman, 1980). These therapists seemed to take both approaches and meld them together. They had many procedures, treatment modalities, and strategies that were frequently used with most persons who had the same sort of injury. What they cared most about, however, was not the precise application of the "correct procedure," but finding the best way for this person to function. This meant that they wanted to find activities that would "motivate" or challenge patients to try something new, and in which they would have some well-earned success. The integration of concern for the patient and concern to resolve the problem seemed to be a common, but not always harmonious, way of thinking about and conducting therapy. It required many ways of thinking and rapid, sometimes awkward, shifts from one mode of thinking to another, and from one form of interaction to a very different one. The practice is one that requires a mode of operation where the "occupational therapist, during a single treatment session enters into the patient's life-world and simultaneously controls and manages the treatment process" (Crepeau, 1991, p. 1016). The degree to which and the finesse with which therapists are able to make these shifts varied from therapist to therapist and from situation to situation. Sometimes it seemed that experience contributed to the development of this ability. At other times we thought that this skill might be linked to the therapist's personal abilities or style. The extent to which therapists were comfortable with the interactive and meaning-making aspects of therapy seemed to be very strongly linked to this ability.

PATIENTS ARE INCLUDED IN THE DECISION-MAKING PROCESS

Another common assumption is that decision making is something that involves only the clinician or the experts. The knowledge, skill, and thinking capacity of the clinician are brought to bear on the information given, and the ensuing analysis results in problem identification and treatment selection. Who the patient is, or how he or she participates in the diagnostic and treatment process is usually considered of little consequence (except in cases of poor information or noncompliance). In occupational therapy we did not find this to be so. Therapists' thinking was not limited to how they might identify or solve problems. Rather, it was more focused on how they could get patients to recognize their own problems and develop ways to go about tasks that they wanted to accomplish. Treatment success was quite dependant upon the patient's participation. The therapists needed to engage people in the physical and sometimes psychological aspects of evaluation and treatment activities in order to frame and define the problems, and to conduct the treatment. Therapists typically engage their patients in what they call the "problem-solving process." There seemed to be two reasons for this. One was that therapists needed the participation to help identify what the patient saw as problems and preferred solutions. Two, they believed that the ability to "problem-solve" was critical to the patient's future ability to function independently. Therapists viewed teaching the patient problem-solving skills as an essential part of their role. They typically asked the patients, "What do you think is your biggest problem?" or "What do you want to work on first?" or "How do you feel about that?" Problem-solving activities were a typical part of most occupational therapy treatment sessions. Problem identification and problem solving were a joint effort between patient (and often the family) and therapist.

OFFERING CHOICES RATHER THAN MAKING DECISIONS

A common assumption is that the professional makes the decisions and informs the patient as to the best solutions or options. However, in medical practice today many practitioners now offer patients choices of possible solutions, complete with a cost-benefit analysis (Weinstein and Stason, 1977). Patients can decide what sorts of treatment they want, given the risks involved in various choices. They can make decisions in light of the quality of life that may result if a given procedure is successful.

Occupational therapists are interested in giving people choices, and are also interested in choice making itself. In our study, we found that they felt that choice making was a part of the process of regaining one's ability to be independent. They offered people choices, often from a predetermined list of possibilities, and also encouraged them to invent their own. They did not assume that the core of the problem was a concrete entity, in the patient's body, in the disease, and that therefore the trick was simply to find the right answer—to pinpoint the culprit—and make a diagnosis. Rather, the situation was seen to involve a problem complex comprised of multiple aspects of the patient's mind, body, social situation, and environment. The solution was not perceived as a concrete choice to be made; it was something to be developed between the patient and therapist, a solution for the therapist and patient to figure out and to refine. The treatment was often something that the therapist and the patient invented together.

IMAGINING POSSIBILITIES RATHER THAN GENERATING PROBABILITIES

Much of the decision-making literature in both medicine and psychology focuses on the improvement of the clinician's ability to generate hypotheses and assign probabilities to various hypothesized outcomes (Kassirer, Kuipers, and Gorry, 1982). While experienced occupational therapists are able to make quite accurate predictions about the probable "functional status" or therapeutic outcome, or of when the patient would be discharged and where the patient would be at that point, determining probability was not the major focus. Therapists frequently seemed to focus on the possibilities. On a day-to-day basis this took the form of generating a number of ways that a person could exercise a muscle, or accomplish a task, or meet some part of a goal. On a long-term basis, therapists often hoped that a person would find a new and better life than the one that could be predicted simply by interpreting the diagnostic and prognostic statistics. It is not that they expected miracles—far from it. But they hoped and aimed for a possible solution that would make this person's life a little easier, or more meaningful. So, rather than generating hypotheses and settling on probabilities, they imagined possibilities and tried to create ways in which they would be actualized.

VALUES GUIDE RATHER THAN INTERFERE WITH REASONING

Another common assumption is that decision making should be value-free. The clinical problem is considered to be a scientific problem and therefore should be addressed in an objective manner. No prior assumptions, values, or preferences of the clinician should intervene between the problem and the scientific mind of the practitioner. The objective, scientific point of view is adopted to prevent the practitioner from making negative value judgments against the person because the condition represents some behavioral or social condition that is distasteful to the practitioner. The separation of moral judgment and clinical judgment has advantages for both the patient and the practitioner when it prevents social prejudice from interfering with care. However, the converse also seems to be true.

Occupational therapists used their values to guide, promote, and defend care and quality of life for their patients. Often, therapists seek a better treatment of, or attitude toward, patients than was being granted to them. However, there is no formal system or model that is explicitly promoted for making these decisions and that addresses the decision-making process itself. We found that the point of view and the ethics and values of the therapists influenced them in many useful ways. There were several important assumptions, values, and ideals that operated as underlying structures in the process of thinking about problems. These assumptions and values were widely and strongly held among the therapists in the group. The philosophy often influenced decisions as to what was interpreted as a problem and assisted therapists in setting priorities and sequencing problems to be addressed. Far from obscuring problems, or interfering with reaching the best decision, these values, aspirations, and insights led the therapists to useful and often unique solutions to individual patients' problems. Values such as the belief in personal dignity and functional independence, and personal identity and choice making were very influential in the practice. It is tempting to say that rather than being a practice profession with an ethical code, occupational therapy is a practical ethic.

EXPERTISE RATHER THAN AUTHORITY

Therapists said that one of their roles was to "empower the patient," by which they meant that they helped the person see herself or himself as an individual with rights, skills, abilities, and a sense of self-worth. These issues are usually not addressed in the decision-making literature. However, these issues did seem to be central to the therapists' daily concerns, and therefore influenced their thinking. Some of the strategies and characteristics of occupational therapy practitioners that were identified above (such as valuing the person's independence and point of view, including the patient in problem identification, imagining possibilities, and making choices) were used as ways of bringing about this "empowering" of the patient. Perhaps as a result of this, or perhaps as an implicit or tacit function of the practice, the therapist separates expertise from authority. The therapist has expertise based on knowledge about human function and dysfunction and how to improve performance when it becomes difficult, but the therapist is not in a position of authority over the patient. Nor is the therapist an authority on the patient or the medical condition. In this relationship the patient becomes neither subject nor object, but rather a collaborator in thinking about and executing treatment. The therapist assists in examining the problem and offering potential resolutions; but ultimately the patient defines the problem and makes the choices.

CONFLUENCE OF INQUIRY AND ACTION

Typically, thought and action are considered to be separate entities. In these occupational therapists, thought and action were intertwined. The feasibility of a possible solution was often directly tested in action. Similarly, actions often produced ideas about solutions. Thought and action were not independent. They were interdependent. The primary role of the occupational therapist is to evaluate and improve the patient's functional performance. Therefore, the patient's actions are an important source of data. The therapist's attentive observations of the patient's actions, and subtle variations and change in actions, are an important part of therapeutic knowledge and skill.

Similarly, the therapist's own actions and careful interpretations of sensations, were sensitive instruments used to collect such data, for example, when doing manual muscle testing. The therapist's actions, the patient's actions, and the patient's response to the therapist's actions were all dynamic essential data and cues for the therapist's reasoning process. Fine variations in actions gave therapists immediate information, or confirmation, or a basis for further hypothesis making. This active judgment (Buchler, 1955) was not simply an intellectual judgment made as a result of some analysis of a former action. It was judgment *in* action. The action or data-gathering process was confluent with the interpretation of the quality of that action; it was both judgment in action and action based on judgment (Hayes, 1978). This requirement for action on the part of both therapists and patients may account, at least in part, for the phenomenon of continuous hypothesis modification mentioned earlier. The confluence of action and judgment may also be the basis for the therapists' conviction that evaluation and treatment are reciprocal and continuous, not distinct, processes.

Appendix of Clinical Stories*

■ JOHN ■
by Kathy Thurmond

John's chart told me he was a 58-year-old white male presenting with right hemiparesis and expressive aphasia. His diagnosis was noted as "?CVA." John had been admitted to the hospital through the emergency room 3 days ago. Determination of his diagnosis was actually still in progress, with MRIs [magnetic resonance images] and angiograms still being conducted. His chart included notes from various physicians, nursing records, and an intake note from a social worker. In some notes, John was described as having expressive aphasia, in others as being globally aphasic. Some notes offered more detail by stating that John was responding appropriately to simple, one-step directions but was having trouble with more complicated instructions and was unable to express himself verbally. The social worker's note said that John was self-employed as a building contractor, was married, and had several grown children in the area.

I was an OT student halfway into my first affiliation at a small community hospital. The OT department at the hospital was quite small and had been cut back to the point where it now included one full-time outpatient therapist and one part-time inpatient therapist. Although I had been at the hospital affiliation for 6 weeks, there was not a strong OT presence in inpatient care, and John was only the third person with a stroke to be referred to the department since I had been there.

I first saw John when I accompanied Marie, the speech therapist, to observe her eval [evaluation] of him. He was a big man, sitting somehow stiffly in a plastic armchair at the foot of the bed, in his hospital room. He had on a hospital johnnie that, as he sat, came almost to his knees. He had no shoes or socks on. Each elbow rested on an armrest, and each hand hung down from the wrist at the end of the armrest. His head hung down and he seemed to be gazing at the floor. He looked

---

*Names of patients and places have been changed to protect the anonymity of those concerned.

343

up and straightened himself in the chair as we entered the room. He nodded as Marie called his name. He was a good-looking man. He looked neat, well-kept; he wore square, metal-framed glasses; his hair was wavy, graying blond, neatly trimmed and brushed; and his body looked strong, physically fit, with only a slight belly.

Marie introduced us both, and began her exam. John watched her intently. It was quickly apparent that he was unable to respond to her questions verbally. He would nod and say, "Yeah," but he could not find the words to count to 10. He could not find the words to say where he was, what town he lived in, or what his first name was. He could say words and he would try a word or two at each question, then shake his head, grip his chair, strain forward, try another word, clearly recognizing he was not coming up with the right words. Shortly, he sagged back against the chair, shaking his head no. Marie tried some instructions. He responded appropriately. Or did he? For an instruction like "Raise your right hand," he responded; but for an instruction like "Take this pencil, make an 'X' on the paper, then put the pencil on the shelf," he looked up puzzled and did not proceed in the task.

Marie moved on to a swallowing eval, during which she probed in John's mouth with a swab, a stick, a spoonful or two of applesauce. She explained as she went along, but John's puzzlement seemed to expand to frustration, despair, even anger. His body tightened and sagged repeatedly. He vocalized, "Yeah, yeah," "No," "No good, no good."

Marie finished her exam and stepped back to let me approach. I went over and squatted down in front of John's chair to look into his face. I reminded him of my name. I wanted to reassure him, or me, so I told him he was doing okay. I told him I needed to work with him for a little while but that I wanted to give him a little break. I told him I would leave for a bit and then be back to work with him in 10 minutes.

I left the room with Marie. I had to catch my breath, to compose myself. This condition of John's was brand new to him; it was also new to me. I spoke briefly with Marie about what we had seen. Then I reviewed the eval sheets I needed to fill out on John. I believed I could contain the sea of sorrow within me long enough to get through at least a range of motion and manual muscle test this afternoon.

I returned to John's room. He looked up, nodded as I entered. I approached him. I spoke slowly, quietly. "I'm from occupational therapy. I'm going to be working with you on everyday activities. Today we'll work for just a little while. I want to see how you move and how strong you are." He watched me. I demonstrated as I gave the first instruction. He followed me. I used fewer words, more slow demonstration as we proceeded. I smiled, nodded, watched his face for questions. He demonstrated full range of motion, and his strength was good, though perhaps slightly decreased from what I would expect on his right side. He sagged a little bit to the right. He moved slowly but he had full, adequate movement. No facial sagging, no visual tracking problems. He appeared alert. Appeared . . . oriented. But then how could I tell that, with the language problem?

That was all I could do the first day. I told him I would see him tomorrow and said good-by. He looked in my eyes and nodded.

I returned the following day, having discussed John's case with my supervisor. I still needed to complete an ADL eval and a cognitive eval. My supervisor had said, "Start with something familiar. Don't overwhelm him with complicated conversation, try some simple ADLs first." I thought I would see him after breakfast to do some hand- and face-washing, maybe some toothbrushing. I also carried a cognitive eval kit in case we could use that. When I got to his room he was sitting alone and disheveled in the armchair. He was unshaven, his hair uncombed, again in only a johnny. His breakfast tray was pushed to the side, with some of the food eaten.

He looked up and smiled when I entered. "Hi, kiddo," he said. I greeted him. I asked about his beard. "No," he said. "No," and shook his head. I asked if he would like to clean up. He watched me. I elaborated and mimicked face-washing. "Yeah, yes," he said. Finding supplies took a few minutes. His nurse vigorously approved the shaving idea, telling me he was not on any bleeding precautions due to anticoagulant meds. It was just that she hadn't yet had time to "do him," she told me. John's chart said he needed two people to assist in walking due to decreased balance and a question of dyspraxia. The nurse said, "Just shave him at bedside, dear." So I set up the supplies on the tray table in front of John, trying to think of everything we would need. Then I stood back.

Slowly he took the cloth from the water and squeezed it out with both hands. It was awkward action, but I thought, "This is an odd setup for him, unfamiliar." He wiped his face, watching himself in the mirror. He dropped the cloth back on the table, then looked around him. I lifted the little can of shaving foam and identified it for him, thinking again this is an unfamiliar setup. He reached slowly to take the can with his right hand and overshot it. With some effort he got hold of the can, but then could not get the button pushed to release the foam into his waiting left hand. I helped him. Foam in hand, he began to spread it on his face. Again he was awkward, as if having trouble finding his face.

"Well, I'll be goddamned," he said. The phrase was complete, the first complete, natural phrase I had heard him use. "The damnedest thing," he said.

I leaned down to face him. "It's okay," I said. "We're just gonna work through it." He switched to using his left hand to spread the foam. It was awkward but not nearly as awkward as his right hand. Then he reached for the razor. His right hand got caught under the table as he brought it up from his lap. He looked surprised. He struggled and brought the hand out and up over the razor. Struggling throughout to position his hand appropriately, he managed to pick up the razor and bring it near his face. I watched, my breath caught in my chest, unable to shift my gaze, as I might watch the trapeze artist in midair reaching for the swing.

There was no tremor, no loss of range, no problematic weakness. John's hand just didn't know what to do. But it was apparently only his right hand, his right side. His left hand, though awkward, clearly knew how to move, to do what John wanted to do; his right hand seemed lost to him.

We got through the shaving and toothbrushing and hairbrushing with similar awkwardness, and growing amazement. John repeated several times his exclamation, "I'll be goddamned." At one point he sat back and laughed. But it was not a good laugh.

We finished. I squatted down in front of him. "We have some things to work on," I said. "That's what we're going to be doing. There's a team of people, doctors, and nurses, and therapists, and we're all going to work with you on this thing."

He stayed with me. He watched me talk. "Yes, yeah," he said. I put my hand on his shoulder. "Okay," he said.

"That's enough for now," I said. "I'll be in again this afternoon."

He met my eyes. "Okay," he said and nodded.

I walked from the room on shaky knees, thinking of how such simple things can hold such awful discoveries. Thinking there were more such discoveries to come for John, and hoping that soon, as soon as possible, some of the discoveries would begin to be those of hope and accomplishment.

Discussion Questions

1. What did the student therapist identify as problems for this person?
2. What were some of the conflicts that the student therapist experienced in coming to her decisions about intervention?
3. How do you feel about the resolution of the problem(s)?
4. Can you identify features of procedural, interactive, conditional, or narrative reasoning?
5. What implicit or explicit occupational therapy values emerge in this story?

■ MARY ■

by Gretchen Braun

Mary G. is a 72-year-old woman hospitalized with depression and posttraumatic stress disorder; she had been abused by a friend of her father's and her brother when she was very young. She is very close to her son and his daughter, from whom she receives a great deal of love and support. Before she entered the hospital, she had been planning a camping trip by herself in the mountains and was very concerned that she would not be able to make her trip if she was not out of the hospital by the next weekend.

Mary was a very sociable person around the unit and found great comfort in talking with others. She often dressed as a little girl would dress, and many times she behaved in the same manner—as if she was regressing to the time that she had been abused. My supervisor identified Mary as a typical alcoholic because of the characteristic dark circles under her eyes, but we never found that she had such a problem. Some days, Mary had a wild look in her eyes and she would act rather impulsively and without boundaries. Other days, it was easy to see that there was goodness in her heart, and that she had a desire to get help and to take part in helping others.

Mary was often very emotional on the unit, and demanded a lot of attention at times. One day, Mary "cornered" me on the unit and proceeded to discuss her fears and feelings about her son going away on a business trip, and leaving his daughter at home and her in the hospital. She was concerned that something might happen to him and that no one would know how or where to contact her. She grabbed my arm desperately and began to talk about how much her granddaughter needed him. I could see the tears come to her eyes as she began to talk about the past and how it was to feel alone as a child. I watched her unravel in front of me as her memories of abuse came to mind, though she said nothing specific about them; and I just stood and listened. I did not discourage but tried to comfort her and help her to see that her son would be all right. I felt helpless and heartsick as I encouraged her to talk with her "key person," who I thought would be more equipped to help her. As quickly as these thoughts flooded her, they subsided and she returned to the discussion of her son and granddaughter. Her eyes lit up as she spoke of her granddaughter and I saw this as a sign that she was feeling better. I made her promise to check in with her "key person" before I returned to the OT clinic, exhausted and frustrated that I felt so incapable of helping her.

The next day, Mary joined the gardening group in a terrible mood.

Something had just happened with one of the unit nurses and Mary had no desire to be in OT. When she first entered the room, she made an unnecessary and inappropriate comment to another of the group's members; but once a limit was set, she responded immediately and apologized. She then turned her initially negative energy into positive energy that filled the room. She was cheerful, smiling, full of compliments, and interested in making everyone else feel good for the rest of the session. It was as if she realized that making someone else feel bad had the same effect on her, so she turned around and did the opposite. She did not care about the activity we were doing, yet her presence in the room made the group so light and so much fun for everyone that I did not care that she chose not to join the activity. The woman who had been so upset and desperate the day before was now cheerful and smiling. Toward the end of the group, Mary asked why the OT clinic was the only room on the unit where she felt like herself again, and that she always felt so good in the clinic. I asked her if she could tell me why and we found that neither one of us really knew; but it made me feel like I had helped her in some way.

A couple of weeks ago, I was outlining some of the neurologic problems and deficits that Mary had; it was more of a medical model case study for the neuroanatomy students. After I completed my discussion, one of the students in the class asked me how I knew that she had all the deficits that I was outlining. I told her that I would usually think through and describe the things that I saw before I realized what clinical significance they had; and that the longer I was in the setting, the easier it became to see the functional deficits "clinically." I thought about that question for a while later, and realized that I would respond to what I had seen [in the patient] before I truly identified what it was. Maybe that was why Mary was so comfortable in the clinic—I responded to her needs as a person and a patient before I took the time to really think about what those needs should be; it was automatic. Maybe that was why she chose to open up to me that afternoon instead of her "key person," because I was willing to give her what she needed, an ear to listen and a place to feel safe and comfortable.

I have always thought of Mary as one of the patients that will always be with me, but I never realized how much of an impact she had on my feelings of what being an occupational therapist means to me. I feel as if I enabled Mary to be herself in some ways, just by acknowledging her as a person. There are so many aspects of a hospital unit that take away a person's ability to be who they really are, but the OT clinic gave Mary a place where she could be that person and not have to be aware of all her thoughts and behavior. One of the most striking things about OT is that it places such an emphasis on getting to know and meet the patient's wants and needs. Mary made me realize that I was trying to help her do just that—be herself again.

Discussion Questions

1. What did the student therapist identify as problems for this person?
2. What were some of the conflicts that the student therapist experienced in coming to her decisions about intervention?
3. How do you feel about the resolution of the problem(s)?
4. Can you identify features of procedural, interactive, conditional, or narrative reasoning?
5. What implicit or explicit occupational therapy values emerge in this story?

■ WANDA ■
by Rebecca Reis

For some unknown reason, people named Wanda usually have a lot of character. The Wanda in this story is certainly no exception. I met her during my Level II physical dysfunction affiliation in the out-patient department of a large general hospital in Boston.

I spend the first 6 weeks of my affiliation working on the spinal cord injury (SCI) unit and had recently transferred to the outpatient department. I was experiencing some difficulty adjusting to the faster pace of the world of outpatient therapists. Patients arrived on the hour for their appointments, and left an hour later after their treatment. If someone was a half-hour late for a treatment session, that patient might end up being treated simultaneously with another patient. It could really turn into a juggling act, and did quite regularly. This was notably different to life on the (SCI) unit, where patients lived in the hospital for months on end.

This new environment into which I was struggling to assimilate lacked the intimacy of the SCI unit. My caseload was twice the size and all the hand and wrist injuries seemed to blend together. I felt as if the patients were coming to me for an hour of service and they wanted to leave feeling like they had gotten their money's worth. My supervisor seemed to manage it all so easily; she could do all the procedural necessities and still manage to have personal and interesting conversations with each patient she treated.

I was feeling quite challenged and in conflict because of all of this when my supervisor informed me that I would be picking up one of her patients named Wanda. She told me, "I've been seeing Ms. _____

for a few weeks now; she had a Colles' fracture and is doing fairly well. You should have no problems with her. Take a look at her chart when you get a chance.'' I looked at her chart and her treatment plan seemed relatively straightforward: "Begin with fluidotherapy, followed by some range of motion exercises, retrograde massage, strengthening exercises on the BTE, and finish up with a few minutes of cryostim." That seemed simple enough. I would see her twice a week for 45 minutes.

When Wanda first walked into the clinic, she certainly made an impression. She is a tall, middle-aged, black woman with "big" hair. She was wearing red, heart-shaped sunglasses, tight polyester slacks, a bright floral blouse, and an exceptionally supportive brassiere, which lifted her chest, causing it to be quite conspicuous. We politely introduced ourselves, and I escorted Wanda to the treatment table, where we sat down and began to discuss her course of treatment.

My supervisor had informed her that I would be taking over her treatment and she seemed to have no qualms about this. She was a pleasant woman, quiet, and courteous. I inquired about how she was managing at home in her current condition. She indicated that she was having no major problems, just minor inconveniences with things like opening jars and carrying heavy items. I examined her wrist, trying to get a sense of her abilities and limitations, and then proceeded to carry out the rest of her usual treatment. We ended the session with the customary formalities, and she went out to the reception area to schedule her next appointment. I wrote up a quick progress note and continued with the rest of my day.

This scenario was typical of the next five or six sessions I had with Wanda. She always wore some sort of bizarre outfit, and our conversations usually centered around her wrist and the progress she was making with her treatment program. This was interspersed with some small talk, but we never really had a conversation that made a significant impression on me until my last appointment with Wanda.

I had informed all of my patients that the last week of my affiliation was approaching. As for Wanda, I knew that she did not require much more therapy for her wrist. She would probably be seen one or two more times by my supervisor after I left, then be discharged. The last week arrived, as did my last appointment with Wanda.

It was a relatively quiet day at the clinic. Wanda walked in making her usual fashion statement. I got her set up in the fluidotherapy tank and stood next to her making some light conversation. I cannot recall how the conversation started, but before I knew it, Wanda had begun this tremendous story.

She told me about a time when she was going on a trip and she was in a bus station. She said, "A girlfriend of mine always told me that I should write a book about all that I have been through. So I went into the ladies room at the bus station and took a huge stack of paper towels out of the dispenser and went out to get on the bus. I started writing on the paper towels about when I was a little girl and how my daddy and my uncle used to come into my room late at night, and how I always thought that my mother hated me. I thought this all my life." She proceeded to tell me all about her family and her past. She talked about being an alcoholic and a drug addict and being in rehab for a very long time. She described feeling like she was going to die and what an awful experience this was for her. She talked at great length about her mother and how she felt that her mother hated her. She talked of the moment that she confided this to her mother, only to find out how much her mother had truly loved her all those years. She talked and talked just like she had probably written for miles that day. I was stunned. I couldn't get a word in, nor did I know what to say anyhow.

The story finally tapered off, and we segued into a discussion of how the whole "family values" political campaign rhetoric was such a joke. We had reached this completely different level of communication. Here we were talking about politics and our feelings about important issues. I am still perplexed about what prompted this catharsis.

I was struck by the insignificance of a Colles' fracture in the scheme of this woman's life. It began to make sense why she had always seemed so indifferent to my questions about how she was managing at home with her wrist. We ended our session. I thanked Wanda for talking with me and expressed how much I had enjoyed working with her. I wished her luck and she went on her way.

I didn't know what to do with all this information in my head and I'm still not quite sure what to make of it.

Discussion Questions

1. What did the student therapist identify as problems for this person?
2. What were some of the conflicts that the student therapist experienced in coming to her decisions about intervention?
3. How do you feel about the resolution of the problem(s)?
4. Can you identify features of procedural, interactive, conditional or narrative reasoning?
5. What implicit or explicit occupational therapy values emerge in this story?

■ BINGO ■

by Kristen Hick

Bingo. This was the game of the week, or shall I say the game of every day of the week. A favorite of clients, abhorred by staff, these groups were the domain of the student OTs. Not only did the clients have the chance to join the weekly bingo group on Friday afternoons, but if they were in the Socialization Focus group, bingo was the rule every Wednesday morning. The purpose of this focus group was to promote interaction among clients during the group, throughout their day at the center, and in their free time. Wednesday meetings had traditionally been set aside for interactive games, and bingo had become the favorite and expected game of the members. (Enter new, energetic, going-to-change-the-world OT student from Tufts.)

Well, here I was, the new face in the group, one who had decided to observe and keep quiet—for a little while at least. As I observed these weekly sessions of bingo in the socialization group, it struck me that really no interaction was occurring between clients. In fact, the only person in the room who was vocal was the one client in charge of calling out the numbers. As in any traditional bingo game, the participants must keep quiet in order to hear the correct numbers being called. So much for interaction! The silence in the room became deafening to me.

Finally, I broached this subject with the two other staff members who had been running this group for 2 years. I voiced my concerns that bingo was not a social game and it was defeating the purpose of this focus group and the individual goals of the clients. I was shaking in my shoes. I had just questioned the methods used by two experienced therapists to promote interaction in their group, methods that had never been questioned or changed since the formation of the group 2 years before. (Of course I didn't know this at the time.)

My premise was this: Socialization is important for the members of this group, yet it is extremely difficult for these individuals, even in the protection of their peers. If the goal for the group as a whole was to increase interaction and promote socialization within the group, so that these could be carried over into their individual private lives, activities should revolve around communication and working together. I proposed that activities for this group should have a two-level purpose: to provide individuals with the opportunity to work on their personal goals around socialization, and to provide the group as a unit the chance to work on a group goal to promote interaction, group unity, and peer support.

As everyone knows, change is not usually welcomed and can create anxiety. In this instance, both staff members agreed with the reasoning behind my suggestions, but neither wanted to be responsible for "rocking the boat" with the clients. We even had discussions as to who this change was for—was it for the therapists, to make us feel better that we were really "doing our jobs," trying to promote change, and helping clients to function better in the community? Were we neglecting the fact that the clients were happy with the way the group was being run and that they enjoyed their bingo and it was their group? Should we let the status quo rule? Personally, I felt the change needed to be made. Of course, it was much easier for the leaders of the group to let bingo continue—they didn't have to do anything during that group time because the clients did the calling and played the game independently! What could be easier for a group leader than to sit back and observe? That's a pretty enticing way to spend Wednesday mornings for "overworked" staff. Of course, now they had to deal with the newest co-leader of their group . . . a budding OT student fresh out of group theory class and dying to try some new activities with their perfectly happy bingo crowd. Anyway, I got my first chance to design an activity to change the bingo tradition of Wednesday mornings.

Of course, the catch to this seemingly great opportunity was that I had to break it to the clients and suffer their wrath. This was OK with me, because I figured since I was new and not real familiar yet, these clients would at least humor me initially. I figured I could handle the moans and groans and protests because they would love my activity! I was half right.

What better activity to promote interaction, group unity, creativity, communication, socialization and fun, than a scavenger hunt?! This was my activity. I spent a week devising lists of items and scoring techniques for each item retrieved. I even picked out prizes for each team as an incentive to really participate. I knew this was going to be a hit!

Doomsday arrived and I walked into the room with a manila file of papers and a handful of pens—no bingo cards, marker bottles, or calling squares. The clients became restless. A few pointedly asked where the bingo materials were. The other staff members looked at me with wary eyes. I flashed the biggest, brightest smile I could.

As I introduced the activity of the day and explained why there would be no bingo, the expected moans and groans arrived, but I was determined. I asked the clients to try this new activity, and proposed that we end group 10 minutes early so that they would have the opportunity to give me some feedback on the activity, and their feelings about it, and then we could discuss the continuation of bingo.

With a little prodding and verbal cuing, the scavenger hunt began and most of the clients participated—actually more than I had anticipated seemed to enjoy the game. Some openly refused to do anything, but they expressed their opinions and that was a form of communication. So though I tried to get them involved, I eventually accepted their verbal refusal—for that week. Actually, I was pleasantly surprised with the outcome and had high hopes of ridding this group of bingo forever.

After the items were collected, scores given, and prizes awarded, it was time for feedback. I held my breath and asked the clients for their honest opinions on the activity (not an easy task). Many voiced their approval, a few said nothing, and some enjoyed the change on this day but wanted bingo back. There was no mutiny, no walk-outs, and few raised voices. I was thrilled! We discussed the possibility of doing different activities each week and finally came up with a compromise with the die-hard bingo players. (This whole process took more than 1 week of negotiating). Bingo would be held twice a month, but members had to sit at different tables each session and the game would end 10 minutes early for socialization time with the players at each table. The other two Wednesdays in the month would be left open for different activities planned, in part, by the clients themselves. Needless to say, I was very pleased with this outcome. My co-leaders were satisfied and offered support as Wednesday activities became my project. I was able to bounce ideas off them (although I should add, they were not OTs so they didn't always follow my reasoning for some activities!), and they were present on Wednesdays to help handle the occasional refusals and general discontent.

The summer continued with few revolts about the lost bingo sessions. Some of our activities included making murals, going out for coffee, and planning and giving a party. Not every activity was a hit, and I learned how to better handle criticism and use feedback. I don't know if this new tradition continued after I left, but it was great to see the interaction among members increase during these different activities. For me, this change in protocol for the socialization focus group was a chance worth taking.

Discussion Questions

1. What did the student therapist identify as problems for this group?
2. What were some of the conflicts that the student therapist experienced in coming to her decisions about intervention?
3. How do you feel about the resolution of the problem(s)?
4. Can you identify features of procedural, interactive, conditional or narrative reasoning?
5. What implicit or explicit occupational therapy values emerge in this story?

■ BILLY ■
by Stephanie Foster

I was sitting in the subway station waiting for the train when I recognized a familiar face. In a city where I travel on the subway daily and remain anonymous, running into a person with whom I had constant contact for 3 months is a rare occurrence. However, I immediately recognized this person as a former patient from Oak Hill Hospital, and one whose case I had grown to know quite well during my affiliation there last summer.

Knowing this person as I did—his vulnerabilities, strengths, and weaknesses—I waited for him to recognize me, and feel comfortable with acknowledging me.

Billy B. saw me and in his reserved manner said, "Hello, are you still working at Oak Hill?" Relieved, I explained to him that I was at Oak Hill last summer doing my 3-month affiliation and that I was currently still in school. I sensed his unease in running into me, and was in touch with my discomfort as well. The subway rumbled into the station and I said good-by, losing sight of him in the crowd of people that gathered around the door.

Last summer, as a fledgling occupational therapist, my judgment would not have been as good. Some of the discomfort I felt toward this patient stemmed from the fact that I had indeed identified with him somewhat last summer, and struggled with setting boundaries, separating myself from his mental illness, and treating him as a patient.

Billy was a 20-year-old African-American undergraduate student at the National Technology Institute, hospitalized at Oak Hill because he attempted suicide. He was diagnosed with major depression and obsessive-compulsive disorder, and his treatment included a medication evaluation, psychotherapy, and rehabilitation. He was an unusual patient in that his insurance covered him for 365 days of hospital care, and he was struggling with issues surrounding his major in school, independence and separation from his family, and his father's values and ideas of what was good for him, problems with isolation and social withdrawal, and his racial identity.

While on the unit, Billy was expected to partake in all occupational therapy activities, although attendance in groups was not mandatory for any patient. At one point, since it was believed he was progressing, Billy had gained the privilege of walking on the grounds alone. This privilege was taken away when he revealed ways in which he was considering hurting himself on the grounds of the hospital.

During the time he was confined to the locked unit, Billy isolated himself by refusing to attend any groups, to complete projects, or to interact with others on the unit. He was often found alone, in his room, reading. Attendance in group activities would treat his isolation, obsessive-compulsive behavior, and depression since he would be identifying with others, moving on by completing projects, and identifying a wider range of social and leisure skills and activities.

At one point in his hospitalization, Billy had continued to refuse to partake in any activities on the unit. One afternoon I approached him, while he was alone reading in his room, to explain the benefit he would gain from attending occupational therapy groups. At the end of our conversation, which lasted about 20 minutes, Billy, who was always reserved and quietly behaved, mumbled a plan he was devising to leave the unit. I could barely ascertain from his mumbling that he was planning to walk down the hill to Barclay Square and catch the bus which would take him to Glenside Square. At that point, he continued, he could walk across the bridge to the National Technology Institute and go to his fraternity, where he was living while at school.

When Billy expressed this plan, I was alerted and explained to him that he did not have ground privileges and was confined to the unit. Furthermore, I told him that if he wanted to leave the hospital, he could apply for off-ground privileges the next morning in rounds. I thought the issue was settled and it did not occur to me to report any threat of elopement to the nursing staff or to my supervisor.

The next morning when I arrived at work, I was notified that Billy had lost all privileges, was on 5-minute checks, and confined to one wing of the unit because he had eloped the night before. He had managed to leave the locked unit and proceed with his plan to go to the National Technology Institute. Once there, someone in authority there notified Oak Hill as to Billy's whereabouts and he was safely returned to the unit.

In rounds the next morning, I learned that no one on the unit, including professional nursing staff and mental health workers, had taken Billy's plan and threats to elope seriously. Apparently, he had gone as far as to approach the nursing station with a map in his hand and had stood in front of nurses and staff asking directions and mumbling about his plan.

I felt relieved to learn that nursing staff on the unit had also learned of Billy's plan to elope and believed they had dealt with him adequately. Nevertheless, I felt terrible because I had not reported his plan to the staff or my supervisor, and felt compelled to confess in rounds the conversation I had with Billy the day before.

Luckily, Billy survived the elopement unharmed and was safely back at Oak Hill. In retrospect, I see that I was inclined to treat Billy as a "person" and not view him as a diagnosis. Perhaps I was partially unable to accept the fact that this affable, bright young man, who attended the National Technology Institute, had a serious illness and was involved with issues of life and death. In retrospect, by staging his elopement, I believe he was crying out for attention, perhaps something he perceived he was not getting from staff at Oak Hill Hospital.

Billy remained on the unit at Oak Hill for some weeks after my affiliation ended. When I left, he was partaking in more occupational therapy groups, interacting, and broadening his repertoire of leisure activities. In addition, he was taking a semester off from school, and making a transition back to his regular activities by living in a halfway house.

When I met Billy on the subway 3 months later, he was, in fact, free to travel in the city, as he was living in the halfway house. It was good to see him, although I was still uncertain as to how to separate myself from him professionally.

Discussion Questions

1. What did the student therapist identify as problems for this person?
2. What were some of the conflicts that the student therapist experienced in coming to her decisions about intervention?
3. How do you feel about the resolution of the problem(s)?
4. Can you identify features of procedural, interactive, conditional or narrative reasoning?
5. What implicit or explicit occupational therapy values emerge in this story?

■ ANNA ■
by Beth Bernstein

I met Anna Krementz (not her real name) in August of 1992, when she was admitted to M1, a locked inpatient psychiatric unit. She was a 42-year-old divorced white woman, diagnosed with bipolar disorder.

She was admitted after overdosing on her meds. Her depression was exacerbated by financial pressures. Her 17-year-old son was expecting to start college in the fall, and she had not been able to raise the money to send him. She had asked her father to lend her some money, but he had refused, apparently perpetuating a lifelong pattern of letting her down.

Anna had worked in the state mental system for years as a counselor and was pursuing a master's degree at that time. She had thought of herself as creative and had enjoyed various crafts in the past. At that point, she had not felt creative or resourceful for quite a while, and instead she was overwhelmed with feelings of incompetence and a lack of control over her life—especially in the financial realm.

I did the initial interview when Anna was admitted. We tried to do some problem solving about how she could start to regain control

of her life and her feelings. She had immediate concerns that her medications were affecting her memory, and I helped her to contact her
doctor immediately to investigate that possibility. This seemed to help
build an initial bond—that I took her concerns seriously and helped
her to take some action.

I identified with her in many ways. She was a professional woman
with vocational and avocational interests similar to my own. She was
trying to juggle the roles of mother/worker/student, and had a problem
with overcommitting and then feeling guilty about not being able to
follow through. She was also rather quiet, gentle, and caring—a pleasant
person to be with. There were parts of her background that came out
that I was fortunate not to have shared, such as parental physical and
substance abuse. The fact that she was usually able to function as well
as she did filled me with a sense of awe, and of hope that things would
improve again for her.

We began to meet informally and chat. She was initially quite
isolative. She felt out of place, self-conscious, embarrassed about what
she had done, and the fact that she was hospitalized. She didn't want
any part of going to groups or interacting with other patients on the
unit. I reminded her each day that we would like to see her in groups
when she was ready. I had tailored her group schedule to her needs as
I saw them, and had discussed my rationale with her. I tried to minimize
the pressure, but make the options clear.

Considering her past interest in crafts, I had especially hoped that
she would attend a rather new "crafts group" that I was running. This
was the first group that she showed up for. We were decorating painter's
caps with fabric markers that day. I explained the project and she initially declined to participate. Eventually, after I left the supplies in
front of her and tended to some other patients for a while, she quietly
became engrossed in the task. She drew a garden scene with bright
flowers growing, roots to blooms, and delicate greenery.

When I spoke to her as the group was ending and commented on
the positive theme, she expressed surprise. She said that it was the first
art work she had done in a few years in anything besides grays and
browns. She got lots of reinforcement from the group about her project
and seemed truly pleased by her accomplishment. She opted to take it
to her room immediately. It seemed symbolic of her hope . . . that she
would blossom as well.

This marked the beginning of a dramatic difference in her behavior
on the unit. She began to attend all of her assigned groups and became
an active participant on the unit, encouraging her peers to participate.
She became a strong ally in rallying support for OT's efforts in particular, and the welfare of the unit in general.

Certainly other factors were at work here as well: her meds were
better stabilized each day and she had time to become acclimated and

come to terms with her situation. However, the task did tap into an existing strength and start her on what seemed to be a healing path to increased satisfaction, self-confidence, and self-expression.

Discussion Questions

1. What did the student therapist identify as problems for this person?
2. What were some of the conflicts that the student therapist experienced in coming to her decisions about intervention?
3. How do you feel about the resolution of the problem(s)?
4. Can you identify features of procedural, interactive, conditional or narrative reasoning?
5. What implicit or explicit occupational therapy values emerge in this story?

Bibliography

Aristotle. (1985). *Nicomachean ethics.* Indianapolis, IN: Hackett Publishing.

Arendt, H. (1958). *The human condition.* Chicago: University of Chicago Press.

Argyris, C., & Schön, D. A. (1981). *Theory in practice: Increasing professional effectiveness.* San Francisco: Josey-Bass.

Ayres, A. J. (1972). *Sensory integration and learning disorders.* Los Angeles: Western Psychological Services.

Barthes, R. (1975). An introduction to the structural analysis of narrative. *New Literary History,* 6:237–272.

Barthes, R. (1977). Introduction to the structural analysis of narrative. In: S. Heath (Ed. and Trans.), *Image, music, text.* New York: Hill & Wang.

Bateson, G. (1972). *Steps to an ecology of mind.* New York: Ballantine Books.

Bauman, R. (1986). *Story performance and event.* Cambridge, UK: Cambridge University Press.

Bauman, Z. (1978). *Hermeneutics and social science.* New York: Columbia University Press.

Belenky, M. F., Clinchy, B. M., Goldberger, N. R., & Tarule, J. M. (1986). *Woman's ways of knowing.* New York: Basic Books.

Benner, P. (1984). *From novice to expert: Excellence and power in clinical nursing practice.* Reading, MA: Addison-Wesley.

Benner, P., & Tanner, C. (1987). Clinical judgement: How expert nurses use intuition. *American Journal of Nursing,* 87:23–31.

Berger, P. L., & Luckmann, T. (1967). *The social construction of reality.* Garden City, NY: Doubleday.

Bernstein, R. J. (1971). *Praxis and action.* Philadelphia: University of Pennsylvania Press.

Bing, R. (1981). Occupational therapy revisited: A paraphrastic journey. *American Journal of Occupational Therapy,* 35:499–518.

Bourdieu, P. (1977). *Outline of a theory of practice.* Cambridge, UK: Cambridge University Press.

Bradburn, S. L. (1992). *Psychiatric occupational therapists' strategies for engaging patients in treatment during the initial interview.* Unpublished master's thesis, Tufts University, Medford, MA.

Bruner, J. (1986). *Actual minds, possible worlds.* Boston: Harvard University Press.

Bruner, J. (1990). *Acts of meaning.* Cambridge, MA: Harvard University Press.

Buchler, J. (1955). *Nature and judgement.* New York: Grosset & Dunlap/Solidus Columbia University Press.

Bunge, M. (1967). *Scientific research I: The search system.* New York: Springer-Verlag.

Burke, K. (1945). *A grammar of motives.* Berkeley, CA: University of California Press.

Burrell, D., & Hauerwas, S. (1977). *From system to story: An alternative pattern for rationality in ethics.* In T. Engelhardt & D. Callahan (Eds.), *Knowledge value and belief.* Hastings-on-Hudson, NY: The Hastings Center.

Christiansen, C. (1991). Occupational therapy intervention for life performance. In C. Christiansen & C. Baum (Eds.), *Occupational therapy: Overcoming human performance deficits.* Thorofare, NJ: Slack Incorporated.

Christiansen, C., & Baum, C. (Eds.). (1991). *Occupational therapy: Overcoming human performance deficits.* Thorofare, NJ: Slack Incorporated.

Crepeau, E. B. (1991). Achieving intersubjective understanding: Examples from an occupational therapy treatment session. *American Journal of Occupational Therapy, 45:*1016–1025.

Cohn, E. S. (1989). Fieldwork education: Shaping a foundation for clinical reasoning. *American Journal of Occupational Therapy, 43:*240–244.

Coughlin, L., & Patel, V. (1987). Processing of critical information by physicians and medical students. *Journal of Medical Education, 62:*818–828.

Csikszentmihalyi, M. (1975). *Beyond boredom and anxiety: The experience of play in work and game.* San Francisco: Jossey-Bass.

Cutter, P. (1979). *Problem solving in clinical medicine: From data to diagnosis.* Baltimore: Williams & Wilkins.

DelVecchio Good, M. J., Good, B., Schaffer, C., & Lind, S. E. (1990). American oncology and the discourse on hope. *Culture, Medicine and Psychiatry, 14:*59.

DelVecchio Good, M. J. et al. (1992). *Oncology & narrative time.* (in press).

DelVecchio Good, M. J., Hunt, L., Manakato, T., & Kobayashi, Y. (in press). A comparative analysis of the culture of biomedicine: Disclosure and consequences for treatment in the practice of oncology. In P. Conrad & E. Gallagher (Eds.), *Medical care in the developing world.* Philadelphia: Temple University Press.

Dewey, J. (1915). The logic of judgements of practice. *Journal of Philosophy. 12:*505.

Dewey, J. (1916). *Essays in experimental logic.* New York: Dover Publications.

Dewey, J. (1929). *Experience and nature.* New York: W. W. Norton.

Dewey, J. (1934). *Art as experience.* New York: Minton, Balch & Co.

Dreyfus, H. L. (1972). *What computers can't do.* New York: Harper Colophon Books.

Dreyfus, H., & Dreyfus S. (1986). *Mind over machine: The power of human intuition and expertise in the era of the computer.* New York: The Free Press.

Elstein, A. S., Shulman, L. S., & Sprafka, S. A. (1978). *Medical problem solving: An analysis of clinical reasoning.* Cambridge, MA: Harvard University Press.

Engelhardt, T. (1977). Defining occupational therapy: The meaning of therapy and the virtues of occupation. *American Journal of Occupational Therapy, 31:*666–672.

Erikson, E. (1968). *Identity use and crisis.* New York: W. W. Norton.

Feinstein, A. (1973a). An analysis of diagnostic reasoning, I. *Yale Journal of Biology and Medicine, 46:*212–232.

Feinstein, A. (1973b). An analysis of diagnostic reasoning, II. *Yale Journal of Biology and Medicine, 46:*264–282.

Feinstein, A. (1974). An analysis of diagnostic reasoning, III. *Yale Journal of Biology and Medicine, 1:*5–32.

Fidler, G., & Fidler, J. (1963). *Occupational therapy: A communication process in psychiatry.* New York: Macmillan.

Fidler, G. & Fidler, J. (1978). Doing and becoming: Purposeful action and self-actualization. *American Journal of Occupational Therapy. 32:*305–310.

Fleming, M. H. (1989). The therapist with the three-track mind. *The AOTA Practice Symposium Program Guide.* Rockville, MD: The American Occupational Therapy Association, Inc.

Fleming, M. H. (Ed.). (1990). Proceedings of the institute on clinical reasoning for occupational therapy. *Educators.* Meford, MA: Clinical Reasoning Institute, Tufts University.

Fleming, M. H. (1991a). Clinical reasoning in medicine compared with clinical reasoning in occupational therapy. *American Journal of Occupational Therapy,* 45:988–996.

Fleming, M. H. (1991b). The therapist with the three-track mind. *American Journal of Occupational Therapy,* 45:1007–1014.

Foucault, M. (1972). *The archeology of knowledge.* (A. M. Sheridan Smith, Trans.). London, England: Tavistock Publications.

Foucault, M. (1973). *The birth of the clinic: An archeology of medical perception.* New York: Pantheon Books.

Foucault, M. (1979). *Discipline and punish: The birth of the prison.* New York: Vintage Books.

Freda, M. (1990) *The Story of Ann.* Medford, MA: Clinical Reasoning Institute, Tufts University.

Gardner, H. (1985). *Frames of mind: The theory of multiple intelligences.* New York: Basic Books.

Geertz, C. (1983). *Local knowledge: Further essays in interpretive anthropology.* New York: Basic Books.

Gilligan, C. (1982). *In a different voice.* Cambridge, MA: Harvard University Press.

Goffman, E. (1963). *Stigma: Notes on the management of spoiled identity.* Englewood, NJ: Prentice-Hall.

Goldberg, L. R. (1970). Man versus model of man: A rationale, plus some evidence for a method of improving on clinical inferences. *Psychological Bulletin,* 73:422–432.

Good, B. (1977). The heart of what's the matter: The semantics of illness in Iran. *Culture, Medicine and Psychiatry,* 1:25–28.

Good, B. (in press). Medicine, rationality and experience: An anthropological perspective. Cambridge, UK: Cambridge University Press.

Good, B., & DelVecchio Good, M. J. (1985). *The cultural context of diagnosing and therapy.* Unpublished manuscript.

Good, B., & Delvecchio Good, M. J. (1980). The meaning of symptoms: A cultural hermeneutic model for clinical practice. In: I. Eisenberg, & A. Kleinman (Eds.), *The relevance of social science for medicine.* Norwell, MA: D. Reidel.

Greeno, J. G. (1989). A perspective on thinking. *American Psychologist,* 44:134–141.

Hammond, K. R. (1988). Judgment and decision making in dynamic tasks. *Information and Decision-Making Technologies,* 14:3–14.

Hayes, M. F. (1978). *Toward a theory of clinical judgement.* Unpublished doctoral dissertation. Boston University, Boston, MA.

Heidegger, M. (1962). *Being and time* (E. Robinson & J. Macquarrie, Trans.). New York: Harper & Row.

Hopkins, H. L., & Smith, H. D. (1990). *Willard & Spackman's occupational therapy* (7th ed.). Philadelphia: J. B. Lippincott.

Hunt, L. (1992). *Practicing oncology in provincial Mexico: A narrative analysis.* Manuscript submitted for publication.

Iser, W. (1978). *The act of reading.* Baltimore: Johns Hopkins University Press.

Kassirer, J. P., Kuipers, B. J., & Gorry, G. A. (1982). Toward a theory of clinical expertise. *American Journal of Medicine,* 73:251–259.

Kegan, R. (1982). *The evolving self: Problems and process in human development.* Cambridge, MA: Harvard University Press.

Kermode, F. (1966). *The sense of an ending: Studies in the theory of fiction.* London: Oxford University Press.

Kessera, J. (1989) Diagnostic Reasoning. *Annals of Internal Medicine,* 110:893–900.

Kestenbaum, V. (1982). *The humanity of the ill: Phenomenological perspectives.* Knoxville: University of Tennessee Press.

Kestenbaum, V. (1977). *The phenomonological sense of John Dewey: Habit and meaning.* Atlantic Highlands, NJ: Humanities Press.

Kielhofner, G., & Burke, J. (1977). Occupational therapy after 60 years: An account of changing identity and knowledge. *American Journal of Occupational Therapy,* 31:675–689.

Kleinman, A., Eisenberg, L., & Good, B. (1978). Culture, illness, and care: Clinical lessons from anthropologic and cross-cultural research. *Annals of Internal Medicine,* 88:251–258.

Kleinman, A. (1980). *Patients and healers in the context of culture.* Los Angeles: University of California Press.

Kleinman, A. (1988). *The illness narratives: Suffering, healing, and the human condition.* New York: Basic Books.

Koestler, A. (1948). *Insight and outlook: An inquiry into the common foundations of science, art and social ethics.* Lincoln, NE: University of Nebraska Press.

Koestler, A. (1967). *The ghost in the machine.* Chicago: Henry Regnery.

Kuhn, T. (1962). *The structure of scientific revolutions.* Chicago: University of Chicago Press.

Labov, W., & Waletzky, J. (1967). Narrative analysis: Oral versions of personal experience. In: J. Helm (Ed.), *Essays in the verbal & visual arts.* Seattle: University of Washington Press for the American Ethnological Society.

Langthaler, M. (1990). *The components of therapeutic relationship in occupational therapy.* Unpublished master's thesis. Tufts University, Medford, MA.

Lau, J., Kassirer, J. P., & Pauker, S. G. (1983). Decision maker 3.0: Improved decision analysis by personal computer. *Medical Decision Making,* 3:39–43.

Leder, D. (1984). Medicine and paradigms of embodiment. *Journal of Medicine and Philosophy,* 9:29–44.

Levine, R. (1987). The influence of the arts and crafts movement on the professional status of occupational therapy. *American Journal of Occupational Therapy,* 41:248–254.

Llorenz, L. A., & Rubin, E. Z., (1967). *Developing ego functions in disturbed children.* Detroit, MI: Wayne State University Press.

Lusted, L. B. (1968). *Introduction to medical decision making.* Springfield, IL: Charles C Thomas.

Mattingly, C. (1989). *Thinking with stories: Story and experience in a clinical practice.* Unpublished doctoral dissertation, Massachusetts Institute of Technology, Cambridge, MA.

Mattingly, C. (1991). The narrative nature of clinical reasoning. *American Journal of Occupational Therapy,* 45:998–1005.

Mattingly, C., & Gillette, N. (1991). Anthropology, occupational therapy, and action research. *American Journal of Occupational Therapy,* 45:972–978.

Mauss, M. (1967). *The gift: Forms and functions of exchange in archaic societies* (I. Cunnison, Trans.) New York: W. W. Norton.

Meehl, P. E. (1954). *Clinical versus statistical prediction.* Minneapolis: University of Minnesota Press.

Merleau-Ponty, M. (1962). *Phenomenology of perception.* London: Routledge & Kegan Paul.

Merleau-Ponty, M. (1963). *The structure of behavior.* (A. L. Fisher, Trans.) Boston: Beacon Press.

Meyer, A. (1977). The philosophy of occupational therapy. *American Journal of Occupational Therapy,* 31:639–642.

Mosey, A. C. (1970). *Three frames of reference for mental health.* Thorofare, NJ: C. B. Slack.

Murphy, R. (1987). *The body silent.* New York: Henry Holt & Company.

Newell, A., & Simon, H. (1972). *Human problem solving.* Englewood Cliffs, NJ: Prentice-Hall.

Nussbaum, M. (1990). *Love's knowedge.* New York: Oxford University Press.

Paget, M. A. (1988). *The unity mistakes.* Philadelphia: Temple University Press.

Papa, F. J., Shores, J. H., & Mayer, S. (1990). Effects of pattern matching, pattern discrimination and experience in the development of diagnostic expertise. *Academic Medicine,* 65:21–22.

Parham, D. (1987). Toward professionalism: The reflective therapist. *American Journal of Occupational Therapy,* 41:555–561.

Perry, W. (1979). *Forms of intellectual and ethical development in the college years.* New York: Holt, Rinehart & Winston.

Pierce, C. S. (1931–1935). *Collected papers of Charles Sanders Pierce* (Vols. 1–6). (C. Hartshorne & D. Weiss, Eds.). Cambridge, MA: Harvard University Press.

Polanyi, M. (1966). *The tacit dimension.* Garden City, NY: Doubleday.

Polanyi, M. (1958). *Personal knowledge: Towards a post-critical philosophy.* Chicago: University of Chicago Press.

Polanyi, M. (1974). *Personal knowledge: Towards a post-critical philosophy.* (Fifth Impression). Chicago: University of Chicago Press.

Propp, V. (1968). *Morphology of the folk tale.* Austin, TX: University of Texas Press.

Raiffa, H. (1970). *Decision analysis: Introductory lectures on choices under uncertainty.* Reading, MA: Addison-Wells.

Ricoeur, P. (1981). *Hermeneutics and the human sciences: Essays on language, action, and interpretation.* In: John B. Thompson (Ed.), *The function of narrative.* Cambridge, UK: Cambridge University Press.

Ricoeur, P. (1984). *Time and narrative:* Vol. 1. Chicago: University of Chicago Press.

Ricoeur, P. (1985). *Time and narrative,* vol III. Chicago: University of Chicago Press.

Rogers, C. (1961). *On becoming a person.* Boston: Houghton-Mifflin.

Rogers, J. C. (1982a). Educating the inquisitive practitioner. *Occupational Therapy Journal of Research,* 2:4–11.

Rogers, J. C. (1982b). The spirit of independence: The evolution of a philosophy. *American Journal of Occupational Therapy,* 36:709–715.

Rogers, J. C. (1983). Clinical reasoning: The ethics, science, and art. *American Journal of Occupational Therapy,* 37:601–616.

Rogers, J. C., & Holm, M. B. (1991). Occupational therapy diagnostic reasoning: A component of clinical reasoning. *American Journal of Occupational Therapy,* 45:1045–1053.

Rogers, J. C., & Kielhofner, G. (1983). Treatment planning. In G. Kielhofner (Ed.). *A model of human occupation: Theory and Application* (pp. 136–146). Baltimore: Williams & Wilkins.

Rogers, J. C., & Masagatani, G. (1982). Clinical reasoning of occupational therapists during the initial assessment of physically disabled patients. *The Occupational Therapy Journal of Research*, 2:195–219.

Sacks, O. (1984). *A leg to stand on*. New York: Summit Books.

Sacks, O. (1987). *The man who mistook his wife for a hat and other clinical tales*. New York: Perennial Library.

Schön, D. (1983). *The reflective practitioner: How professionals think in action*. New York: Basic Books.

Schön, D. (1987). *Educating the reflective practitioner*. San Francisco: Jossey-Bass.

Schutz, A. (1975). *On phenomenology and social relations*. Chicago: University of Chicago Press.

Siegler, C. C. (1987). *Functions of humor in occupational therapy*. Unpublished master's thesis, Tufts University: Medford, MA.

Smith, J. E. (1971). Being immediacy and articulation. *Review of Metaphysics*, 24:593–613.

Sontag, S. (1988). *Illness as metaphor*. New York: Farrar, Strauss & Giroux.

Starr, P. (1982). *The second transformation of American medicine*. New York: Basic Books.

Swets, Tanner, Birdsall (1961). Decision process in perception. *Psychological Review*, 68:3–1–340.

West, W. (1989, June 9–11). *Keynote address*. Directions for the Future Workshop, Chapel Hill, NC.

Yankelovich, D., & Barrett, W. (1970). *Ego and instinct: The psychoanalytic view of human nature—revised*. New York: Random House.

Index

Action. *See also* Activity(ies)
episodes within clinical encounter, structured into coherent plot, 246
inquiry and, confluence of, 342
judgment and, 25, 332–333, 342
meaning and, 16, 94, 198–201. *See also* Meaning(s)
phenomenological sense of, 224
observation and, interpretation and, 320–322
occupational therapy's view of, problems with, 210–212
phenomenology and, 65, 224
practical theory guiding, 23
reasoning and, 316
thinking in, 322–324
Action-centered therapy, 264–265
Action research, 7
ethnographic approach combined with, 5–6
Active collaboration. *See* Collaboration
Active judgments, 25, 332–333, 342
Activity(ies). *See also* Action
choice and
intentionality and, 201–212
multiple reasons and, 201–202
common, in uncommon world of clinic, 111–112
engagement in, 16, 97. *See also* Engagement
everyday, meaning of, 105–108
focus on, 97
habit re-creation through, 215
meaningful, 218–221. *See also* Meaning(s)
as metaphors, 221–226
as metaphors, 221–226
motives for use of, 202–204
purposeful, processes versus, 101–102
selection of, 217–218

therapeutic, integrating phenomenological and biomechanical frames, 91–92
Adaptations, of common objects and activities, 111–112
American Occupational Therapy Association (AOTA), Clinical Reasoning Study and, 3. *See also* Clinical Reasoning Study
American Occupational Therapy Foundation (AOTF), Clinical Reasoning Study and, 3. *See also* Clinical Reasoning Study
American Pragmatist philosophy, legitimacy of practical theories and, 22–23
Analytical reasoning, intuitive reasoning versus, 123
Answer recognition, solution seeking versus, 143
AOTA. *See* American Occupational Therapy Association
AOTF. *See* American Occupational Therapy Foundation
Appraisal, 325–327
inference and, 329, 330–332
tacit, 327–328
Aristotle, practical reasoning concept of, 10–12
Artificial intelligence, 139
Arts and crafts movement, 68–70
Assessment, functional, treatment of whole person and, 74–75
Association, hypothesis postulating, 149–150
Assumptions
about decision making, occupational therapists' reasoning versus, 333–342
about patients, 8–9
Atomistic check-list approach, 49

Atomistic check-list approach—*Continued*
professional role dilemma and, 303
Authority, expertise versus, 341–342

"Because" motive, "in-order-to" motive versus, 202–204
Behavior(s)
interactive, 194–196
occupational, 48–49
Biomechanical view, 42–43
case presentation and, 61–63
in medicine, 43–46. *See also* Biomedical culture
phenomenological framework and, integration of, 91–92
treatment approaches and, 53–59
Biomedical culture
biomechanical view in, 43–46
chart talk and, 59–63
diagnostic emphasis of, 49–51. *See also* Diagnosis
case example of, 51–53
disease versus illness experience and, 37–40
case example of, 40–42
historical perspective on, 42–43
institutionalization of, 45
occupational therapy relationship to current concepts of practice and, 48–49
shifts in, 46–48
orientation of, 42–46
in occupational therapy, 46–53
professional role dilemma and, 300
prospective stories framed by, clashes with phenomenologically framed stories, 273–275
treatment approaches in, 53–59
values of, conflict between OT values and, 4
Biomedical metaphors, 42–43
Body
lived. *See* Lived-body paradigm
mechanistic view of. *See* Biomechanical view
Body space, medical problem solving and, 142

Calculation, rational, 11–12
Case examples, 343–359. *See also* specific topic

Causal relationship, hypothesis of, 149
Chart talk, 59–60
story talk and, 60–61
Check-list approach
atomistic, 49
professional role dilemma and, 303
Choice(s)
activity and
intentionality and, 201–212
multiple reasons and, 201–202
central importance of, 205–206
creation of, collaboration and, 184–186
criteria for, 204–205
offering of, rather than making decisions, 339–340
Clients. *See* Patients
Clinic, uncommon world of, 108–112
Clinical cases, description of, role of, 59–63
Clinical prediction, statistical prediction versus, 138
Clinical reasoning. *See also* Reasoning
characteristics of, common assumptions about decision making versus, 333–342
defined, 9–13
instrumental perspective and, 319
in medicine, research on, 138–139
narrative nature of, 239–269. *See also* Narrative reasoning
scientific method and, 317–324
theoretical reasoning versus, 9–10
viewed as process, 4
Clinical Reasoning Study, 3. *See also* specific topics of study
data analysis in, 7–9
data collection in, 6
definition of clinical reasoning and, 9–13
innovative features of, 5–6
phases of, 6–7
research design of, 4
sequence of events in, 6–7
site of, 6
Clinical revision, 270–271
changing stories in midstream and, 282–291
prospective stories and, 271–275
search for story and, getting lost and, 279–282
therapeutic role and, 275–279
Clinical session
demarcation into "work" and "nonwork," 299

"keeping on track," 131–132
Clinical stories, 343–359. *See also specific topic*
Cognitive processes, in clinical reasoning, 138
Cognitive space, medical problem solving and, 142
Collaboration. *See also* Interactive reasoning
  action research and, 5–6
  creation of choices and, 184–186
  encouragement of, strategies for, 184–194
  with others, 182–184
  with patient, need for, 178–182
Common objects and activities, in uncommon world of clinic, 111–112
Common sense, 16–17, 114–115
  cultural values and, 96–97. *See also* Cultural values
  Howard Gardner's notion of, 112–113
  as legitimate mode of reasoning, 112–114
  transporter role and, 114
Communication, with patients, 78–84
Community, transporting patient back to, common sense in, 114
Competing formulations, 152F
  case examples of, 160–165, 165T, 173–174
Computers, in research on clinical reasoning in medicine, 138–139
Conditional reasoning, 17–18, 121, 133–136, 197–198
  action and meaning and, 198–201
  activity, choice, and intentionality and, 201–212
  habits and meaning and, 212–221
  meaning and metaphor and, 221–226
  treatment of whole person and, 226–234
"Connected knowing," 123
Consciousness, intentionality and, 208
  engagement and, 101–102
Construction, concept of, 104–105
Continuous reasoning, sequential reasoning versus, 335–336
Cue(s)
  acquisition of
    case example of, 172
    in four-stage model of medical inquiry, 148–149, 159
  interpretation of
    case example of, 173, 174–176, 175T
    in four-stage model of medical inquiry, 150, 159–160
    in medical problem solving, 139
    nonexclusive, 156–159
Cue identification, 172
  skills in, 148–149
Cultural contexts, 37–63. *See also* Biomedical culture; Phenomenology
Cultural values
  common sense and, 96–97
  implicit and explicit, in occupational therapy, 97–98
  in practice, case example of, 98–99

Data analysis
  final stage of research and, 7
  strategies for, 7–9
Data collection, 6
Decision analysis, 138–139
Decision making
  common assumptions about, occupational therapists' reasoning versus, 333–342
  offering of choices versus, 339–340
  process of, patient inclusion in, 338–339
Deficits, discrete, emphasis on "fixing," 49, 53–59
Depth dilemma, 304–305
  case examples of, 305–307
Desire, narrative time governed by, 255–257, 265–266
Diagnosis
  accuracy of, pattern recognition and, 143–144
  biomechanical view and, 44–45
  emphasis on, 49–51
  as not separate from treatment, 335–336
  as purpose of medical problem solving, 139–140
Diagnostic confusion, clinical revision and, 279–282
Diagnostic puzzles, case example of, 51–53
Disability. *See also* Injury; Therapeutic problem(s)
  definition of, biomechanical view and, 54–55
  description of, chart talk and, 59–63
Discontinuous hypothesis generation, 336

Disease
  categorization of, biomechanical view
    and, 44
  illness experience and, 37–42. *See also*
    Illness
  patients viewed as separate from, 44–
    45. *See also* Biomechanical view
Disease-centered therapy, action-centered therapy rather than, 264–265
Distal tacit knowledge, 29
"Double binds" of good practice, 295–
  297
Dualism, chart talk and story talk and,
  60–61
Dysfunction-centered therapy, action-
  centered therapy rather than, 264–
  265

Emplotment, five elements of, 253–260
  case example of, 260–268
Empowerment, of patient, 341–342
Ending
  time dominated by, 257
  unknown, 259–260, 268
Engagement
  focus on, 97
  intentionality and, 101–102
  interactive strategies and, 124
  meaning of term, 16
Environment, task, problem space and,
  141–142, 151–153
Espoused theories, 23
Ethnographic approach, 5. *See also* Clinical Reasoning Study
  language development in, 14
Evaluation process, during treatment,
  130–133
Everyday activities. *See also* Activity(ies)
  meaning of, 105–108
Existential meaning, reframing of, in biomechanical terms, 58–59
Experience(s)
  defined, 30
  as *an* experience, 218–221
  illness. *See* Illness experience
  meaningful
    creation of. *See* Conditional reason-
      ing
    "having," 218–221
  significant, narrative and creation of,
    244–247
  tacit knowledge acquisition through,
    30

thinking in action and, 322–324
Expertise
  authority versus, 341–342
  development of, factors contributing
    to, 33–34
  professional, practical theories and,
    23–24

Fabrication, labor versus, 70
Field observations, open-ended, 6
Four-stage model of medical inquiry,
  147–150
  application to occupational therapy,
    159–160
Functional assessment, treatment of
  whole person and, 74–75
Functional limitations, addressing,
  137–173. *See also* Procedural reasoning
Functional performance, 106
Functional relationships, of initial problem formulations, 152F
Future
  function in, focus on, rather than on
    past history, 337
  narrative reasoning and. *See* Narrative
    reasoning

Gardner, Howard, common sense notion
  of, 112–113
Generalization, individualization versus,
  338. *See also* Individual, focus on
Generate-and-test method, in problem
  solving, 145–146, 146T
"Getting stuck" analyses, 8
Gift exchange, collaboration and, 190–
  193
Goals, problem solving and, 140–141
  in occupational therapy, 151–153
Good practice, "double binds" of, 295–
  297
Grand theories, 23, 24

Habits
  activity selection and, 217–218
  disruption of, in illness or injury, 214–
    217
  meaning and, 212–213
  phenomenological concept of, 213–
    214
Heuristic search, 147

Hierarchical organization, of problem formulations, 152F

History, future function versus, focus on, 337

Hospital
  institutional context of, professional image dilemma and, 297–299
  medical model and, 108
  as temporary world, 109–110

Hypothesis(es)
  competing, 152F
    case example of, 173–174
    in occupational therapy, 160–165, 165T
  evaluation of
    case example of, 176
    in four-stage model of medical inquiry, 150, 159
  generation of
    case example of, 173
    discontinuous, 336
    in four-stage model of medical inquiry, 149–150, 159

Hypothetical reasoning, example of, analysis of, 166–176, 175T

Identity, interactive reasoning and, 124–125

Illness
  habit disruption in, 214–217
  intentionality and, 207–210

Illness experience, 12, 64–66. See also Phenomenology
  diagnosis and, biomechanical view and, 44
  disease and, 37–42. See also Disease
  making sense of, narrative reasoning in, 18–21

Image, professional, dilemma of, 297–299

Images, narrative, creation of, 239–242

Implicit knowledge. See Tacit knowledge

Implicit meaning-making, 32–33

Individual, focus on, 97, 338
  collaboration and, 186–187
  intuitive reasoning and, 123
  narrative and, 247

Ineffable knowledge, 28. See also Tacit knowledge

Inference, 328–330
  appraisal and, 329, 330–332

Initial problem formulations, structural features of, 150–151, 152F

case example of, 176
in occupational therapy, 160–165, 165T

Injury. See also Disability; Illness
  habit disruption in, 214–217

"In-order-to" motive, "because" motive versus, 202–204

Inquiry, 324–325
  action and, confluence of, 342
  appraisal and, 325–328
  four-stage model of, 147–150. See Four-stage model of medical inquiry
  application to occupational therapy, 159–160
  inference and, 328–332

Institutional context, professional image dilemma and, 297–299

Instrumental rationality, 319

Intelligence
  artificial, 139
  interpersonal, 124

Intelligibility
  appraisal, 325–328
  inference, 328–332
  inquiry and, 325

Intelligible knowledge, 28. See also Tacit knowledge

Intentionality
  action and meaning and, 198–201
  choice and, activity and, 201–212
  engagement and, 101–102
  illness and, 207–210
  occupational therapy's view of, problems with, 210–212
  as strong but implicit value, 206–207

Interaction, perception of other reasoning styles during, 130–133

Interactive behaviors, 194–196

Interactive reasoning, 17, 119–120, 121–125
  active collaboration and
    with others, 182–184
    with patient, 178–182
    strategies for encouragement of, 184–194
  interactive behaviors and, 194–196
  procedural reasoning and, integration of, 125–130

Interpersonal intelligence, 124

Interpretation, 324
  of cues
    case example of, 173, 174–176, 175T

Interpretation—*Continued*
  in four-stage model of medical in-
    quiry, 150, 159–160
  observation and, action and, 320–322
Interviewing, second phase of research
    and, 6–7
Intuitive reasoning, analytical reasoning
    versus, 123

Joint problem solving, collaboration and,
    194
Judgments, active, 25, 332–333, 342

Kinesiological model, 48
Knowledge
  ineffable, 28
  intelligible, 28
  stock of, 26
  symbolic, 28
  tacit, 14–15
    search for, 22–34

Labor, fabrication versus, 70
Language
  chart talk, 59–63
  role of, 3–22
  tacit knowledge and, 28–29
Life
  quality of
    engagement and, 16
    focus on, 97
  reconstruction of, 102–105
Life-world, 100–101. *See also* "Real
    world"
  clinic world versus, 108–112
Lived-body paradigm, 64–93. *See also*
    Illness experience
  phenomenology and, 71–74
  rehabilitation of lived body and, 73–74

Machine, body viewed as. *See* Bi-
    omechanical view
Meaning(s)
  action and, 94, 198–201
    phenomenological sense of, 224
  conditional reasoning and. *See* Condi-
    tional reasoning
  of everyday activities, 105–108
  existential, reframed in biomechanical
    terms, 58–59

formulation of, 224–226
habits and, 212–213. *See also* Habits
metaphor and, 221–226
Meaningful experience, "having," 218–
    221
Meaning-making, 15–16, 94
  implicit, 32–33
Means-end rationality, 11
Mechanistic view of body. *See* Bi-
    omechanical view
Medical culture. *See* Biomedical culture
Medical inquiry, four-stage model of,
    147–150
  application to occupational therapy,
    159–160
Medical model, hospital operation and,
    108
Medical problem solving, 138–140. *See
    also* Problem solving
  problem space in, 142
Medicine, focus of, occupational therapy
    focus versus, 95–98
Meetings, importance of, chart talk and,
    59–60
Mental illness, occupational therapy
    movement and, 69–70
Metaphor(s)
  biomedical, 42–43
  meaning and, 221–226
Model of Human Occupation, 48
Monitoring process, during treatment,
    130–133
Moral Treatment movement, 46
  phenomenology and, 68–69
Motive(s)
  centrality of, human time and, 254–255
  for use of activity, 202–204
Movement, possibility of, lived-body par-
    adigm and, 72
Multiple modes of reasoning, 119–121
Multiple reasons, choices of activity and,
    201–202
Multiple subspaces, of problem formula-
    tions, 152F

Narrative images, creation of, 239–242
Narrative modes of analysis, 7–9
Narrative reasoning, 18–21
  case example of, 247–253
  clinical revision and, 270–291. *See
    also* Clinical revision
  creation of narrative images and, 239–
    242

five elements of emplotment and, 253–
260
case example of, 260–268
prospective stories and, 241–243
changing, 271–275
treatment structure and, 243–247
Narrative time, features of, 253–254
case example of, 260–268
centrality of motive, 254–255
domination by ending, 257
government by desire, 255–257
trouble, 258–259
unknown ending, 259–260
Neurological model, 48
Null hypothesis, 150

Objects, common, in uncommon world of
clinic, 111–112
Observation
action and, interpretation and, 320–
322
first phase of research and, 6
Occupation, meaning of term, 15–16, 94
Occupational behavior, 48–49
Occupational therapist(s) (OT). See also
Occupational therapy
assumptions made by, 8–9
"doing for," 190
interviews with, 6–7
observations of. See Observation
professional image dilemma of, 297–
299
reasoning of, common assumptions
about decision making versus,
333–342
role perception of, reasoning influenced by, 125–127
as transporter, 110–111
common sense and, 114
understanding of, as people, 128–130
values of, conflict between biomedical
culture values and, 4. See also Biomedical culture
videotaping of, 6
Occupational therapy. See Occupational
therapist(s) (OT); Treatment
biomedical orientation in, 46–53
cultural values in, implicit and explicit, 97–98
ethnographic study of clinical reasoning in. See Clinical Reasoning
Study
phenomenological roots within, 68–71

procedural reasoning in, 151–165,
165T. See also Procedural reasoning
as reconstruction, 102–105
shifting conceptions of, 46–48
as therapeutic practice rather than
medical profession, 95–98
as two-body practice
body as machine and, 37–63
lived body and, 64–93
validation of, language development
and, 15
view of action and intentionality in.
See also Action; Intentionality
problems with, 210–212
Occupational therapy movement, 69–70
Open-ended field observations, 6
Operations, values and, as basis of common sense, 96
Organ system, medical problem solving
and, 142
OT. See Occupational therapist(s)

Participant observation
action and, interpretation and, 320–
322
first phase of research and, 6
Participation, willing, importance of,
101–102
Past history, future function versus, focus
on, 337
Patients
assumptions about, 8–9
collaboration with. See Collaboration
communication with, 78–84
"doing for," 190–193
empowerment of, 341–342
good, for occupational therapist versus
doctor, 77
inclusion of, in decision-making process, 338–339
individual. See Individual
problems of. See Therapeutic prob-
lem(s)
returning to "real world," 84–91
treated as whole person, 74–78, 226–
234
understanding of, as people, 128–
130
viewed as separate from disease, 44–
45. See also Biomechanical view
Pattern recognition
case example of, 155–156

Pattern recognition—*Continued*
  nonexclusive cues and patterns and,
    156
    case example of, 156–159
  in problem solving, 143–145
  in occupational therapy, 153–159
Perception
  of other reasoning styles, 130–133
  role, reasoning influenced by, 125–127
  sensory, lived-body paradigm and, 72
Personality style, strategies employed re-
    gardless of, 127–128
Personal stories, exchange of, collabora-
    tion and, 193
Phenomenology
  action and meaning in sense of, 224
  "being-in-the-world" and, 106
  biomechanical framework and, 57
    integration of, 91–92
  case example of, 66–67
  communication with patients and, 78–
    84
  conditional reasoning and, 134
  consciousness in, 101
  in current practice, 71–74
  defined, 64–65
  habit concept in, 213–214
  prospective stories framed by, clashes
    with biomedically framed stories,
    273–275
  returning patients to "real world" and,
    84–91
  roots of, within occupational therapy,
    68–71
  therapeutic practice versus medical
    profession and, 95–96
  treatment of whole person and, 74–78
Philosophy, American Pragmatist, legiti-
    macy of practical theories and, 22–
    23
Physiological process, medical problem
    solving and, 142
Positivism, instrumental rationality and,
    319
Possibilities, imagining, rather than gen-
    erating probabilities, 340
Practical reasoning, Aristotle's concept
    of, 10–12
Practical theories
  explication of, 22–24
  legitimacy of, 22–23
  professional expertise and, 23–24
Practice(s). *See also specific practice-re-
    lated topics*

active judgments of, 25
basis in action rather than language, 25
current concepts of, 48–49
efficient elegance of, 27–28
expert, thinking in action and, 322–324
familiar, unfamiliar names for, 13–21
language related to, 3–22
models of, biomedical framework and,
    48
phenomenology in, 71–74
in tacit dimension, 30–33
underground, 4, 295–315. *See also* Un-
    derground practice
values in, case example of, 98–99
Praxis, 23
Prediction. *See also* Prognosis
  clinical versus statistical, 138
Probabilities, generation of, imagining
    possibilities versus, 340
Problem formulations, initial, structural
    features of, 150–151, 152F, 160–
    165, 165T, 176
Problem identification, 137–138. *See
    also* Therapeutic problem(s)
  pattern recognition in, 143
  problem solving and, 140–142
Problem representation, problem-solving
    skills and, 142
Problem solving. *See also* Procedural rea-
    soning; Therapeutic problem(s)
  answer recognition in, solution seeking
    versus, 143
  best reasoning method and, 333–335
  case example of, 166–176, 175T
  defined, 137–138
  four-stage model of, 147–150
    application to occupational therapy,
      159–160
  generate-and-test method in, 145–146,
    146T
  goals and, 140–141
  heuristic search in, 147
  initial problem formulations and, 150–
    151, 152F
  inquiry and, 324–325
  joint, collaboration and, 194
  medical, 138–139
    four-stage model of inquiry for, 147–
      150
    problem space in, 142
    purpose of, 139–140
  pattern recognition in, 143–145
  in occupational therapy, 153–159
  problem identification and, 140–142

problem space and, 141–142
  in occupational therapy, 151–153
  skills in, problem representation and,
    142
  task environment and, 141, 142
  types of, 143–151
Problem space
  in medical problem-solving literature,
    142
  task environment and, 141–142
  in occupational therapy, 151–153
Procedural reasoning, 17, 119, 121
  four-stage model of medical inquiry
    and, 147–150
  interactive reasoning and, integration
    of, 125–130
  in occupational therapy, 151–165,
    165T
    case example of, 166–176, 175T
  selection of procedures to suit problem
    in, 137–138. See also Problem
    identification; Problem solving
Process(es)
  clinical reasoning as, 4
  decision-making, patient inclusion in,
    338–339
  physiological, medical problem solv-
    ing and, 142
  purposeful activity versus, 101–102
Professional(s), different types of. See
    also specific type
  relevance of clinical reasoning for, 5
Professional expertise, practical theories
    and, 23–24
Professional image, dilemma of, 297–299
Professional rationality, 319
Professional role, dilemma of, treatment
    of whole person and, 299–304
Prognosis. See also Prediction
  focus on, rather than on past history,
    337
  as purpose of medical problem solving,
    140
Prospective treatment stories, 241–242.
    See also Narrative reasoning
  biomedically versus phenomenologi-
    cally framed, 273–275
  changing shape of, 242–243
  revision of, 271–275. See also Clinical
    revision
Proximal tacit knowledge, 29–30
Psychoanalytic model, 48
Purposeful activity, processes versus,
    101–102

"Putting it all together," 132–133, 226,
    227

Quality of life
  engagement and, 16
  focus on, 97

Rational calculation, 11–12
Rationality
  instrumental, 319
  means-end, 11
  technical, 11, 319
"Real world," returning patients to, 84.
    See also Life-world
  case example of, 85–91
Reasoning. See also Clinical reasoning;
    Thinking
  action and, 317
  best method of, 333–335
  common sense as legitimate mode of,
    112–114
  conditional, 17–18, 121, 133–136,
    197–235. See also Conditional rea-
    soning
  continuous versus sequential, 335–
    336
  disparate modes of, integration of, 17–
    18
  hypothetical, example of, 166–176,
    175T
  interactive, 17, 119–120, 121–125,
    178–196. See also Interactive rea-
    soning
    integrated with procedural reason-
      ing, 125–130
  intuitive versus analytical, 123
  multiple modes of, 119–121
  narrative, 18–21, 239–269. See also
    Narrative reasoning
  perception of other styles of, 130–133
  practical, 10–12
  procedural, 17, 119, 121, 137–173,
    137–177. See also Procedural rea-
    soning
    integrated with interactive reason-
      ing, 125–130
  role perception influencing, 125–127
  scientific, 9, 317–318
  theoretical, clinical reasoning versus,
    9–10
  values guiding rather than interfering
    with, 340–341

Reasons, multiple, choices of activity
and, 201–202
"Reciprocity of motives," 123
Recognition method. *See also* Pattern
recognition
in problem solving, 143
Reconstruction, therapy as, 102–105
"Reflection-in-action," 244
Rehabilitation, of lived body, 73–74
Rehabilitation unit, as transitional world,
109–110
Research. *See also* Clinical Reasoning
Study
action, 7
ethnographic approach combined
with, 5–6
on clinical reasoning in medicine,
138–139
design of, 4
Revision, clinical, 270–291. *See also*
Clinical revision
Role
professional, treatment of whole person and, 299–304
therapeutic, reframing of, 275–279
Role perception, reasoning influenced
by, 125–127
Routines, meaning of, 105–108

Scientific method, clinical reasoning
and, 317–320
action, observation, and interpretation
and, 320–322
interpretation and, 324
thinking in action and, 322–324
Scientific model, clinic world and, 109
Scientific reasoning, 9, 317–318
Search, heuristic, 147
Self, sense of
activity selection and, 218
interactive reasoning and, 124–125
meaning and metaphor and, 221
Self-esteem, everyday activities and,
107–108
Self-movement, lived-body paradigm
and, 72
Sensory perception, lived-body paradigm and, 72
Sequential reasoning, continuous reasoning versus, 335–336
Session
demarcation into "work" and "non-
work," 299

"keeping on track," 131–132
Set-predicate formulation, generate-and-
test method as, 145–146
Situational relationship, hypothesis of,
150
Social construction, 104–105
Solutions. *See also* Problem solving
seeking of, answer recognition versus,
143
Statistical prediction, clinical prediction
versus, 138
Story talk, chart talk and, 60–61
Storytelling
clinical stories, 343–359. *See also specific topic*
data analysis using, 7–8
narrative reasoning and, 18–21. *See
also* Narrative reasoning
personal story exchange, collaboration
and, 193
prospective treatment stories and, 241–
242
changing shape of, 242–243
Success, structuring of, collaboration
and, 187–190
Surface orientation, professional role dilemma and, 302–303
Suspenseful time, unknown ending and,
259–260, 268
Symbolic knowledge, 28. *See also* Tacit
knowledge
Symbolic meaning-making, 32–33

Tacit appraisal, 327–328
Tacit dimension, 13–15
practice in, 30–33
Tacit knowledge, 14–15
access to, 26–27
acquisition of, 30
distal, 29
efficient elegance of practice and, 27–
28
knowing more than can be told, 24–27
practical theories and, 22–24
proximal, 29–30
search for, 22–34
types of, 28–30
Tacit teaching, 30–32, 34
Task environment, problem space and,
141–142
in occupational therapy, 151–153
Tasks, used as therapeutic activities,
multiple reasons for choice of, 202

"Teachable moment," 132
Teaching, tacit, 30–32, 34
Technical rationality, 11, 319
Temporary world, 109–110
Terminology, 3–22
Thematic analysis of data, 7–9
Theoretical reasoning
  clinical reasoning versus, 9–10
  limitations of, 10
  usefulness of, 9–10
Theories
  definition of term, 23
  espoused, 23
  grand, 23, 24
  practical. See Practical theories
Theories-in-use, 23
  professional expertise and, 24
Therapeutic activities. See also Activity(ies)
  habit re-creation through, 215
  integrating phenomenological and biomechanical frames, 91–92
  tasks used as, multiple reasons for choice of, 202
Therapeutic problem(s). See also Disability; Problem identification; Problem solving
  construction of, 104–105
  definition of, 54–55
  elements of, 141
  selection of procedures to suit, 137–138. See also Procedural reasoning
Therapeutic role, reframing of, 275–279
Therapeutic story. See Storytelling
Therapist. See Occupational therapist(s) (OT)
Thinking. See also Reasoning
  in action, 322–324
  forms of, 9
"Three-track" mind, 119–136
Time, narrative, 253–268
Transformation, time of, 257, 266–267
Transition, assisting patients with, 84–91
Transitional motive state, 204
Transitional world, 109–110
Transporter role, 110–111
  common sense and, 114
Treatment
  action-centered, rather than disease- or dysfunction-centered, 264–265
  biomedical approach to, 53–59
  diagnosis as not separate from, 335–336

individualization of. See also Individual, focus on
  collaboration and, 186–187
  Moral, 46, 68–69
  prospective stories of, 241–242
  changing, 271–275
  changing shape of, 242–243
  selection of, as purpose of medical problem solving, 140
  significant experiences in, narrative and creation of, 244–247
  structure of, 243–247
  of "two bodies," integration of, 91–92
  of whole person, 74–78, 226–227
  case examples of, 227–234
  professional role dilemma and, 299–304
Trouble, narrative time and, 258–259, 267–268

Underground practice, 4
  depth dilemma and, 304–307
  "double binds" of good practice and, 295–297
  professional image dilemma and, 297–299
  professional role dilemma and, treatment of whole person and, 299–304
  values dilemma and, 308–315
Understanding
  of patient and therapist as people, 128–130
  phenomenology and, 65
  problem of, 65–66

Value(s)
  cultural, 4
    common sense and, 96–97
    implicit and explicit in occupational therapy, 97–98
  guiding rather than interfering with reasoning, 340–341
  interactive reasoning and, 124
  in practice, case example of, 98–99
  strong but implicit, intentionality as, 206–207
Values dilemma, 308–315
Videotapes
  analysis of, 7–8
  second phase of research and, 6

Whole person, treatment of, 74–78, 226–227
case examples of, 227–234
professional role dilemma and, 299–304

Willing participation, importance of, 101–102
"Work cures," 70